USEFUL INDIAN HERBS

An Ethnobotanical Handbook

USEFUL INDIAN HERBS

An Ethnobotanical Handbook

By

Dr. (Mrs.) Sudha Prakash

Reader in Botany (Retired)

Daulat-Ram College

University of Delhi

DELHI

BIOTECH

2008

Biotech Books

Delhi - 110 035

ISBN10 81-7622-200-3
ISBN13 978-81-7622-200-6

Published by : **BIOTECH BOOKS**
1123/74, Tri Nagar,
DELHI – 110 035
Phone: 27383999
e-mail: biotechbooks@yahoo.co.in

Showroom : 4760-61/23, Ansari Road, Darya Ganj,
New Delhi - 110 002
Phone: 23245578, 23244987

Laser Typesetting : **Classic Computer Services**
Delhi - 110 035

Printed at : **Chawla Offset Printers**
Delhi - 110 052

PRINTED IN INDIA

Dedicated to the Memory
of
MY PARENTS
Mr. SHAM SUNDAR GARG and
Mrs. BHAGWATI GARG

for
their Love, Encouragement and Kindness

Preface

In our ancient literature and carvings in stone on the walls of various monuments and temples lies a hidden treasure of knowledge on the economic value of plants. In Hindu, Buddhist and Jain scriptures mention has been made of the beauty and bounty of mother nature as the provider for humanity in general, and life in particular on our planet called 'Prithvi' or the Earth, and hence our obligation to protect it. The concept of protection of our environment and its importance was known to our ancient sages. The vast knowledge of plant resources for various purposes was passed orally from the 'Guru' to the 'Shishya' or disciples and later compiled into texts or depicted on temple walls and monuments for visual aid. One of the Ajanta frescoes shows very clearly the sugarcane plants with typical barrel-shaped internodes, denoting the particular species of sugarcane being cultivated in India for centuries. Sugarcane as a source of sugar was being used in India, at a time when the rest of the world depended completely on honey, and until the invasion of India by Alexander the Great, the West had no idea that sugar could be derived from a plant source. Numerous ancient texts have been credited regarding the knowledge of a large number of medicinal and other economic plants *viz.*, Rigveda, Atharvaveda, Charaka samhita and Susruta samhita besides their casual mention in the sacred Ramayana, Srimad Bhagawata and Bhagvadgita educating the masses about not only their aesthetic and economic value but also our total dependence on plant life. Many modern eminent scholars have brought forth extremely valuable works on economic plants of India, a few in dictionary form, arranging the information according to the universally accepted international Latin botanical names of plants alphabetically, with other details. Out of the total useful plants about 20 per cent are medicinal and many authors have restricted themselves to only details of medicinal plants. However, useful plants include cereals, pulses, oil crops, fruits, nuts, vegetables, and spices for food, timber for shelter and other purposes, fibre for clothing, fodder for animal feed and latex, resins, gums, dyes, tannins and other miscellaneous plant products for innumerable other purposes. The latest amongst the list are many plants identified as petro-crops which after development of proper technology, offer immense potential as infinite renewable sources of diesel and ethanol to supplement the ever increasing fuel requirement of the world.

India has a rich flora of medicinal plants of which more than 3,000 have already been authentically listed. There is a need to integrate western and traditional remedies. It is therefore, very encouraging that many government and private research organisations are now taking keen interest in folk and tribal medicine. Traditional Indian medicine has captured the interest of private institutions like Academies of Ayurveda which are making serious effort for qualitatively testing and analysing Ayurvedic raw drugs, mixtures and 'bhasmas' by modern techniques. Experts in the Central Council for Research in Ayurveda and Siddha (CCRAS) and its regional Ayurvedic research centres, University of Health Sciences, and centres for experimental science of many medical colleges in different states of India are now concentrating to find out the ways to adapt the traditional indigenous medicinal systems to modern medical needs. The days when traditional folk and tribal medicine was just dismissed cursorily are over, and the World Health Organisation is now closely monitoring worldwide developments in local traditional medicinal systems. This is in view of the fact that in the Third World countries traditional medicinal systems developed over centuries, are often the only form of treatment available to the rural masses and in the interior regions. Further, traditional tribal medicines are much more readily available to the tribals. Another distinct advantage of Ayurvedic and other traditional indigenous medicinal treatments is their use of natural herbal products which have negligible side effects, low cost and ready availability. The resurgence of research in traditional herbal treatment of innumerable diseases holds out a ray of hope for the suffering poor people. The only way to repay the kindness of mother nature which abounds in providing for us almost everything from the top three essentials of food, clothing and shelter to everything else that we need for our existence, sustenance and comfort is by protecting our environment.

Mention has been made in our ancient texts about 'Kalpa vriksha' and 'Soma rasa'. Although nothing can be said with certainty some authors have advocated that *Adansonia digitata* L., the Baobab tree known in Hindi as 'Gorak amli' is the real Kalpa vriksha. Others feel the reference is to *Cocos nucifera* L., the coconut called 'Narial' in Hindi. Similarly the term 'Soma rasa' is clouded in mystery and except that it was a very nutritious drink, nothing more can be said as to its authentic and definite plant source.

With the recent awareness of people in general, about the importance of natural herbs in almost all walks of life and the harmful effects of chemicals in medicines, drugs, cosmetics, hair dyes, perfumery, preservatives, insecticides and various other materials of daily use by us, people all over the world are preferring to go back to natural products. The key words today are herbal and natural herbs, and hence the importance of indigenous plant resources available to us. The need for writing this text and the inspiration for it, was received from friends who were sending their requests very often regarding information about the botanical names and other details such as family, habit, climate where a particular plant grows, plant part used and economic uses of many Indian herbs about which they were familiar with the Hindi name only. The requests were from people with a keen interest in gardening, people interested in traditional Indian plant products used as home remedies and people engaged in various industrial enterprises. Thus began an endeavour to start the compilation of an exhaustive data on useful Indian herbs, and list them in dictionary form according to their Hindi and Sanskrit names arranged in English alphabetical order. The common Hindi name is followed by other Hindi names available and then by its Sanskrit name if available after which a capital letter S is written in brackets. This is followed by the universally accepted Latin botanical name and the name of the author who validated the name, and then the common English name if available, again followed by the letter E in brackets. This sequence has been kept throughout the text. This is followed by the name of the family to which the plant belongs, its habit, and details of its economic importance along with the plant-part used and any important chemical constituents present such as alkaloids. Care has been taken to incorporate and emphasize medicinal uses of many Indian plants in alternative systems of medicine prevalent in India specially the ancient Ayurvedic system and also tribal medicines and home-made remedies. Care has also been taken to highlight the traditional usage of our plant resources from time immemorial, associated with our way of life, rituals, traditions and culture of India comprising diverse ethnic groups. Mention has also been made about the habitat, in case the plant distribution is limited to a particular area or to high altitude. Attempt has been made to include as many Hindi and Sanskrit names as could be possibly included and in case several names exist, the name by which the plant is most commonly known is described and the rest of the names given in alphabetical order are again referred back to its first prevalent name in Hindi for the convenience of the reader. However, the compilation work is by no means claimed to be absolutely complete. Further the term 'Indian Herbs' has been used in a broader sense to include all plant wealth of India.

For the convenience of the readers who wish to know Hindi and Sanskrit names of those plants of which they know only the botanical names or just the common English names, a comprehensive index of botanical names with page number and another of common English names with page number of their Hindi/ Sanskrit equivalent is provided at the end of the text.

The author will welcome and appreciate suggestions for improvement of the text from all friends, which can be incorporated in future editions.

In the preparation of this work, data has been collected from numerous sources of which the important ones have been cited in the select bibliography. I wish to express my thanks to all the authors whose publications have been consulted. My grateful thanks are also due to Prof. H.Y. Mohan Ram for his invaluable suggestions and to all my colleagues in the Department of Botany, Daulat Ram College, University of Delhi for their encouragement. Last but not the least I wish to express my sincere thanks to my husband Prof. I.P.

Gupta and my children who prompted me to undertake the present work, and their constant cooperation and patience throughout the preparation of this text. I owe special thanks to my daughter Dr Abha Prakash Campourcy for her help in editing the final script.

Dr. (Mrs.) Sudha Prakash

A

Aamli, Amari, Dhakki, Kali khatai – *Antidesma diandrum* Hayne. ex Roth.; Stilaginaceae; small tree. Fruits and acidic leaves are edible. Seeds yield a fatty oil.

Aamra (S) – *see* Am.

Aamrataka (S) – *see* Amara.

Aaraar – *see* Abhal.

Abhal, Aaraar, Haubera; Vapusha (S) – *Juniperus communis* L.; Juniper (E); Cupressaceae; evergreen tree. Bark is the source of tannin. Roots and fruiting bodies yield a dye. Fruiting bodies are aromatic and are rich in fermentable sugars, an essential oil and a fatty oil. Essential oil called juniper oil is used to flavour liquors, cordials and food products. It is considered to be a stimulant, carminative and diuretic and is also used for cutaneous infections. Young twigs and wood are used as incense.

Abnus, Ebans – *Diospyros ebenum* Koenig; Ebony persimmon (E); Ebenaceae; evergreen tree. Dark coloured wood yields precious timber, which is used for decorative panelling, veneers, cabinets, turnery articles, keys of musical instruments, sports goods, and handles. Fruits are edible.

Ach – *see* Al.

Adhaki (S) – *see* Arhar.

Adhasisi, Banokra, Chhota gokhru; Arishta (S) – *Xanthium strumarium* L.; Cocklebur (E); Compositae; herb. Seeds yield a semi-drying oil called 'Adhasisi' oil, which is used for bladder infections and herpes; it is also used in the manufacture of soaps and paints. Decoction of the leaves is reportedly used for curing urinary troubles and chronic malaria. Root extract is applied locally to boils and ulcers. Fruits are a rich source of vitamin C, and also contain β-D glucoside of β-sitosterol, and are used in pharmaceuticals for the treatment of urinogenital diseases, regulation of hormonal activity, and as an anti-inflammatory.

Adiphala (S) – *see* Amla.

Adityabhakta (S) – *see* Hulhul.

Adityavalli (S) – *see* Surajmukhi.

Adrak; Ardraka (S) – *Zingiber officinale* Rosc.; Ginger (E); Zingiberaceae; perennial herb. Cultivated for its rhizomes (underground modified stem) which are very widely used as a spice, condiment, digestive stimulant and in medicine. Fresh rhizomes and dried rhizome powder are used in many culinary preparations and to flavour liqueurs. Oil of ginger is used for flavouring and is rich in gingerol. The rhizomes are also rich in an oleo-resin called gingerin. Fresh rhizome juice helps in reducing nausea and vomiting in motion sickness and improves function in people suffering from arthritis.

Adulasa – *see* Arusha.

Afim, Post, Khas; Ahifen (S) – *Papaver somniferum* L.; Opium poppy (E); Papaveraceae; herb. Cultivated as a medicinal plant for the opium derivatives, strictly under government control. Drug opium is the dried latex obtained by making gashes or incisions on the ripe green capsules. It is a narcotic, habit forming and is much abused. It induces sleep and relieves pain. Chief alkaloids present in the latex are morphine, codeine, narcotine and papaverine of which morphine is a powerful narcotic and stimulant, and is used medicinally as a sedative and pain killer. Seeds called 'khas' are free from narcotic principles and contain a fatty oil. Seed paste is used in culinary and skin-care preparations, and poppy-seed oil is used in remedies for diarrhoea and dysentery.

Agar; Agaru (S) – *Aquilaria agallocha* Roxb.; Eagle wood (E); Thymelaeaceae; tree. Plant is the source of an incense obtained from patches of dark-coloured wood in the older parts of stem containing an oleo-resin. Wood is aromatic and yields an essential oil called 'agar attar' or otto of agar which is used in perfumery. Agar incense is used in the manufacture of incense-sticks called 'agarbattis' and in fumigators; it is also used in medicine as a tonic and carminative. Wood is used for inlay work and cabinets, and bark yields a fibre used for cordage and home-made paper.

Agaru (S) – *see* Agar.

Agasti, Agastoya, Bak; Agati (S) – *Sesbania grandiflora* (L.) Poir.; Agati Sesbania (E); Papilionaceae; tree. Tender leaves and young fruits are edible. Bark yields a fibre; bark juice is used for toughening fish nets and colouring mats. Trees are cultivated as live-support and shelter for betel-vines and pepper-vines and to provide shade for coconut seedlings. They are also used as wind breaks for banana plantations.

Agastoya – *see* Agasti.

Agati (S) – *see* Agasti.

Agetha, Arani, Ustabunda; Agnimantha (S) – *Premna obtusifolia* R. Br.; Verbenaceae; tree. Roots comprise as one of the constituents of the Ayurvedic preparation 'Dasamula'. Chief alkaloids present are premnine, ganikarine and ganiarine. Leaf decoction is used for flatulence and colic. Wood is used for knife handles and leaves are lopped for fodder.

Aggai, Kallai – *Dillenia pentagyna* Roxb.; Dilleniaceae; large tree. Wood is used for timber. Flower buds and fruits are edible. Bark yields a fibre used for cordage and tannin which is used in tanning industry.

Aghya ghas – *see* Agin ghas.

Agia – *Striga lutea* Lour.; Scrophulariaceae; scabrid herb found as partial root parasite. Herb is considered to be an appetizer.

Agin ghas, Aghya ghas, Sugandha-rohisha; Bhustriana (S) – *Cymbopogon citratus* (DC.) Stapf.; Lemon grass (E); Gramineae;

perennial herb. Cultivated for its fragrant leaves, rich in an essential oil called lemon grass oil which is used in cosmetics and perfumery. Residual spent leaves after extraction of the essential oil are used for paper manufacture.

Agni-jal – *Clausena excavata* Burm f.; Wampee (E); Rutaceae; small tree. Cultivated for its orange flavoured edible fruits. Infusion of roots, leaves and flowers is used for colic. Wood is used for tool-handles.

Agnijwala (S) – *see* Dawi.

Agnimantha (S) – *see* Agetha.

Agnimanthini (S) – *see* Arni.

Agnimukhi (S) – *see* Kalihari.

Agnishikha (S) – *see* Kalihari.

Agumaki, Bilari – *Melothria maderaspatana* (L.) Cogn.; Gwala kakri (E); Cucurbitaceae; Wild climbing herb. Root decoction is used for flatulence and roots are chewed to relieve toothache.

Aguru (S) – *see* Shisham.

Ahifen (S) – *see* Afim.

Aila – *Acacia intsia* Willd. (syn. *Acacia caesia* Wight & Arn.); Mimosaceae; large scrambling shrub. Bark is used for washing hair and as a soap substitute. Bark extract is used for coating fishing nets and boats. Plant serves as a host to lac insect.

Ainta, Hartho – *Securinega leucopyrus* (Willd.) Muell.-Arg.; Euphorbiaceae; thorny shrub. Fruits are edible, and slender twigs are used for basketry. Leaf paste mixed with tobacco is used for destroying maggots in open sores. Bark yields tannin, and is also used as a fish-poison.

Ajabhakshya (S) – *see* Damahan.

Ajagara (S) – *see* Bhangra.

Ajaka (S) – *see* Tulsi.

Ajapriya (S) – *see* Baer.

Ajakarna (S) – *see* Safed-damar.

Ajmoda (S) – *see* Ajwain.

Ajmot – *see* Ajmud.

Ajmud, Ajmot; Randhuni – *Trachyspermum roxburghianum* (DC.) Craib; Indian celery (E); Umbelliferae; herb. Cultivated for its fruits which are used as a spice. Fruits act as a carminative and cardiac tonic and are used for treating asthma and bronchitis.

Ajowan – *see* Ajwain.

Ajwain, Ajowan; Ajmoda (S) – *Trachyspermum ammi* (L.) Sprague ex Turril; Ammi (E), Lovage (E); Umbelliferae; herb. Cultivated for its fruits which are used as a spice. Fruits are carminative, tonic and antispasmodic and are used for flatulence and as an ingredient of cough mixtures. They are reported to exhibit antifungal activity. Essential oil from the fruits yields thymol used as a carminative, antiseptic and aromatic. Aquous residue after distillation of essential oil, called omum, is used for gripe and flatulence. Fruits also yield a fatty oil which is used externally for rheumatic inflammation and in vinyl industry as a plasticizer.

Ak; Arka (S), Mandara (S) – *Calotropis gigantea* Ait.; Madar (E); Asclepiadaceae; undershrub. Floss from seeds is used for stuffing purposes. Root bark is medicinal. Flower paste is used for controlling cough, colds and asthma. Stem bark is the source of fibre used for making fishing-nets. Fermented mixture of madar, salt and starch is used for dehairing sheep and goat skin in the processing of leather.

Akada, Madar, Safed-ak – *Calotropis procera* (Ait.) R. Br.; Akund (E), Swallow-wort (E); Asclepiadaceae; evergreen undershrub. Floss from seeds and fibre from stem are used similar to 'Ak' or *Calotropis gigantea*. Powdered flower paste is used for curing cough and asthma. Root bark is used to treat dysentery and leprosy.

Akalber – *see* Akalbir.

Akalbir, Akalber – *Datisca cannabina* L.; False hemp (E); Datiscaceae; bushy herb. Roots are the source of a dye used for dyeing cottons and wool.

Akanadi, Harjori, Palat-ki-bel; Ambashtha (S) – *Cissampelos pareira* L.; False pareira (E); Menispermaceae; twining shrub. Roots are used medicinally for cough, diarrhoea, colic, dysentery and urinary disorders. Roots and stem are rich in the alkaloid hayatine, and are used as a muscular relaxant and a good substitute for curariform drugs.

Akarkara, Pokarmul – *Spilanthes acmella* Murr.; Compositae; herb. Roots, leaves and flower-heads are used in Ayurvedic medicine for gums and throat infections and toothache. Active principle spilanthol extracted from the flowers, acts as a local anaesthetic, powerful insecticide and fish poison. Plant decoction is an effective diuretic and is used in scabies and psoriasis. Another plant *Anacyclus pyrethrum* DC. is also known by the same Hindi name.

Akarkara – *Anacyclus pyrethrum* DC.; Spanish pellitory (E); Compositae; annual hairy herb. Roots are long, thick, rough, finger-like and aromatic with pungent taste, and are used for toothache and in tooth powders and gargles. Alcoholic extract of roots is used to treat Mange disease of horses. Active principle present is called pellitorine. Roots also contain an essential oil.

Akasbel; Amarvela (S) – *Cuscuta reflexa* Roxb.; Convolvulaceae; twining, slender leaf-less total parasite on trees and shrubs. Stems are purgative, and are also used in treating flatulence and itch. Seeds are rich in pigments cuscutin and amarbelin, and are considered as a tonic and demulcent.

Akasgaddah, Rakasgaddah; Patalagaruda (S) – *Corallocarpus epigaeus* (Rottl. & Willd.) Clarke; Cucurbitaceae; climbing herb. Roots are used in the indigenous system of medicine for combating dysentery and rheumatism.

Akashvalli (S) – *see* Amarbeli.

Akasneem, Neem-chameli, Mini-chambelli – *Millingtonia hortensis* L.f.; Indian cork tree (E); Bignoniaceae; tall tree. Cultivated in parks and also as an avenue tree. Wood is used for furniture and tea-chests. Bark is rich in tannin and is used as an antipyretic.

Akhrot – *Juglans regia* L.; Walnut (E); Juglandaceae; tree. Plant is cultivated for its nutritious seed kernels which are used as a dry fruit and source of walnut oil. Shells are used for making activated carbon. Pulverized shells find extensive usage as an ingredient of linoleum and for the manufacture of moulded wood products, plywood, and roofing paper; they are also used as an abrasive for plastics and extender in synthetic resin adhesives. Wood provides valuable timber used for cabinet work, carving, furniture, musical instrument bodies e.g. piano, and rifle parts. Leaf extract exhibits bactericidal properties. Bark is used for cleaning teeth and also yields a dye.

Akola, Dhera; Ankola (S) – *Alangium salviifolium* (L.f.) Wang; Sage-leaved Alangium (E); Alangiaceae; small tree. Fruits are edible. Wood is used for cabinet, inlay and ornamental work. Root bark is used as an astringent, purgative, anthelmintic, and for cutaneous infections; also used for biliousness and colic. Active principle present is the alkaloid alangine. Root extract is hypotensive in action. Seeds are tonic and source of a fatty oil used for illumination.

Akra, Akta, Chatri matri – *Vicia sativa* L.; Common vetch (E); Papilionaceae; annual herb, cultivated for fodder and green manure.

Akri, Punir – *Withania coagulans* (Stocks) Dunal; Vegetable rennet (E); Solanaceae; undershrub. Fruits are used for coagulating milk for the preparation of cheese. Fruits are used medicinally for indigestion, liver complaints and asthma.

Aksota (S) – *see* Jangli Akhrot.

Akta – *see* Akra.

Al, Ach, Bartundi; Ashyuka (S) – *Morinda citrifolia* L.; Indian mulberry (E); Rubiaceae; small tree. Cultivated for its roots which yield a yellow-orange dye present in the bark in the form of morindin, and used for dyeing cottons. Fruits are used for dysentery, leucorrhoea and throat disorders; they are also the source of an essential oil. Wood is used for toys and turnery articles. Leaves are used for rearing silkworms and also lopped for fodder. Another species *Morinda tinctoria* Roxb. is also known by the same Hindi name and its roots yield a red dye.

Alabu (S) – *see* Ghia.

Alarka; Alarka (S) – *Solanum trilobatum* L.; Solanaceae; climbing shrub found in S. India. Leaves are used as pot-herb. Flowers and berries are used for cough and they contain an active principle called solasodine.

Alarka (S) – *see* Alarka.

Aliar, Sinatha – *Dodonaea viscosa* (L.) Jacq.; Jamaica switch sorrel (E); Sapindaceae; evergreen shrub. Plant is usually cultivated for hedges. Bark and leaves are a rich source of tannin used for giving light colour to leather. Wood is used for making walking-sticks and tool-handles. Seeds yield a semi-drying oil.

Alkusi – *see* Kawanch.

Alla, Awa, Bichua – *Girardinia palmata* (Forsk.) Gaud.; Himalayan nettle (E); Urticaceae; perennial herb. Stem fibre is used for ropes, twines and rough cloth.

Alpa marisha (S) – *see* Van natya.

Alsi, Tisi; Atasi (S) – *Linum usitatissimum* L.; Flax (E); Linaceae; annual herb. Cultivated as an oil-seed crop. Seeds yield a drying oil used in paints, varnishes and printer's ink. Oil cake is used as fertilizer and stock-feed. Linseed mucilage is used as a demulcent in pharmaceuticals and in cosmetics. Stem fibre which is extracted at blooming time yields flax fibre which is used in the manufacture of linen, oil cloth, high grade paper and cigarette paper. Crushed seeds poultice is applied to ulcers, boils and inflammations.

Alu – *Solanum tuberosum* L.; Potato (E); Solanaceae; annual herb. Cultivated for its starchy stem-tubers formed underground. Tubers are nutritious and also contain the protein tuberin and several enzymes; they are used as staple food in certain parts of the world. In India tubers are used as vegetable and for preparing many dishes and fast foods. Tubers are used extensively for the manufacture of starch and ethyl alcohol.

Alubalu – *Prunus cerasus* L.; Sour cherry (E), Dwarf cherry (E); Rosaceae; tree. Fruits are edible but acidic, and are used for making preserves. Fatty oil from kernels and bark is used in pharmaceuticals. Bark also contains tannin. Tree yields a gum similar to gum-tragacanth in usage.

Alubukhara – *see* Alucha.

Alucha, Alubukhara – *Prunus domestica* L. ssp. *insititia* (L.) Schneid.; Plum (E), Bullace (E); Rosaceae; tree. Cultivated in the hills for its juicy and nutritious edible fruits.

Aluka (S) – *see* Aru.

Am, Amb; Aamra (S) – *Mangifera indica* L.; Mango (E); Anacardiaceae; large evergreen tree. Cultivated for its delicious, highly prized edible ripe fruits which are much relished and are a rich source of vitamins A and C. Raw fruits are preserved into pickles, jams, chutneys and squashes. Mango kernels yield a fatty oil used for edible purposes and the residual spent kernel is used as cattle-feed. Kernels are used medicinally for asthma, and the bark in uterine haemorrhage. Many popular varieties are grown in different parts of India. Plant is considered sacred by the Hindus and festoons of leaves hung on auspicious ceremonies, are reported to possess antimicrobial activity. Mango branches with fruits have been carved in many ancient sculptures like the 'Sanchi stupa' denoting its importance in Indian life. Important cultivated varieties are Langra, Dassehri, Bombai, Safeda, Chausa, Totapari, Himsagar, Malda, Fazli, Bangalora, Panseri and many others. Many new varieties have been added such as the dwarf mango Amrapali and the hybrid variety Mallika. Ethnobotanical uses claim medicinal properties for the 'Tukhmi' variety which can cure early stages of cancer, and prevent cancer if taken regularly in the two summer months.

Amahaldi; Karpura-haridra (S) – *Curcuma amada* Roxb.; Mango-ginger (E); Zingiberaceae; perennial herb. Cultivated for its aromatic rhizomes with raw mango like flavour used as a spice and condiment; it is also used medicinally in ointments and poultices for external application on sprains and inflammations.

Amalaka (S) – *see* Amla.

Amal-bel, Ramchana; Aranyavasini (S), Atyamlaparni (S) – *Cayratia carnosa* (Wall.) Gagnep (syn. *Vitis carnosa* Wall.); Foxgrape (E);

Vitaceae; climbing shrub. Roots are considered to be astringent. Leaf poultice is used for treating yoke-sore in bullocks.

Amaltas, Girimalah; Rajataru (S), Suvarnaka (S) – *Cassia fistula* L.; Indian laburnum (E), Golden shower (E), Purging Cassia (E); Caesalpiniaceae; large tree. Cultivated as an ornamental for its beautiful bright yellow flowers on a pendant inflorescence. Wood provides good timber which is used for furniture. Fruit pulp is used as a purgative and dried pods are used in medicine.

Amara, Amra, Jangli-am, Aamrataka (S) – *Spondias pinnata* (L.f.) Kurz.; Hog plum (E); Anacardiacdeae; small tree. Often cultivated for its raw green acidic fruits made into pickle, jams and chutneys. Wood is used for packing-boxes, boats, plywood and in match industry. Bark is rich in tannin. Gum from the tree is used as a demulcent and for fumigation.

Amarbeli; Akashvalli (S) – *Cassytha filiformis* L.; Lauraceae; twiner. Stem is the source of a brown dye. Plant is used in dysentery, indigestion, urethritis and skin ailments.

Amari – *see* Aamli.

Amarkand, Goruma; Balakanda (S), Manya (S) – *Eulophia nuda* Lindl.; Orchidaceae; terrestrial herb with fleshy tubers. Tubers are mucilaginous and are used for treating scrofulous glands in the neck and also as a vermifuge.

Amarphal – *Monstera deliciosa* Liebm.; Ceriman (E); Araceae; robust epiphyte. Plant is cultivated widely as an ornamental for its beautiful evergreen foliage. Ripe fruits are edible and have banana and pineapple flavour.

Amarvela (S) – *see* Akasbel.

Amb – *see* Am.

Ambari – *see* Patsan.

Ambari palak – *see* Chuka.

Ambarvel, Shingrota – *Pentatropis capensis* (L.f.) Bullock; Asclepiadaceae; slender, twining undershrub. Plants are used in indigenous Ayurvedic medicine as a cooling agent.

Ambashtha (S) – *see* Akanadi.

Ambavah, Amrule, Jangli palak – *Rumex dentatus* L.; Polygonaceae; herb. Leaves are rich in minerals and vitamin A, and are used as vegetable. Roots yield a red dye and are also used for skin ailments.

Ambavati – *Rumex scutatus* L.; French sorrel (E); Polygonaceae; herb. Leaves are succulent and are used in salads, sauces and soups; they are also used to treat dysentery.

Amburuha (S) – *see* Ratanpurus.

Amelvet – *Garcinia pedunculata* Roxb.; Guttiferae; large tree. Often cultivated in E. India for its fruits with red coloured acid-pulp. Fruits are considered to be useful in indigestion, constipation, loss of appetite, colds, cough, hiccups and rheumatism. They are used fresh or made into a refreshing cordial. Pulp is also used as a mordant for saffron dye.

Amla, Aonla; Adiphala (S), Amalaka (S), Dhatri (S) – *Emblica officinalis* Gaertn; Emblic myrobalan (E), Indian goose-berry (E); Euphorbiaceae; deciduous tree. Cultivated for its fruits in parks and near farm boundaries. Ripe fruits are acidic and one of the richest sources of vitamin C, and are used fresh or preserved into jam, chutneys and syrups. Fruits are laxative, diuretic and liver tonic and are used in dry powder form for diarrhoea and dysentery. They are used as an important ingredient of indigenous ancient health preparations, *viz.*, 'Triphala', 'Chyawanprash' and many others. Fruit pulp contains phyllembin, a mild depressant of the central nervous system. It is reported to show antibiotic activity against several micro-organisms. Fruit juice and dried fruit powder are used as hair-tonic, dye and shampoo mixed with other herbs, and are used in several hair oils. Bark and leaves yield tannin. Seeds contain both a fatty oil and an essential oil. Fermented fruit liquor is considered diuretic and used medicinally in anaemia, jaundice, indigestion and certain heart complaints.

Amladandi – *see* Sarai.

Amlanch – *see* Baikunti.

Amli – *see* Imli.

Amlika (S) – *see* Imli.

Amlok – *Diospyros lotus* L.; Date plum persimmon (E); Ebenaceae; tree. Fruits are edible, and seeds act as a sedative. Rooted cuttings are used as a stock for grafting 'Halwa tendu' or *Diospyros kaki* L.f.

Amlosa – *Bauhinia malabarica* Roxb.; Malabar mountain ebony (E). Caesalpiniaceae; tree. Tender leafy tips are edible and also used to flavour food. Bark is the source of tannin. Tender seeds are edible.

Ampich – *see* Ashok.

Amra – *see* Amara.

Amrita (S) – *see* Giloe.

Amrit-phala (S) – *see* Bihi.

Amroda – *see* Pathurchur.

Amrool – *see* Jamrul.

Amrud, Jamphal, Mansala (S) – *Psidium guajava* L.; Guava (E); Myrtaceae; tree. Fruits are edible, delicious and are considered to be a rich source of vitamin C. They are eaten fresh or preserved into jams and jellies. Seeds yield a fatty oil. Bark and leaves are used for tanning. Bark decoction is used for diarrhoea. Wood is used for tool handles, engraving and lac-turnery.

Amrul, Chuka tripatti, Khatti-buti – *Oxalis corniculata* L.; Indian sorrel (E); Oxalidaceae; herb. Leaves are rich in vitamin C and carotene but oxalate content is high. Fresh juice of plant is considered to be useful in dyspepsia, piles and anaemia. Leaf infusion is reported to cure opacity of cornea.

Amrule – *see* Ambavah.

Ananas – *Ananas comosus* (L.) Merr.; Pineapple (E); Bromeliaceae; biennial herb. Fruits are consumed fresh or preserved as jam, juice, and canned slices, or mixed with ice-cream and confectionery. Pineapple waste is used for the preparation of vinegar and oxalic acid or used as a cattle feed. Leaf fibre is used for making fishing nets, cords and pina cloth. Juice from unripe fruits acts as a purgative and abortifacient.

Anantamul, Kapuri, Magrabu; Sariva (S) – *Hemidesmus indicus* (L.) Schult. Indian sarsaparilla (E); Periplocaceae; slender twining undershrub. Roots are tuberous but slender. Dried aromatic roots, source of the drug called 'anantmul' or hemidesmus are used as a diuretic, blood purifier, diaphoretic and demulcent, and are prescribed in rheumatism. Roots contain an essential oil rich in coumarine, hemidesmine, saponin and tannin.

Anar; Dadima (S) – *Punica granatum* L.; Pomegranate (E); Punicaceae; small tree. Fruits with juicy edible seeds are rich in vitamin C, iron and sugars. Fruit rind and bark are used for tanning. Rind is also used for diarrhoea and dysentery and the bark to expel tapeworms. Flowers yield a dye and flower-buds are used in bronchitis.

Anasphal – *Illicium verum* Hook f.; Star anise (E); Illiciaceae; tree. Fruit is fragrant, and used as a condiment. Oil from the fruit is used in perfumery and in medicine as a carminative, expectorant, stomachic and to treat dysentery. It is also used locally on rheumatic joints and scabies.

Anchhu, Hinsalu – *Rubus ellipticus* Smith; Himalayan yellow raspberry; Rosaceae; shrub. Fruits are edible.

Andachampa, Himchampa – *Magnolia grandiflora* L.; Bull bay (E), Great laurel Magnolia (E); Magnoliaceae; evergreen tree. Flowers and bark are aromatic, and most parts contain an essential oil. Bark is stimulant and tonic and is used for rheumatism and malaria; wood is considered suitable for unbleached paper-pulp.

Aneta – *see* Madhavi lata.

Angan – *Fraxinus floribunda* Wall.; Oleaceae; deciduous tree. Wood is considered useful for ploughs, oars, poles, tool handles and walking-sticks.

Angaru – *Diospyros ferrea* (Willd.) Bakh. (syn. *Maba buxifolia* Pers.); Ebenaceae; small tree. Fruits are edible. Wood is used for rafters, boats, anchors and tool handles.

Angoor, Draksha (S) – *Vitis vinifera* L.; Wine grape (E) European grape (E), Vitaceae; woody shrubby climber. Cultivated for its fruits, consumed both fresh and dried, the latter are called 'kishmish' and 'munakka' or raisins. Fruits of many varieties are seedless, juicy, refreshing, delicious, and rich in sugars, minerals, and vitamins. Fruits are widely used in Ayurvedic tonic preparations like 'Drakshasav' and 'Chyawanprash'. By-products include tannins and grape-seed oil.

Angurshefa, Sag-angur – *Atropa belladonna* L.; Deadly nightshade (E), Belladonna (E); Solanaceae; coarse perennial medicinal herb. Cultivated to some extent in Kashmir. Dried roots are marketed as belladonna radix, and the dried leaves as belladonna folium. The drug acts as a sedative, tonic and antispasmodic. Leaves act as a narcotic, and are rich in extremely toxic alkaloids *viz.*, atropine and hyoscyamine. Atropine is used as eye-drops for ophthalmic treatment and eye-sight testing as it has the property of dilating the pupils of the eye. Atropine is also used as an antidote to certain poisons. Roots are used in the manufacture of belladonna plaster and tincture.

Anhuri – *see* Bakla.

Anjan – *Memecylon umbellatum* Burm. f. (syn. *M. edule* Roxb.); Iron-wood tree (E); Melastomataceae; small tree. Fruits are edible, leaves and flowers are the source of a dye used to colour cotton fabrics and mats. Root decoction is prescribed to check excessive menstruation. Leaves are astringent and their infusion is used in gonorrhoea and leucorrhoea. Wood is used for rafters, posts, decorative work, walking-sticks, tool handles and for making good quality charcoal.

Anjir; Anjira (S) – *Ficus carica* L.; Fig (E); Moraceae; small tree. Cultivated for its fruits used fresh and dried. Fruits are also used in the preparation of fig-wine. Fresh fig latex yields ficus–rennet which is used in the preparation of cheese and it is also used for getting rid of warts.

Anjira (S) – *see* Anjir.

Anjiri, Bedu – *Ficus palmata* Forsk. (syn. *F. virgata* Roxb.); Moraceae; small tree. Fruits are edible; they are also used medicinally for diseases of bladder and lungs. Young leaves and tender shoots are used as vegetable. Latex is used for curdling of milk.

Anjun – *Hardwickia binata* Roxb.; Caesalpiniaceae; large tree found in S. India. Wood is very hard and is used for making bridges, beams, cart-wheels and oars; it is also used for carving. Heartwood when tapped, yields an oleo-resin used for varnishes. Stem is the source of a fibre used for ropes and leaves are lopped for fodder.

Ankola (S) – *see* Akola.

Anshphal, Wumb – *Euphoria longan* (Lour.) Steud; Longan (E); Sapindaceae; tree. Cultivated as an ornamental and shade tree. Fruits are edible with succulent aril, and are consumed either fresh or dried or canned. Seeds are the source of saponin and a fatty oil. Wood is used for furniture and agricultural implements.

Antamul, Jangli pikvam – *Tylophora indica* (Burm. f.) Merr.; Emetic swallow-wort (E); Asclepiadaceae; twining undershrub. Leaves and roots are emetic, expectorant and diaphoretic, and are used for cough, bronchitis, diarrhoea and dysentery. Fresh leaves are used to treat some types of asthma. Leaves and roots are also used as a substitute for ipecacuanha.

Anu – *see* Cheen.

Aonla – *see* Amla.

Apamarga (S) – *see* Latjira.

Apang – *see* Zarga.

Aparjit, Gokurni, Aparajita (S) – *Clitoria ternatea* L.; Papilionaceae; rambling perennial undershrub. Cultivated as an ornamental for its beautiful showy blue-coloured flowers and evergreen foliage. Seeds are purgative and source of a fixed oil and tannin. Roots are diuretic and cathartic. Flowers yield a blue dye.

Aparajita (S) – *see* Aparajit.

Apavisha (S) – *see* Jadwar.

Aparang, Hiradukhi – *Daemonorops kurzianus* Becc & Hook. f.; (syn. *Calamus grandis* Kurz.); East Indian dragon's blood (E); Palmae;

tall, slender spinous climbing palm found in the Andaman islands. Fruit exudate is resinous, and is used for colouring varnishes and lacquers.

Aragvadha – *see* Kachlora.

Araka (S) – *see* Pitpapara.

Arandi – *see* Errandi.

Arangaka (S) – *Melia composita* Willd.; Malabar Nim-wood tree (E); Meliaceae; medium sized tree. Wood is used for the manufacture of cigar-boxes, packing cases, pencils, plyboard, match-boxes and match-sticks; it is also used for making catamarans and musical instruments. Fruit pulp is anthelmintic and is also used for colic and in ointments for skin diseases.

Arani – *see* Agetha.

Aranyadhanya (S)–*see* Janglidal.

Aranyavasini (S) – *see* Amal-bel.

Ararut, Tikhor – *Maranta arundinacea* L.; West Indian arrowroot (E); Marantaceae; perennial herb or undershrub. Cultivated for its edible starchy rhizomes, which are the source of commercial 'ararut' or arrowroot starch, used in infant foods and culinary preparations such as puddings, jellies and confectionery. Fibrous residue left after extraction of starch is used as cattle feed. Rhizomes are also eaten boiled or roasted.

Archaka – *Sonneratia caseolaris* (L.) Engl. (syn. *S. acida* L.f.); Sonneratiaceae; tree found in marshy tidal waters. Raw fruits are used for flavouring chutneys and for making vinegar. Ripe fruits are edible and the pericarp is considered as a vermifuge. Wood is used for general carpentry. Stem bark yields tannin. Vertical spongy respiratory roots or pneumatophores are used as a substitute for cork in the preparation of shoe soles, floats for nets, artificial flowers and fancy articles.

Ardanda, Gitoran, Karambha (S) – *Capparis zeylanica* L.; Capparidaceae; thorny climbing shrub. Cultivated as a hedge plant. Fruits are made into pickle. Root bark acts as a stomachic and sedative.

Ardraka (S) – *see* Adrak.

Arhar, Tur; Adhaki (S), Tuvari (S) – *Cajanus cajan* (L.) Millsp.; Pigeonpea (E), Red gram (E); Papilionaceae; shrub. Cultivated extensively as a pulse crop. Split seeds are used as a popular pulse. Globulins *viz.*, cajanin and con-cajanin are present. Husk of pods and leaves are used as stock-feed and slender straight branches are used for basketry and thatching. Plants are also used for green manuring and as a cover crop in plantations.

Arinj – *see* Safed kikar.

Arimeda (S) – *see* Safed kikar.

Arishta (S) – *see* Adhasisi; *see also* Neem.

Arishtha (S) – *see* Reetha.

Arjun, Kahu; Arjuna (S) – *Terminalia arjuna* (Roxb.) Wight. & Arn.; Arjun Terminalia (E); Combretaceae; large tree. Cultivated as an avenue tree. Wood is used as timber for building boats and agricultural implements. Powdered and pulverized bark is used for curing hypertension and cirrhosis of the liver. Bark contains tannin which is used for dyeing and tanning. Leaves are used to feed 'tassar' silkworms.

Arjuna (S) – *see* Arjun.

Arka (S) – *see* Ak.

Arkakanta (S) – *see* Hulhul.

Arkapushpi (S) – *see* Chhirvel.

Arkapushpika (S) – *see* Hulul.

Arkavallabha (S) – *see* Dopahariya.

Arlu, Saona, Son-patti; Shyonaka (S) – *Oroxylum indicum* (L.) Vent. (syn. *Calosanthes indica* Blume.); Bignoniaceae; deciduous tree. Root bark comprises as one of the constituents of the Ayurvedic preparation 'Dasamula'. Roots are used in diarrhoea, dysentery and rheumatism. Leaf decoction is used for stomach ache and leaves are also used for external application in ulcers, headache and spleen enlargement. Seeds are purgative and tender fruits are stomachic. They are also the source of a semi-drying oil. Wood is used for match boxes and bark yields tannin. Young shoots and fruits are consumed as vegetable.

Arni; Agnimanthini (S) – *Clerodendrum multiflorum* (Burm. f.) Kuntze; Verbenaceae; shrub. Roots are astringent and aromatic. Root decoction is used in gonorrhoea and leaf decoction is administered in syphilitic complaints.

Arsaghna (S) – *see* Zamin-kand.

Aru, Shaftalu; Aruka (S), Aluka (S) – *Prunus persica* (L.) Batsch.; Peach (E), Nectarine (E); Rosaceae; small tree. Cultivated for fruit with its soft and juicy flesh which is rich in sugars, ascorbic acid and thiamine, and used as a dessert fruit. Kernels yield a fatty oil used for cooking and as an illuminant and the kernel shells yield charcoal. Roots are the source of a black dye. Decoction of the leaves and bark is used in whooping cough.

Arua – *see* Maharuk.

Aruka (S) – *see* Aru.

Arusha, Adulasa, Bansa, Basaka; Vasaka (S) – *Adhatoda vasica* Nees; Malabar nut (E); Acanthaceae; evergreen shrub. Leaves are rich in the alkaloid vasicine and an essential oil, and are used in the preparation of cough syrups which are used chiefly as an expectorant and for giving relief in bronchitis. Leaves also possess a resin which is toxic to insects and is used as a weedicide and anthelmintic. Seeds yield a fatty oil and roots, flowers and leaves yield an essential oil reported to be active against tuberculosis bacteria. Plant is also found useful for reclamation of soil.

Aruskaara (S) – *see* Bhilawa.

Arvi, Ghuiyan, Kachalu; Kachu (S) – *Colocasia esculenta* (L.) Schott; Arum (E), Taro (E); Araceae; perennial rhizomatous herb. Cultivated for its edible tuberous rhizomes which are used as a vegetable. Rhizome is rich in starch and its flour is used for the preparation of taro-lactin, malt and alcohol. Mucilage in rhizomes is used for sizing impermeable paper.

Asalrai, Rai – *Brassica juncea* (L.) Czern. & Coss.; Indian mustard (E); Cruciferae; annual herb. Cultivated as an oil-seed crop. Seeds yield a fatty oil called mustard oil used as a cooking medium. The oil has very low content of saturated fatty acids, high content of monounsaturated fatty acids and 9-15 per cent of polyunsaturated fatty acids with the desirable ratio of linolenic and linoleic acids. Oil cake is used as cattle feed. Tender shoots and leaves are used as vegetable. Seeds are used as a condiment, and for making pungent mustard sauce and some pickles.

Asan, Sain, Saj – *Terminalia alata* Hayne ex Roth; Combretaceae; tree. Cultivated for timber which is used for rafters, beams, telegraph and electric poles, furniture, bodies of carts, plywood, and manufacture of paper. Bark is used for dyeing and tanning and the residue is used for the extraction of oxalic acid. Bark is also used medicinally as a cardiotonic. Leaves are used to rear 'tassar' silkworms. Tree exudes a gum which is used as a purgative and adhesive.

Asana (S) – *see* Ekdania.

Asar – *Microcos paniculata* L. (syn. *Grewia microcos* L.); Tiliaceae; large, shrub. Leaves are used as cigar wrappers. Plant is also the source of a fibre.

Asbarg, Gul-jalil; Trayamaana (S) – *Delphinium zalil* Aitch & Hamsl; Zalil larkspur (E); Ranunculaceae; herb found in Kashmir. Flowers are used for the extraction of 'asbarg', which is considered as an anodyne and diuretic and is used in spleen disorders, dropsy and jaundice. Flowers also yield 'asbarg' dye which is used for colouring cotton and silk fabrics.

Asgandh; Aswagandha (S), Aswarohika (S) – *Withania somnifera* (L.) Dunal; Winter cherry (E); Solanaceae; undershrub. Roots are smooth, tapering, plump and of a yellow brown colour and are reported to exhibit antibiotic and antibacterial activity. Roots are source of the drug 'asgandh' which has been used in traditional Ayurvedic medicine from ancient times for treating cough, hiccups, consumption, dropsy, rheumatism, general debility and certain female ailments; it is also used externally for ulcers and inflammations. Roots contain several alkaloids and leaves contain withaferin A and are applied to painful swellings and sore eyes.

Ashok, Ampich; Asok (S) – *Saraca asoca* (Roxb.) de Wilde (syn. *Saraca indica* auct. non L.); Asoka tree (E); Caesalpiniaceae; tree. Cultivated as an ornamental for its beautiful scarlet red flowers and handsome foliage. Bark is astringent and is used in the indigenous Ayurvedic system of medicine for treating excessive menstruation; it is also used for treating diarrhoea, dysentery, leucorrhoea and kidney stones.

Ashoke, Debdari – *Polyalthia longifolia* Thw.; Mast tree (E); Annonaceae; evergreen tree. Cultivated as an avenue tree along road-sides and pathways. The tree has straight stem and branches almost at right angles forming a symmetrical pyramidal crown with downward sweeping branchlets and glossy green beautiful leaves. Wood is soft, light and flexible and is used for pencils, match industry and packing boxes. Bark yields fibre. Festoons of leaves are used at festivities and ceremonies to decorate daises, gates, pillars and arches.

Ashta – *see* Kachnal.

Ashvaghna (S) – *see* Peeli kaner.

Ashvaghra (S) – *see* Badrang.

Ashvashakota (S) – *see* Ban-nimbu,

Ashvattha (S) – *see* Peepal.

Ashwagandha (S) – *see* Asgandh.

Ashwakatri (S) – *Drynaria quercifolia* (L.) J. Smith (syn. *Polypodium quercifolium* L.); Polypodiaceae; perennial evergreen fern. Poultice of fronds is used for inflammation. Rhizomes astringent, and their aqueous extract is used for treating pulmonary tuberculosis, cough and dyspepsia, and exhibits antibacterial properties.

Ashyuka (S) – *see* Al.

Asmantaka (S) – *see* Bistendu.

Asmarighna (S) – *see* Bilasi.

Asok (S)–*see* Ashok.

Asphota (S) – *see* Nwari.

Aspurk – *Melilotus officinalis* (L.) Lamk; Yellow sweet-clover (E); Papilionaceae; herb. Cultivated for fodder in some parts of India. Plant is used fresh and as hay, and provides nutritious fodder which is rich in proteins and minerals. Herb is also used as an emollient and carminative.

Asrel – *see* Sarpagandha.

Asthisanhara (S) – *see* Hadjora.

Astmabayota (S) – *see* Gorakh booti.

Asumodhagam (S) – *see* Methi.

Asvarohika (S)–*see* Asgandh.

Aswagandha (S)–*see* Asgandh.

Atamagupta (S)–*see* Kiwach.

Atasi (S) – *see* Alsi.

Atavi-jambira (S)–*see* Jangli nimbu.

Atibala (S) – *see* Kanghi.

Atiguha (S)–*see* Pithvan.

Atirasa (S) – *see* Rasna.

Atis; Ativisha (S) – *Aconitum heterophyllum* Wall. ex Royle (syn. *A. atees* Royle); Atis root (E); Ranunculaceae; tall perennial herb. Cultivated in the hills and also found wild in high altitudes of W. Himalayas. Roots are used to treat hysteria, cough, dyspepsia, diarrhoea, vomiting and abdominal pain. Several alkaloids are present *viz.*, heterophylline, heterophyllidine, atidine, atisine and histisine.

Atitejani (S) – *see* Badrang.

Ativisha (S) – *see* Atis.

Atrilal – *Peristrophe bicalyculata* (Retz.) Nees; Acanthaceae; annual much branched herb. Plants are used as fodder for horses. Essential oil from the plant is reported to exhibit tuberculostatic activity *in vitro*. Macerated plant mixed with rice infusion is considered as an antidote to snake-poison.

Attah-bar – *see* Bor.

Attardana – *see* Madanmohan.

Atyamlaparni (S) – *see* Amal-bel.

Avachirayeta – *Exacum tetragonum* Roxb.; Gentianaceae; branched herb. Plant is considered to be a tonic and stomachic and is used as a substitute for 'chirayeta' or *Swertia chirayita* (Roxb. ex Flem) Karst.

Avartani (S) – *see* Marorphali.

Avighna (S) – *see* Karaunda.

Awa – *see* Alla.

Ayapana – *Eupatorium triplinerve* Vahl. (syn. *E. ayapana* Vent.); Ayapana tea (E); Compositae; small undershrub. Often cultivated for aromatic aerial parts, which are the source of an essential oil. Aqueous extract of the shoots is a cardiac stimulant. Leaf juice is used to check internal haemorrhage. Hot infusion of the herb acts as a tonic, emetic, diuretic and diaphoretic and is used in jaundice and scurvy and for fomentation of ulcers and sores.

B

Babchi, Bukchi; Bakuchi (S), Kushth-nashini (S), Sugandha-kantak (S) – *Psoralea corylifolia* L.; Babchi (E); Papilionaceae; herb. Seeds are diuretic, laxative and anthelmintic and their paste is considered to be very useful for leucoderma, leprosy and the inflammatory diseases of skin. Active principles present are psoralen and iso-psoralen. Seeds contain both a fixed oil and an essential oil. Seed cake is used as manure

Baberang; Wawrang; Vrishanasana (S) – *Embelia ribes* Burm. f.; Myrsinaceae; shrub. Fruits are stomachic, anthelmintic and tonic and are used specifically to expel tapeworms. Active principle present is emblin. Tender fruits and leaves are used as vegetable. Fruit decoction is administered in chest and skin disorders. Dried fruit is used to adulterate black pepper.

Babni – *see* Babui.

Babui, Babni, Bhabar – *Eulaliopsis binata* (Retz.) C.E. Hubb. (syn. *Andropogon binatus* Retz.); Baib-grass (E), Sabai grass (E); Gramineae; tufted perennial herb. Plants are used for the manufacture of paper, ropes and mats.

Babui tulsi – *see* Ban tulsi.

Babul – *see* Kikar.

Babuna – *Cotula anthemoides* L.; Compositae; herb. Plant decoction prepared in oil is used externally for painful rheumatic swellings. Decoction of the plants in water is used for treating colds and infusion is used for washing eyes. Another species *Matricaria chamomilla* L. is also known by the same Hindi name.

Babuna, Sutei-gul – *Matricaria chamomilla* L.; German chamomile (E); Compositae; herb. Plant is considered to be a gastric stimulant, carminative, expectorant, antispasmodic, anthelmintic, diuretic and sedative, and is used in remedies for flatulent colic, general debility, and children's ailments. Plant infusion is applied to sores, bruises, eczema and inflammation. Plant also yields an essential oil called German chamomile oil which is used for flavouring liqueurs, cosmetics and tobacco, and is also valued in perfumery.

Bacchang – *see* Bish.

Bach, Safed-bach; Vacha (S) – *Acorus calamus* L.; Sweet flag (E); Araceae; aromatic marshy herb. Rhizomes are branched, aromatic, and used in mental ailments as a stimulant to the central nervous system; they are also used medicinally as a tonic, expectorant and carminative, and in treating diarrhoea and dysentery. Essential oil from the rhizomes is used to flavour liqueurs and foodstuffs and in perfumery. Alcoholic extract of the rhizomes is analgesic, blood-pressure depressant and sedative.

Bachita, Lapetua, Pithia, Unga, Van-bhenda – *Urena lobata* L.; Aramina (E), Cadillo (E); Malvaceae; small shrub. Stem yields a fibre which is used as a jute substitute; it is also used for coarse cloth, carpets, linoleum, ropes, and cordage. Plant cuttings are used for paper pulp, and the mucilaginous seeds for making soap. Roots are considered to be diuretic.

Bacho – *Rubia tinctorum* L.; Alizari (E), European madder (E); Rubiaceae; herb found in Kashmir. Roots yield a red dye used for dyeing and printing cloth, and also used for colouring food products and cosmetics. Plants are also used as fodder. Roots are tonic and astringent and are used for the treatment of arthritis, spleen, liver and gall bladder disorders.

Badam – *Prunus amygdalus* Batsch; Almond (E); Rosaceae; tree. Cultivated in many parts of India for its edible seeds which are used as dry fruit and nerve tonic. Seeds are very nutritious, rich in the protein globulin, minerals iron and calcium, and vitamins. Dry seeds are used as such, roasted, or soaked to activate the enzymes. Oil called 'badam rogan' extracted from the seeds is used extensively in confectionery, pharmaceuticals and cosmetics.

Badar – *see* Paludar.

Badara (S) – *see* Baer.

Badavard, Rissa – *Oligochaeta ramosa* (Roxb.) Wagen [syn. *Volutarella ramosa* (Roxb.) Santapau]; Compositae; herb found in the tropical parts of India in dry, hard and stony places. Plant is considered as a tonic and febrifuge; and is also used for curing cough.

Badhara, Nag-phul; Gopbhadra (S), Vikarini (S) – *Gmelina asiatica* L. (syn. *G. parviflora* Pers.); Verbenaceae; spiny straggling shrub. Cultivated for its bright yellow flowers and for making hedges. Roots are mucilaginous, and are used for treating rheumatism, catarrh of bladder and gonorrhoea. Fruits are edible. Seeds yield a semi-drying oil.

Badian, Saurif; Shetapushpa (S) – *Pimpinella anisum* L.; Anise (E); Umbelliferae; annual herb. Cultivated for its aromatic dried fruits, considered to be carminative, expectorant, diuretic and antiflatulent, and used in pharmaceuticals. Fruits are a rich source of anise oil which is used in perfumery and for the manufacture of soaps and cosmetics.

Badrang; Ashvaghra (S) Atitejani (S), Sutejasi (S) – *Zanthoxylum limonella* (Dennst.) Alston; Rutaceae; tree. Bark, leaves and seeds are aromatic. Fruits are digestive, appetizing and reported to be used in combating asthma, bronchitis, rheumatism and heart trouble. Seeds yield a fatty oil. Wood is used for turnery and carving; mullilam oil, an essential oil obtained from the fruit rind is used as an antiseptic and disinfectant, and also shows antibacterial properties.

Badri (S) – *see* Baer.

Bael; Bilva; Sriphala (S) – *Aegle marmelos* (L.) Correa; Bael tree (E); Bengal quince (E); Rutaceae; thorny deciduous tree. Fruit pulp which is sweet and aromatic is either eaten raw or made into squashes. Half ripe fruits act as an astringent and digestive, and are used for curing diarrhoea and dysentery. Gummy substance around the seeds is used for adhesives, and is mixed with water-colour paints to give shine. Wood pulp is used for paper manufacture and leaves yield an essential oil. Plant is held sacred by the Hindus, and its leaves called 'bael patra' are offered to Lord Shiva, one of the Trinity gods.

Baer, Ber, Ajapriya (S), Badara (S), Badri (S), Madhura-phala (S) – *Ziziphus mauritiana* Lamk. [syn. *Z. jujuba* (L.) Lamk. non Mill.] Indian jujube (E); Rhamnaceae; medium sized spiny tree. Fruits are edible, and a rich source of vitamin C. Dried fruit forms constituent of 'Joshanda' an Ayurvedic mixture of dried herbs for treating colds. Bark is used for tanning and leaves for fodder. Wood is used for multifarious purposes and the plant serves as a host to lac insect.

Bagamushada – *see* Bega.

Bagbherenda, Safed Arand, Ratanjyot; Kananaeranda (S), Parvataranda (S) – *Jatropha curcas* L.; Physic nut (E); Euphorbiaceae; shrub. Seed oil called curcas oil is used as a strong purgative. It is also used in the manufacture of soaps, varnishes and candles and for lubrication. It is used medicinally in treating sciatica and paralysis and externally for rheumatism and skin troubles. The oil has been used for illumination and for lighting 'mashals' or torches since olden times. The seeds contain about 30 per cent oil and superior genotypes are being evolved by The Energy and Resources Institute (TERI), New Delhi, India. With the development of proper technology the oil can be used as a substitute for diesel and a promising biofuel. Bark yields a blue dye and tannin. Leaves also yield a dye.

Baghanulla – *see* Soltraj.

Bahera; Bahira (S), Vibhitaka (S) – *Terminalia bellirica* (Gaertn.) Roxb.; Belleric myrobalan (E); Combretaceae; deciduous tree. Cultivated as an avenue tree. Ripe fruits are rich in tannin and are used as an astringent in combination with chebulic myrobalan. Bark acts as a tonic and diuretic. Fruits are used for dyeing and tanning. Fruit pulp is used in dropsy and diarrhoea and half ripe fruits are used as a purgative. Kernel oil is used in soap manufacture. Wood pulp is considered to be good for the manufacture of wrapping paper.

Bahira (S) – *see* Bahera.

Bahukanda (S) – *see* Kakri.

Bahukantaka (S) – *see* Makoh.

Bahupada (S) – *see* Barh.

Bahuvaraka (S) – *see* Lasora.

Baib – *see* Babui.

Baichi – *see* Bilangra.

Baikal, Kingani, Vingar; Vikangata (S), Sudhavriksha (S) – *Gymnosporia montana* (Roth.) Benth; Thorny staff tree (E); Celastraceae; tree. Wood is used for making beads and leaves are used for fodder. Decoction of shoots is used for curing colic, diarrhoea and dysentery among children.

Baikunti, Amlanch – *Ribes grossularia* L.; European gooseberry (E); Grossulariaceae; shrub. Fruits are edible.

Bailewa – *see* Kuchla.

Baingan, Bhanta; Vartaka (S), Jukutam (S) – *Solanum melongena* L.; Brinjal (E), Aubergine (E), Egg plant (E); Solanaceae; undershrub. Cultivated for its fruit, which is used as a vegetable. Fruit is reported to stimulate interhepatic metabolism of cholesterol. Leaves are used in combating bronchitis and asthma. Roots also act as anti-asthmatic. Seeds yield a fatty oil.

Bairola, Kumpaiman – *Cordia vestita* Hook. f. & Thoms.; Ehretiaceae; tree. Fruit is edible, and is considered to be an astringent and expectorant. Wood is used for wheels, panelling and carving.

Baishi, Bilsa, Sukul bet; Varuna (S) – *Salix tetrasperma* Roxb.; Indian willow (E); Salicaceae; tree. Wood is used for construction work, bent-wood furniture and other articles such as ploughs, cricket-stumps, packing cases, gunpowder charcoal, match boxes and pencils. Branches are flexible, and are used for making baskets.

Bark is rich in tannin, and is used as a febrifuge. Dry leaf-powder is medicinal, and is used for treating rheumatism, epilepsy, stones in bladder and venereal diseases.

Bajarbattu; Sritalam (S), Tali (S) – *Corypha umbraculifera* L.; Fan palm (E), Talipot palm (E); Palmae; tall palm. Cultivated in Bengal and the Andaman islands. Leaves are used for making fans, baskets, mats, umbrellas and for thatching. Strips of leaves were used for writing ancient Buddhist texts. Leaf stalks are used in the manufacture of wrapping paper and the seeds find use as ivory substitute for the manufacture of buttons, beads and small carved ornaments.

Bajra, Lahra – *Pennisetum typhoides* (Burm. f.) Stapf & C.E. Hubb.; Pearl millet (E); Gramineae; tall annual robust grass. Cultivated for its edible grains which are also suitable for making malt. Plant makes good fodder.

Bak – *see* Agasti.

Bakain, Drek; Mahanimba (S) – *Melia azedarach* L.; China tree (E), Pride of India (E), Persian lilac (E); Meliaceae; small tree. Leaf juice is anthelmintic and diuretic. Infusion of bark is used in ascariasis. Wood is used for making musical instruments, handles and toys. Fruit pulp is used in colic pain and seeds yield an oil which is used topically in rheumatism.

Bakal-bip – *Derris elliptica* (Wall.) Benth.; Tuba root (E); Papilionaceae; climbing shrub. Cultivated for its roots, which are used as an insecticide and fish poison. Roots are rich in rotenone.

Bakam, Patang; Pattaranjaka (S) – *Caesalpinia sappan* L.; Sappan wood (E); Caesalpiniaceae; shrub or small tree grown for hedges. Heartwood yields a red dye. Decoction of wood is useful in treating mild diarrhoea and dysentery. Leaves contain an essential oil. Pods and bark contain tannin.

Bakar, Basota – *Premna mucronata* Roxb.; Verbenaceae; deciduous tree. Wood is of inferior quality and used as fuel. Latex from the bark is applied topically to boils, and fed to cattle for colic.

Bakarcha, Dalme, Patala – *Securinega virosa* (Roxb. ex Willd.) Baill.; Euphorbiaceae; large shrub. Grown as hedge plant; ripe fruits are edible. Bark yields tannin. Wood is used for agricultural implements and walking-sticks. Decoction of leaves is given as a laxative. Alkaloids present are securinine and virosecurinine. Leaf juice mixed with tobacco is used to kill worms in open wounds of livestock.

Bakla, Anhuri, Kala matar – *Vicia faba* L.; Broad bean (E), Windsor bean (E); Papilionaceae; herb. Seeds and fresh pods are consumed as vegetable. Also grown for fodder and green manure. Decoction of tender shoots is diuretic.

Bakri-patti – *Trema cannabina* Lour.; Ulmaceae; small tree. Bark yields a fibre used for making fishing-nets. Decoction of roots is used as a cure for sore tongue. Leaves are reported to be toxic.

Bakuchi (S) – *see* Babchi.

Bakul (S) – *see* Maulsari.

Bala – *see* Kungyi.

Balakanda (S) – *see* Amarkand.

Balaya (S) – *Cadaba trifoliata* (Roxb.) Wight & Arn; Capparidaceae; shrub. Roots and leaves act as a purgative and anthelmintic.

Balbasant – *see* Basanti.

Balchir – *see* Jatamansi.

Balhika (S) – *see* Hing.

Bal kunwari – *Ginkgo biloba* L.; Maidenhair tree (E); Ginkgoaceae; evergreen tree native to China. Cultivated as an ornamental tree in very few places in India. Kernels are edible after cooking or roasting; they also serve as an expectorant and sedative. Wood is suitable for making toys and chessboards.

Balmota – *see* Jainti.

Balnag – *Aconitum chasmanthum* Stapf. ex Holmes (syn. *A. napellus* L. var. *spicatum* Duthie); Indian napellus (E); Ranunculaceae; herb found in the hills of W. Himalayas. Rhizomes yield the aconite of commerce which is used in asthma, sore throat, cough, nasal catarrh, gastric disorders, certain fevers of inflammatory origin and as a sedative. Paste is used for topical application in rheumatism. Active principles in rhizomes include chasmaconitine, chasmanine, chasmathinine, homochasmanine and indaconitine.

Balraja – *see* Mandla.

Balsana – *see* Bassant.

Baltanga – *Plantago lanceolata* L.; Plantaginaceae; herb. Seeds are used as a purgative. Leaves and roots are astringent, and are applied to inflamed surfaces and wounds; they are also used in pulmonary diseases.

Balukand (S) – *see* Zamin-kand.

Balu-ka-sag; Valuka (S) – *Gisekia pharnacoides* L.; Aizoaceae; herb found in dry regions. Plant is used as pot-herb; also given to camels and goats as fodder. Leaves are anthelmintic.

Bamna, Hika-gadi, Mathaniya – *Chloris dolichostachya* Lagasca; Gramineae; herb. Plants are used for fodder.

Bamora, Tharbal – *Benthamidia capitata* (Wall. ex Roxb.) Hara (syn. *Cornus capitata* Wall. ex Roxb.); Cornaceae, small tree. Fruits are consumed fresh and also made into preserves.

Ban – *see* Munj.

Banada – *see* Jangli adrak.

Banafshah; Nilapushpa (S) – *Viola odorata* L.; Sweet violet (E); Violaceae; herb. Plant is utilized widely in Ayurvedic, Unani and Homoeopathic systems of medicine. It is used as an expectorant, diaphoretic, diuretic and for throat infections. Rootstocks contain the alkaloid odoratine which is an hypertensive. Violet leaves and flowers yield high grade perfume and a medicinal oil called 'rogan banafshah' is prepared from the decoction of leaves and flowers of *Viola pilosa* Blume.

Banajowan; Vanayamini (S) – *Seseli diffusum* (Roxb. ex Sm.) Santapau & Wagh.; Umbelliferae; herb. Fruits are aromatic, stimulant, carminative, stomachic and anthelmintic, and are used for expelling roundworms. Fruits yield an essential oil called 'ajmod' oil and a fatty oil. Fruits are widely used in veterinary medicine.

Banajwain – *Thymus serpyllum* L.; Wild thyme (E); Labiatae; an aromatic herb. Leaves are used for making an alcoholic beverage. Leaves and floral tops are used for flavouring, they also yield an essential oil which is used for toothache. Seeds act as a vermifuge and their ethanolic extract is used in scalp and hair lotions.

Banamethika (S) – *see* Senji.

Bananiyar, Bhumi-bala – *Sida veronicaefolia* Lamk.; Malvaceae; shrub. Root bark is used in medicines for treating gonorrhoea and leucorrhoea. Root is also used in urinary complaints and fevers. Leaf poultice is used for cuts and bruises. Herb infusion is used for arthritis in animals. Leaves are also used as pot-herb. Stem is the source of a fibre used for cordage.

Banarasi rai, Kali rai – *Brassica nigra* (L.) Koch; Black mustard (E); Cruciferae; herb. Cultivated for its seeds used as a spice and condiment and table-mustard. Seeds also yield an oil used for edible purpose and soap manufacture. Volatile oil obtained after distillation of defatted seeds is used as a rubefacient and as a preservative for apple juice. Pungent constituent of the seeds is a glycoside called sinigrin.

Ban-baer – *see* Unnab.

Ban-bakar, Kasmol – *Cornus oblonga* Wall.; Cornaceae; tree. Wood is used for making pulleys, shuttles, bobbins and gunpowder charcoal.

Banchilla – *see* Kanju.

Banda; Vanda (S), Vriksharuha (S) – *Dendrophthoe falcata* (L.f.) Ettingsh.; Loranthaceae; evergreen leafy semiparasitic shrub, occurring on trees. Tender shoots are rich in tannin. Bark acts as an astringent and narcotic, and is used for treating asthma and menstrual disorders.

Banda – *Viscum album* L.; European mistletoe (E); Viscaceae; semiparasitic shrub. Drug from the plant is used for the treatment of hypertension, hysteria, epilepsy and piles. Berries and bark yield the resin viscin which is used in sticking plasters.

Bandala – *see* Budu.

Bandari ghas – *see* Bandra.

Band-gobi – *see* Patta-gobi.

Bandhuka (S) – *see* Rangan.

Bando, Maula – *Butea parviflora* Roxb.; Papilionaceae; tree. Decoction of the bark is used in bowel complaints. Tree exudes a gum and the bark yields a fibre used for making ropes. Seeds yield a fatty oil.

Bandra, Bandari ghas – *Setaria glauca* (L.) Beauv. (syn. *Panicum glaucum* L.); Cat-tail millet (E), Foxtail millet (E); Gramineae; annual herb. Plant is used as fodder and the grains are consumed as food and for making alcohol.

Banga-gandina – *Allium tuberosum* Rottl. ex Spreng.; Indian leek (E), Chinese chive (E); Alliaceae; herb. Cultivated in a few places, and used as a condiment.

Ban-gulab – *Rosa macrophylla* Lindl.; Rosaceae; deciduous shrub. Grown as a hedge plant. Fruits are edible, and flowers yield a perfume.

Ban-hardi – *Morinda angustifolia* Roxb.; Rubiaceae; climbing shrub or tree, found in E. Himalayas. Roots yield a yellow dye.

Banharria, Khardol – *Trema politoria* (Planch.) Blume; Ulmaceae; shrub or small tree good for aforestation. Fruits are edible. Wood is good for gunpowder charcoal. Leaves being very rough textured are used for polishing ivory, horns and wood, instead of sand paper. Stem yields rough fibre for ropes.

Banj – *Quercus incana* Roxb.; White oak (E); Fagaceae; evergreen tree. Wood is used for implements, tools and firewood. Wood-pulp is considered to be good for making wrapping paper. Bark yields tannin. Acorns are diuretic and astringent, and yield manna which is used in confectionery.

Bankakri – *see* Papra.

Bankalmi – *Ipomoea sepiaria* Roxb.; Convolvulaceae; trailing herb. Tender shoots and leaves are consumed as pot-herb. Juice is diuretic.

Bankapas – *see* Jangli bhendi.

Bankhor, Kanor, Pangar – *Aesculus indica* Colebr. ex Camb.; Indian horse-chestnut (E); Hippocastanaceae; tree. Fruits are edible, leaves are used as fodder, and wood is used for furniture and gunpowder charcoal. Extract of the wood gives a dye used for dyeing silk. Seeds are consumed after boiling. Seed oil is used for the manufacture of soap.

Bankumra, Bidari-kand, Siali – *Pueraria tuberosa* (Roxb. ex Willd.) DC.; Indian kudzu (E); Papilionaceae; climbing shrub found in the hilly regions. Root tubers are edible, and leaves are used for fodder. Tubers are reportedly used in tribal medicine for treating arthritis and as an aphrodisiac.

Banlaunga; Bhulavanga (S) – *Jussiaea suffruticosa* L.; Onagraceae; herb. Reported to be carminative, diuretic, and anthelmintic; decoction of the herb is given in diarrhoea, dysentery, flatulence and leucorrhoea.

Banmallika – *see* Bela.

Banmethi – *see* Senji.

Bannalia, Hunraj; Nisomali (S) – *Polygonum aviculare* L.; Polygonaceae; herb. Used as pot-herb, fodder, and in indigenous system of medicine for treating diabetes, rheumatism, bleeding piles and excessive menstruation. Plant also yields a blue dye and is considered to be rich in vitamin E. Seeds act as a purgative.

Ban-naringa – *Suregada multiflora* (Juss.) Baill. (syn. *Gelonium multiflorum* Juss.); Euphorbiaceae; tree. Grown as a hedge plant. Fruits are edible. Bark is used in gum trouble. Wood is used for making rafters and has waxy odour.

Ban-nil – *see* Sarphonka.

Ban-nimbu; Ashvashakota (S), Vananimbuka (S) – *Glycosmis pentaphylla* (Retz.) DC.; Rutaceae; shrub. Fruit is edible, leaf juice is used as a vermifuge and in liver complaints. Paste of leaves is used as a cure for eczema.

Banokra – *see* Adhasisi.

Banpalas – *see* Moka.

Banpalti, Galion, Mauli – *Sorbus lanata* (D. Don.) Schauer (syn. *Pyrus lanata* D. Don.); Rosaceae; tree. Wood is used for making packing boxes. Fruit is edible.

Banpatara, Keri – *Ligustrum indicum* (Lour.) Merr.; Oleaceae; large shrub. Leaves are made into poultice and used for bruises; their decoction is used medicinally as a diuretic.

Banpindalu – *see* Paphar.

Ban piyazi, Jangli piyaz, safedi-khus; Kolkanda (S), Vanapandan (S) – *Urginea indica* Kunth; Indian drug squill (E), Sea-onion (E); Liliaceae; herb. Drug from the bulbs is used as a stimulant, expectorant and cardio-tonic in small doses. It is also employed in the treatment of rheumatism, dropsy and skin-trouble. Bulbs are the source of a raticide. Their paste is applied externally to warts and corns.

Ban-rhea – *Oreocnide integrifolia* Miq.; Wild rhea (E); Urticaceae; small tree. Stem is the source of a fibre called 'risa', which is strong, lustrous, silky and does not need degumming as in the true rhea or ramie (*Boehmeria nivea* Gaudich). The fibre is used for fishing nets, ropes, sack cloth, and canvas.

Bans; Vansh (S) – *Bambusa arundinacea* Willd.; Thorny bamboo (E) Gramineae; tall woody grass. Stems are used for making rafters for floating heavy timber, and serve as a source of good quality paper-pulp and rayon-grade pulp. Young shoots are pickled and made into curry. Leaves and twigs are used as fodder.

Bansa – *see* Arusha.

Ban-sangli – *Crataegus oxyacantha* L.; English hawthorn (E); Rosaceae; large thorny shrub found in the hills. Fruit juice is considered to be useful in heart disease.

Banshana – *Crotalaria verrucosa* L.; Papilionaceae; herb or undershrub. Leaves are used for treating scabies and other skin ailments.

Bansi – *see* Gunara.

Bansigru; Kananashigru (S) – *Ormocarpum cochinchinensis* (Lour.) Merr.; Papilionaceae; shrub. Roots are considered to be stimulant and are used for treating lumbago. Root bark boiled in oil is used for treating paralysis. Root is also used as a fish-poison.

Bans kaban, Narbans; Vansha (S) – *Dendrocalamus strictus* Nees; Solid bamboo (E); Gramineae; arborescent perennial forming dense clumps. Culms are used for scaffoldings, rafters, furniture, tent-poles, fishing rods, paper-pulp, and also serve as the source of a cellulose gum which is used in the manufacture of paper, textiles, cosmetics, paints, lacquers and leather.

Bans keora, Bara kanwar; Kalakantala (S) – *Agave americana* L.; Century plant (E); Agavaceae; short-stemmed stout shrub with a rosette of leaves. Plant is very hardy and is suitable for fencing the boundary and checking soil erosion. Leaves yield a fibre used for cordage, mats and brushes. Leaves also contain steroidal saponins and an essential oil which is used for termite-proofing of wall paper. Root is diuretic.

Banslochan – *Phyllostachys bambusoides* Sieb. & Zucc.; Giant timber bamboo (E); Gramineae; giant tree-like bamboo found in the hills. Stems are used for walking-sticks. Wood pulp is rich in cellulose and is used for the manufacture of paper and rayon. Calcareous deposit in the stems marketed as 'banslochan' is used in several Ayurvedic preparations.

Bans-pati – *see* Nini.

Ban tamaku, Phulla, Gidar tamaku – *Verbascum thapsus* L.; Common mullein (E), Cow's lungwort (E); Scrophulariaceae; herb. Leaves, flowers and roots are used for treating cough and asthma; their paste is used for local applications in inflammation of mucous membranes and piles. Decoction of the leaves is used as a heart stimulant and that of roots for curing cramps and migraine. Essential oil is bactericidal.

Ban-tulsi, Babui tulsi; Marua; Manjariki (S) – *Ocimum basilicum* L.; Sweet basil (E); Labiatae; herb. Cultivated for its aromatic leaves which yield an essential oil, called basil oil which is used in perfumery and for flavouring foods, pickles, sauces and beverages; also used as an insecticide and insect repellent. Leaf juice is used for curing ringworm. Seeds are used in controlling diarrhoea and chronic dysentery, and in poultices for sores and sinus.

Baphuli; Bhedani (S) – *Corchorus depressus* (L.) C. Chr.; Tiliaceae; herb. Seeds are used as tonic and leaves as an emollient.

Bar – *see* Barh.

Bara-bet – *Calamus viminalis* Willd. var. *fasciculatus* Becc.; Palmae; a large climber found in E. India. The cane is used for making cane-furniture, walking-sticks, umbrella handles and polo-sticks.

Barabi – *see* Gilla.

Barachandrika – *Rauvolfia tetraphylla* L.; Apocynaceae; a small much branched woody shrub. Extract of the plant mixed with castor oil is used for curing chronic skin diseases. Fruits yield a black dye. Roots are often used to adulterate *R. serpentina* roots, marketed as 'sarpagandha' or rauvolfia.

Bara-chirayeta – *Exacum bicolor* Roxb.; Gentianaceae; branched herb found in peninsular India and Orissa. Plants are tonic and stomachic and are often employed as a substitute for 'chirayeta' or gentian.

Bara-gokhru, Kadua gokkru – *Pedalium murex* L.; Pedaliaceae; herb. Mucilage obtained by soaking young twigs, leaves and seeds in water or milk has tonic properties and is used for treating gonorrhoea, and other urino-genital diseases. Decoction of the fruits is used for impotence.

Bara-gorun – *Ceriops decandra* (Griff.) Ding Hou; Rhizophoraceae; small tree, Bark and leaves yield tannin.

Barakanghi – *Abutilon hirtum* (Lam.) Sweet; Malvaceae; branched shrub. Stem yields a fibre and leaves are used for fodder. Other uses are similar to Kanghi (*Abutilon indicum*).

Bara kanwar – *see* Bans keora.

Barakkhanta – *Pericampylus glaucus* (Lam.) Merr.; Menispermaceae; sub-erect shrub. Stem is used for basketry. Mucilage from the leaves is used to check falling of hair. Infusion of the leaves is used for treating asthma and that of root is used as an antidote to snake poison.

Bara-kulanjan; Kulanjan (S) – *Alpinia galanga* (L.) Sw.; Greater galangal (E); Zingiberaceae; robust herb. Rhizomes are used as spice and to flavour food. They are also used medicinally for bronchial catarrh and rheumatism. Essential oil from the rhizomes is used in perfumery and as an insecticide. Seeds are used for curing colic, vomiting and diarrhoea. Flowers are pickled.

Bara-laniya – *see* Kulfa.

Baranal, Narhal, Narsal – *Arundo donax* L.; Spanish cane (E), Great reed (E); Gramineae; woody perennial bamboo. Stems are used for making fishing-rods, musical pipes, mats, baskets, and also used for thatching. Stems yield cellulose-pulp suitable for rayon-grade pulp, and high grade writing paper.

Bara nibu, Jambira, Pahari-nimbu – *Citrus limon* (L.) Burm. f.; Lemon (E); Rutaceae; a small thorny tree. Fruits are used mainly for the preparation of squashes, lemonade, confectionery and for culinary purposes. Pectin, citric acid and lemon oil from the rind are by-products. Lemon oil is used as a carminative. Common variety 'galgal' is cultivated in Punjab, Uttar Pradesh and many other states of India.

Bara pilu, Jhal, Khakan, Pilu – *Salvadora oleoides* Decne.; Salvadoraceae; a small tree with twisted trunk and drooping branches. Fruits are edible. Leaves are used as a purgative for horses, and also given to relieve cough. Fruits are used medicinally in enlarged spleen and rheumatism. Oil from the seeds is also used locally as a rubefacient for rheumatism.

Barasal – *see* Safed damar.

Bara salpan, Bhalia – *Maughania macrophylla* O. Kuntze; [syn. *Flemingia macrophylla* (Willd.) Kuntze ex Prain.] Papilionaceae; undershrub or shrub. Grown as an ornamental plant. Pods are edible, and roots are used in medicine for external application on ulcers and swellings; plant also serves as the principal source of warrus dye.

Bara sem, Safed kadsumbal – *Canavalia ensiformis* (L.) DC.; Jack bean (E), Horse bean (E); Papilionaceae; bushy herb. Pods are consumed as vegetable and the plant is used as green manure after harvesting the pods.

Bara siaru – *Boehmeria macrophylla* D. Don.; Urticaceae; shrub found in North India. Stem fibre is used for making fishing nets, fishing lines and cordage.

Barau, Dulal – *Taraxacum officinale* Weber ex Wiggers; Common dandelion (E); Compositae; herb. Roots and rhizomes yield a drug known as taraxacum which is used as a mild laxative, stomachic, diuretic, and tonic. Leaves are consumed as vegetable and are employed in the preparation of beer and wine along with flower-heads.

Barchar – *see* Karshu.

Bargad – *see* Barh.

Barh, Bar, Bargad; Bahupada (S), Vata (S) – *Ficus benghalensis* L.; Banyan (E); Moraceae; a large spreading evergreen tree with profuse aerial prop roots produced from the branches. Plant is grown for shade and is considered sacred in India. Leaves are lopped for fodder. Infusion of the bark is used for diarrhoea, dysentery and diabetes. Latex is used in rheumatism and lumbago, and the wood is considered to be good for paper pulp and furniture. The largest banyan tree in the world with the widest canopy covering 21 hectares, and propped up by 1100 roots and almost double the size of the banyan tree at the Botanical Garden, Calcutta is situated at Gutibayulu village near the Thimmamma Marrimanu temple in the Anantpur district of the state of Andhra Pradesh in India.

Barhanta; Duhsparsha, Vrishchikali – *Tragia involucrata* L. var. *rheediana* Muell. Arg.; Indian stinging-nettle (E); Euphorbiaceae; perennial straggling herb, with stinging hair. Fruit is an important constituent of the Ayurvedic preparation 'Kshar-guda' which is used for treating enlarged spleen. Root paste is used for getting rid of guinea worms, and mixed with Tulsi (*Ocimum sanctum*) leaf juice is used for skin ailments.

Barhichuda (S) – *see* Bhant.

Bariara, Kharenta – *Sida acuta* Burm. f.; Malvaceae; undershrub. Plant yields rough fibre for making ropes, and is also used as a jute substitute. Leaves are diuretic, and their decoction is used as a remedy for haemorrhoids. Roots are tonic, and are used in nerve and uterine disorders and to expel worms. Leaves boiled in oil are used in preparing ointments used for external application in rheumatism.

Bari chaulai – *see* Lal sag.

Bari chob-chini – *Smilax glabra* Roxb.; Smilacaceae; climbing shrub. Decoction of the roots is used by tribal people for treating sores and venereal diseases.

Bari elaichi – *Amomum subulatum* Roxb.; Greater cardamom (E); Zingiberaceae; rhizomatous herb. Fruits and seeds are considered as a cheaper substitute for true cardamoms. They are used to flavour sweetmeats and medicines. Seed oil is used for inflamed eyelids; also used as stomachic and stimulant. Another species *Amomum aromaticum* Roxb. is also known by the same Hindi name; *see* Morang elaichi.

Bari-ghumchi; Kun-chandan (S) – *Adenanthera pavonina* L.; Bead tree (E), Coral wood (E); Mimosaceae; large tree. Red heartwood is the source of a dye and is also used as a substitute of 'lal chandan', or true red sandalwood. Decoction of the seeds and wood is used for pulmonary disorders. Kernels contain a pale yellow fat. Shining scarlet red, hard seeds are used for making ornaments by the tribals.

Barik chirayeta, Kheta chirayeta – *Centaurium roxburghii* (G. Don.) Druce.; Gentianaceae; herb. Plant is used as a substitute of 'chirayeta'. It is a bitter tonic and stomachic.

Bari-main – *see* Jhau.

Bari-pipli, Gaja-pippali (S), Kari-pippali (S), Kapiballi (S) – *Scindapsus officinalis* Schott.; Araceae; large epiphytic climber. Dried fruits are used as an aromatic adjunct to other medicines. Decoction of the fruit acts as an expectorant, stimulant, carminative and anthelmintic.

Bari-sanwani – *see* Sanwani.

Barkau, Gair – *Olea glandulifera* Wall. ex G. Don; Oleaceae, large tree found in the hills. Wood is used for general carpentry, turnery, construction work and implements. Bark is rich in tannin. Both leaves and bark are astringent and febrifuge. Leaves are lopped for fodder.

Barlai – *Brassica juncea* L. ssp. *integrifolia* (West.) Thell. var. *integrifolia*; Mustard vegetable (E); Cruciferae; herb. Leaves are used as vegetable and are rich in minerals and vitamin B. Leaves are also pickled in brine.

Barna – *see* Bilasi.

Barphali – *see* Kungku.

Barsali, Bhursali – *Rottboellia exaltata* L.f.; Gramineae; annual herb. Plants are used for making both silage and hay; they are also used for making mats.

Bartundi – *see* Al.

Baru, Kala mucha – *Sorghum halepense* (L.) Pers.; Johnson grass (E); Gramineae; perennial grass. Plant is used as fodder. Grains are diuretic and demulcent.

Barus kapur, Bhimsaini kapur – *Dryobalanops aromatica* Gaertn. f.; Borneo camphor (E); Dipterocarpaceae; tree. Camphor resembles true camphor and occurs inside fissures in the wood. It is used in medicine and perfumery.

Basak – *Dichroa febrifuga* Lour.; Hydrangeaceae; an evergreen shrub. Roots and tender shoots are used as an emetic and febrifuge. Roots contain quinazoline derivatives and are used against malaria.

Basaka – *see* Arusha.

Basanti, Balbasant – *Reinwardtia indica* Dum.; Winter flax (E); Linaceae; shrub. Grown as an ornamental for its yellow flowers. Plant is used to treat paralysis. Crushed leaves are applied to open sores infested with maggots.

Basant rani – *Tabebuia spectabilis* Nichols.; Bignoniaceae; tree. Cultivated as an ornamental for its bright yellow flowers.

Basna – *see* Agasti.

Basota – *see* Bakar.

Bassant, Balsana, Dendhu – *Hypericum perforatum* L.; St. John's wort (E), Klamath weed (E); Hypericaceae; herb. Fresh flowers boiled in olive oil are used externally for treating sores, inflammation, rheumatism and lumbago; they are also used in facials. Herb is poisonous to livestock due to the presence of hypericin.

Bastra – *Callicarpa tomentosa* (L.) Murr.; Verbenaceae; small tree. Root and bark are used for skin troubles. Wood is good for carving.

Bathua – *see* Bethu sag.

Battal – *Sorbus aucuparia* L.; European mountain ash (E); Rosaceae; tree found in W. Himalayas. Fruit is edible, and is also used in preserves and as a flavouring agent. Bark is rich in tannin, and its decoction is given for controlling diarrhoea. Leaf infusion is used in bronchitis.

Baunra, Deura, Gonte – *Eurya japonica* Thunb; Theaceae; small tree. Leaf is used as an adulterant of tea; wood is used as fuel.

Bazarmani – *see* Kanocha.

Bebina, Bedina – *Mussaenda frondosa* L.; Rubiaceae; shrub. Flower calyx lobes and leaves are edible. Decoction of dried shoots is used for cough. Roots are used for treating leprosy and eye ailments. Wood is useful for making spoons and ladles.

Bed – *Salix acmophylla* Boiss.; Salicaceae; tree. Leaves are used for fodder. Wood is used for making small articles. Bark decoction is used as a febrifuge.

Bedina – *see* Bebina, *see also* Sarvad.

Bedmushk – *Salix caprea* L.; Goat willow (E), Sallow (E); Salicaceae; large shrub or small tree. Grown as an ornamental, for its fragrant flowers. Essential oil obtained from the leaves is used as a tonic and in perfumery. Bark and leaves are astringent and used in remedies for piles. Wood is considered to be good for making gunpowder charcoal. Bark yields tannin.

Bedu – *see* Anjiri.

Bega, Bagamushada, Karwanth – *Tiliacora acuminata* (Lamk.) Miers.; Menispermaceae; climbing shrub. Cultivated as an ornamental for its fragrant flowers. Root bark is rich in the alkaloid tiliacorine. Plant is used as a cure for snake bite. Tender branches are used for basketry.

Bekkra, Bhekal, Cherara – *Prinsepia utilis* Royle; Rosaceae; thorny shrub. Seeds yield a fatty oil which is used for cooking and soap industry. Oil is also used in rheumatism as a rubefacient. Wood is used for making walking-sticks.

Bela, Mogra, Banmallika; Mallika (S) – *Jasminum sambac* (L.) Ait.; Arabian jasmine (E), Tuscan jasmine (E); Oleaceae; bushy shrub. Cultivated for its extremely fragrant flowers used for making garlands. Flowers are also the source of an essential oil used in perfumery.

Belkamu – *see* Dela.

Bena – *see* Khas-khas.

Ber – *see* Baer.

Berseem – *Trifolium alexandrinum* L.; Egyptian clover (E), Berseem (E); Papilionaceae; herb. Cultivated as an important fodder crop. Plants are considered to be nutritious due to their high protein, calcium and phosphorus content, and are used as fodder, hay and silage. The crop is also valued for reclaiming saline and alkaline soils and for green manuring.

Bet, Vetasa; Vetra (S) – *Calamus rotang* L.; Rattan (E); Palmae; climbing palm. Stem is used for cane-furniture, basketry and wicker-work. Young tender shoots are used as vegetable.

Bethu sag; Bathua; Vastuka (S) – *Chenopodium album* L.; Pigweed (E); Chenopodiaceae; herb. Leaves and tender twigs are used as vegetable.

Bettar – *see* Thelu.

Bhabar – *see* Babui.

Bhada motha; Nirvisha (S) – *Cyperus kyllingia* Endl.; Cyperaceae; perennial herb. Rhizomes are aromatic. Decoction of the rhizomes is diuretic, demulcent and tonic; rhizomes also yield an essential oil which is used similarly as the decoction.

Bhadrabala (S) – *see* Haranpadi.

Bhadradanti (S), Jyotishka (S) – *Jatropha multifida* L.; Coral plant (E); Euphorbiaceae; shrub. Tuberous roots are edible after roasting. Decoction of the roots is used for colic, and that of leaves as a purgative. Seeds contain a fixed oil which is used in criminal poisoning and is dangerously cathartic.

Bhadramunja (S) – *see* Ramsar.

Bhadraparni (S) – *see* Gambhar.

Bhakura, Bislambhi; Vishala (S) – *Cucumis trigonus* Roxb.; Cucurbitaceae; climbing herb. Fruit pulp is a strong purgative and bitter in taste. Seeds yield a fatty oil which is used for illumination.

Bhalia – *see* Bara salpan.

Bhallataki (S) – *see* Bhilawa.

Bhamri – *Ulmus parvifolia* Jacq.; Ulmaceae; evergreen small tree. Leaves are used as fodder for sheep and goats. Wood is scented.

Bhanda – *Geranium nepalense* Sweet; Nepal Geranium (E), Nepalese crane's bill (E); Geraniaceae; perennial herb. Roots yield a red pigment which is used for colouring medicinal oils and is also used for tanning.

Bhang, Ganja, Charas; Vijaya (S) – *Cannabis sativa* L.; True hemp (E), Marijuana (E); Cannabinaceae; herb. Stems yield a fibre which is used for making ropes, canvas and nets. Leaves yield 'bhang'. Flowering tops of female plants yield 'charas' and 'ganja' which are rich in resin, cannabin and an essential oil. 'Ganja' comprises the dried female inflorescences and 'charas' or hashish is the resinous exudate collected from them, when young female flowers are emerging. All three have narcotic effects. The active principle present in the resin exudate is tetrahydrocannabinol (THC), which is an active hellucinogenic compound. Oil from the seeds is used in paint, varnish and soap industries. Drug is used as an antispasmodic, sedative and analgesic, and is also much abused. Other names commonly used for the drug are pot and grass.

Bhangra, Moochkand; Bhringaraja (S), Ajagara (S), Kesaraja (S) – *Eclipta prostrata* L.; Compositae; perennial herb with tiny white flower-heads. Plants considered as an anodyne, antiflatulent and expectorant are used in treating liver and spleen enlargement, cirrhosis of liver, headaches, toothaches, flatulence, eye and ear troubles and skin diseases. Plant leaf juice is the source of a black dye and is used in many herbal hair-dyes and hair oils. Roots are emetic and purgative, and are also applied locally to cure wounds in cattle.

Bhanjira – *Perilla frutescens* (L.) Britton; Perilla (E); Labiatae; herb. Leaves are used for flavouring. Seeds yield an oil used for waterproofing cloth and in the manufacture of printers ink, paints and varnishes.

Bhanjuri, Ponai – *Apluda mutica* L. var. *aristata* Hackel ex Backer; Gramineae; perennial grass. Herb is used as fodder, and stalks are used for making hats. Plant also serves as a good raw material for rayon industry.

Bhanra – *see* Peela bhangra.

Bhant; Barhichuda (S), Bhantaka (S) – *Clerodendrum infortunatum* L.; Verbenaceae; shrub. Leaves are used as a laxative and vermifuge and are also used externally for tumours.

Bhanta – *see* Baigan.

Bhantaka (S)–*see* Bhant.

Bharadvaji (S) – *see* Ulatkambal.

Bharangi; Bhargi (S) – *Clerodendrum indicum* (L.) Kuntze (syn. *Siphonanthus indica* L.); Turk's turban (E), Tube-flower (E); Verbenaceae; tall shrub. Plant is grown as an ornamental. Roots are used for the treatment of asthma and cough; leaves act as a vermifuge.

Bharband, Kateli, Shialkanta – *Argemone mexicana* L.; Prickly poppy (E); Papaveraceae; herb. Seeds yield a bitter semi-drying oil which is cathartic and is used for cutaneous ailments. Edible mustard oil when adulterated with this oil can cause dropsy. Yellow latex from the plant is used for curing scabies. Roots are used in remedies for chronic skin ailments.

Bharbharra – *see* Jawasa.

Bhargi (S) – *see* Bharangi.

Bharija (S) – *see* Chalta.

Bhasma-kand – *see* Dhey.

Bhat, Ramkurthi, Soyabean – *Glycine max* (L.) Merr.; Soyabean (E); Papilionaceae; bushy herb. Seeds are rich source of a semi-drying oil which is used for the manufacture of margarine, oil cloth, paint, printer's ink, soaps, insecticides and disinfectants. Beans are consumed as vegetable and also used for soya sprouts and soya milk. Refined oil is predominantly rich in polyunsaturated fatty acids and is used as a salad and cooking oil. Oil-cake is used as cattle-feed. Soya protein and meal are used in the manufacture of adhesives, leather finish, insecticidal sprays, fire-fighting compounds, and insulating and wall-board coating; meal is also used in the manufacture of plywood glue. Soya protein yields a synthetic fibre which is suitable for blending with rayon and cotton. After extraction of protein the residue left is used in phenolic plastics.

Bhatia – *Dalbergia volubilis* Roxb.; Papilionaceae; tree. Leaves are used as fodder. Juice of the leaves is used for gargles and throat infections.

Bhat-karela – *see* Kakrol.

Bhat-katiya – *see* Kanteri.

Bhatua ghas – *see* Sarsan-banda.

Bhaulan, Kukurkat; Bhramar-chhallika (S) – *Hymenodictyon excelsum* Wall.; Rubiaceae; large tree. Wood is used for making match-sticks, pencils, toys and packing cases. Bark yields tannin. Leaves are used as fodder and for dyeing.

Bhavanbakra – *see* Papra.

Bhedani (S) – *see* Baphuli.

Bhein – *see* Kamal.

Bhekal – *see* Bekkra.

Bhela – *see* Bhilawa.

Bhemal – *see* Bhimal.

Bhendu – *see* Marorphali.

Bhenght, Chhota kanwal, Koka, Koi–*Nymphaea nouchali* Burm. f.; Indian red water lily (E); Nymphaeaceae; aquatic herb with floating leaves. All parts are eaten. Flower are astringent and used as a cardiotonic. Rhizomes are eaten raw or boiled and are also used to provide relief in dysentery and dyspepsia. Seeds have a cooling effect and are used in cutaneous diseases.

Bherenda – *Jatropha gossypifolia* L.; Bellyache bush (E); Euphorbiaceae; much branched shrub. Roots are used for leprosy; the ether extract of the shoots is reported to be active against *Escherichia coli*. Decoction of the leaves acts as a purgative. Bark contains jatrophine an alkaloid similar in action to quinine.

Bhil – *Juniperus wallichiana* Hook. f.; Black Juniper (E); Cupressaceae; tree. Wood is used for construction purposes and for making charcoal. Leaves and twigs are burnt for repelling insects and as incense.

Bhilawa, Bhella; Aruskaara (S), Bhallataki (S) – *Semecarpus anacardium* L.f.; Marking nut (E); Anacardiaceae; tree. Hypocarp of the fruit (orange cup) is eaten when ripe. Pericarp of the fruit abounds in a resin and is used for marking cloth; it is also used for paint, varnish and plastic industries. Chlorinated derivatives of the phenolic constituents of the pericarp juice are used for the manufacture of insecticides, moth-proofs, termite repellents, synthetic herbicides and fire-proof plastics. Semi-drying oil from the seeds is used as a lubricant and wood preservative against white ants. Tree serves as a host to lac insects.

Bhillar – *see* Paniala.

Bhillaura, Khamara; Pindara (S) – *Trewia nudiflora* L.; False white teak (E); Euphorbiaceae; large tree. Wood is used for match-sticks, packing cases, toys, yokes, and carving. Fruit is edible. Seeds yield a fatty oil. Wood pulp is suitable for the manufacture of writing paper. Root poultice is applied topically in rheumatism.

Bhimal, Biul – *Grewia optiva* Drummond; Tiliaceae; small tree. Fruit is edible. Tender twigs with leaves are used as fodder; bark yields a fibre used for cordage. Wood is used for making tools, handles and oar shafts etc.

Bhimsaini kapur – *see* Barus kapur.

Bhindi – *Abelmoschus esculentus* (L.) Moench; Lady's finger (E), Malvaceae; cultivated, erect, branched herb. Tender fruits are consumed as vegetable. Stem yields a fibre. Ripe seeds are rich in protein and oil. Plants yield the okra gum used as a flavouring and thickening agent of soups and gravies. Mucilage obtained from the stem and root is also used as a clarifying agent in the manufacture of jaggery from sugar-cane. Seeds are stimulant and antispasmodic.

Bhirra, Girya – *Chloroxylon swietenia* DC.; East Indian satinwood tree (E); Flindersiaceae; small tree. Wood yields timber which is used for cabinet-work, high class furniture, carving, and decorative panelling. Wood pulp is used for the manufacture of wrapping paper.

Bhissata – *see* Gandhi-buti.

Bhiunli, Lal-berala, Mahabala, Sahadevi – *Sida rhombifolia* L.; Broomjute Sida (E); Malvaceae; undershrub. Stem yields fibre used for making ropes. Stem mucilage is used as a demulcent; it is also used as a diuretic and febrifuge. The alkaloid ephedrine is present in roots and leaves.

Bhojpatra; Bhurjapatrak (S) – *Betula utilis* D. Don. (syn. *B. bhojpatra* Wall.); Himalayan silver birch (E); Betulaceae; tree. Bark which is smooth and peeling in layers, was used for writing manuscripts in ancient times in India. Infusion of the bark is antiseptic and carminative.

Bhojpattra, Bhujpattra; Chitratvak (S) – *Betula alnoides* Buch-Ham.; Indian birch (E); Betulaceae; tree. Wood is extremely good for plywood, furniture, cabinet work, and turnery. Wood pulp is used for the manufacture of paper.

Bholia, Sodh; Lodra (S) – *Symplocos laurina* (Retz.) Wall ex Rehd.; Chunga (E); Symplocaceae; small tree. Powdered bark mixed with honey is used to cure diarrhoea, haemorrhages, gonorrhoea, biliousness and diseases of the eye. Leaves yield a yellow dye.

Bhoree loth – *see* Thoonia loth.

Bhramar-chhallika (S) – *see* Bhaulan.

Bhringaraja (S) – *see* Bhangra; *see also* Peela-bhangra.

Bhringeshtha (S) – *see* Safed gulab.

Bhuichampa, Bhumichampaca (S) – *Kaempferia rotunda* L.; Zingiberaceae; herb. Grown as an ornamental for hanging baskets. Tuberous rhizomes and young leaves are used for flavouring. Rhizomes are also prescribed in stomach complaints and their paste is applied locally on sores and wounds. They are also used to remove blood clots from the body.

Bhujangakshi (S) – *see* Rasna.

Bhujpattra – *see* Bhojpattra.

Bhukamtaka (S) – *see* Jharberi.

Bhulavanga (S) – *see* Banlaunga.

Bhumiari (S) – *see* Hindi-sana.

Bhumi-bala – *see* Bananiyar.

Bhumichampaca (S)–*see* Bhuichampa.

Bhumikushmanda (S) – *see* Bilaikand.

Bhumyamalaki (S) – *see* Jaramla.

Bhurangi, Bharangi (S) – *Clerodendrum serratum* (L.) Spreng.; Verbenaceae; shrub. Roots are used in remedies for combating dyspepsia and rheumatism. Leaves are used as a febrifuge and for external application in ophthalmia. Seeds are used to treat dropsy.

Bhurat – *see* Titbaigan.

Bhurjapatrak (S) – *see* Bhojpatra.

Bhursali – *see* Barsali.

Bhurundi (S) – *see* Hati-sura.

Bhusa – *see* Kanta-alu.

Bhustrina (S) – *see* Agin-ghas.

Bhutaghna (S) – *see* Taramira.

Bhutakesi (S) – *see* Bhutkis.

Bhutankusa (S) – *see* Chucka.

Bhutia-badam, Urni – *Corylus colurna* L.; Turkish hazel-nut (E); Corylaceae; tree found in W. Himalayas. Seeds are edible.

Bhutik (S) – *see* Rousaghas.

Bhutkis; Bhutakesi (S) – *Corydalis govaniana* Wall.; Fumariaceae; herb. Root acts as a diuretic and tonic and is used in the treatment of cutaneous, scrofulous and syphilic infections.

Bhutta – *see* Makka.

Bichhu – *see* Hathajori.

Bichhu booti – *Urtica dioica* L.; Stinging-nettle (E); Urticaceae; robust herb. Plant is used internally to check haemorrhages and externally to excite paralysed limbs. Roots and seeds are used for controlling diarrhoea and to expel intestinal worms.

Bichua – *see* Alla.

Bidari-kand – *see* Bankumra.

Bihi; Amrit-phala (S) – *Cydonia oblonga* Mill.; Quince (E); Rosaceae; small tree. Fruit is used for making jams and marmalades. Mucilage from the seeds is used in cosmetics specially skin lotions.

Bija – *see* Bijasal.

Bijasal, Bija; Pitasara (S) – *Pterocarpus marsupium* Roxb.; Malabar kino (E), Indian kino tree (E); Papilionaceae; large tree considered as an important timber plant. Wood is used for making furniture. Gum obtained from tapping the stem is used in diarrhoea and dysentery, and is also used in dyeing and tanning. Decoction of the wood is given in diabetes. Leaves provide an excellent fodder and manure. Bark is also used for dyeing.

Bijaura, Turanj – *Citrus medica* L.; Citron (E); Rutaceae; shrub or small tree. Fruit is used chiefly for making pickles and marmalades. Preserved rind is used in dysentery and also for flavouring confectionery. Oil of cedrat (citron oil) is obtained from fresh rind.

Bika-kalibel, Pitti; Raktavalli (S) – *Ventilago madraspatana* Gaertn.; Rhamnaceae; climbing shrub. Root-bark yields a red dye (ventilagin) which is used for dyeing cotton, wool and silk. Root bark is used medicinally as a stimulant, tonic, stomachic and mixed with oil is applied for skin ailments, and itch. Seeds are edible when cooked, and also yield a fatty oil which is used for cooking.

Bikhima – *Aconitum palmatum* D. Don.; Ranunculaceae; herb. Tuberous bitter roots are used in combating diarrhoea, fever and rheumatism. They contain several diterpene alkaloids.

Biksa – *Hemarthria compressa* (L.f.) R. Br.; Gramineae; herb. Plant is used as fodder.

Bilaikand; Bhumikushmanda (S), Vidari (S) – *Ipomoea mauritiana* Jacq. [syn. *I. digitata* Auct. (non L.)]; Convolvulaceae; climber. Often cultivated as an ornamental. Tuberous root-powder is considered to be a tonic and is used for curing general debility, liver and spleen disorders and menorrhagia.

Bilangra, Baichi – *Flacourtia indica* (Burm. f.) Merr.; Madagascar plum (E), Flacourtiaceae; thorny bush or small tree. Fruits are edible and digestive. Bark is diuretic, and also used for tanning. Branches and leaves are lopped for fodder.

Bilari – *see* Agumaki.

Bilasi, Barna; Varuna (S), Asmarighna (S) – *Crataeva nurvala* Buch.-Ham.; Capparidaceae; large tree. Bark is used as a digestive stimulant, appetizer and for curing urinary infections. Root bark is rubefacient. Wood is used for making match-sticks.

Bilayati bel, Vilayati bel – *Crescentia cujete* L.; Calabash tree (E); Bignoniaceae; small tree. Fruit acts as a diuretic and febrifuge; fruit-shell takes a fine polish and can be used as a utensil. Seeds yield a fixed oil.

Bilayati gab, Vilayati gab – *Diospyros discolor* Willd.; Mabola persimmon (E); Ebenaceae; evergreen tree. Cultivated as an ornamental.

Bilayati tulsi, Vilayati tulsi – *Hyptis suaveolens* (L.) Poit.; Labiatae; aromatic herb. Tender shoot tips are used for flavouring. Plant is considered to be a stimulant and carminative. Roots act as an appetizer and stomachic and leaf juice is given for getting rid of stomach ache and colic pain. Plants yield an essential oil.

Bililotan; Laghupushpa madhukar (S) – *Melissa axillaris* (Benth.) Bakh. f.; Labiatae; herb. Fruit is considered as a brain tonic Stem and leaves are antipyretic and are used for the treatment of brain, heart and liver ailments.

Bilimbi – *Averrhoa bilimbi* L.; Bilimbi (E), Tree-sorrel (E); Averrhoaceae; small tree. Cultivated for its acid fruits which are used for making pickles, jams and curries.

Bilin – *see* Kavitha.

Bilpat, Chitrabeez – *Melochia corchorifolia* L.; Sterculiaceae; undershrub. Stem bark yields a strong silvery white fibre which is used for making fishing lines; decoction of the leaves is used as a remedy in dysentery.

Bilsa – *see* Baishi.

Bilva – *see* Bael.

Bina, Tivar – *Avicennia officinalis* L.; White mangrove (E); Avicenniaceae; a tree found in salt marshes. Bark is astringent and also yields tannin. Green fruits are made into poultice and used as a cure for boils. Leaves are used for fodder.

Binda, Pansra – *Colebrookea oppositifolia* Sm.; Labiatae; shrub. Decoction of the root is used in epilepsy.

Bindak – *see* Findak.

Bindal, Ghaghrabel; Koshaphala (S) – *Luffa echinata* Roxb.; Cucurbitaceae; twiner. Fruits are used to cure dropsy and chronic bronchitis and are also used as a purgative.

Biranjasif – *see* Gandana.

Birhatta; Vrihati (S) – *Solanum indicum* L.; Poison berry (E), Indian nightshade (E); Solanaceae; spiny herb or undershrub. Roots are medicinal, and are used for curing cough, colic, nasal ulcers and catarrhal disorders. Several glyco-alkaloids are present which are reported to be a good source of cortisone preparations. Roots are an ingredient of the Ayurvedic preparation 'Dasamula'.

Birkubat – *Andrographis echioides* Nees.; Acanthaceae; herb. Plant juice is used as a febrifuge; plant is also used as a substitute for 'kirayat' obtained from *A. paniculata*. Uses are similar.

Birmi – *see* Thuno.

Birsa, Chila, Tilki – *Wendlandia exserta* (Roxb.) DC.; Rubiaceae; ornamental tree. Wood yields timber which is used for building purposes and agricultural implements and is resistant to termites. Leaves are used as fodder. Bark is used for urinary complaints.

Bisar—*see* Kamini.

Bish, Bacchang, Mahoor; Visha (S) – *Aconitum ferox* Wall. ex Ser.; Indian Aconite (E); Ranunculaceae; herb. Tuberous roots are antipyretic and diuretic, and are used in the treatment of nasal catarrh, tonsilitis, and sore throat. Aconite ointment is used in rheumatism and skin troubles. It is also used as a sedative and diaphoretic.

Bislambhi – *see* Bhakura.

Bistendu, Lohari; Asmantaka (S) – *Diospyros montana* Roxb.; Mountain persimmon (E); Ebenaceae; deciduous tree. Wood is used for agricultural implements, carts, rafters and carving; it is also suitable for making match-sticks. Fruit in crushed form is applied to boils and mixed with crushed leaves is used to stupefy fish.

Biswul – *Acacia pennata* (L.) Willd.; Mimosaceae; large thorny shrub. Plant serves as a host to lac insect.

Bithua, Takoli – *Dalbergia lanceolaria* L.; Papilionaceae; tall deciduous tree. Wood is used for making agricultural implements, tool handles, packing boxes and rafters. Decoction of the bark is used for treating dyspepsia; bark also yields tannin. Seed oil is used locally as a rubefacient for rheumatism.

Biul – *see* Bhimal.

Bodula, Samarri – *Firmiana colorata* (Roxb.) R. Br.; Scarlet Sterculia (E); Sterculiaceae; tree. Stem bark yields a fibre which is used for making ropes; leaves are used as fodder for cattle.

Bohira – *see* Rugtrora.

Bol – *see* Guggul.

Boot – *see* Chana.

Boota – *see* Ghiabato.

Bor, Attah bar – *Ficus elastica* Roxb.; India Rubber tree (E); Moraceae; medium-sized tree. Latex obtained from the bark of branches forms a good source of rubber. It is cultivated as a pot plant for interior decoration in its juvenile stage.

Bora, Mothitrina; Gundra (S) – *Typha elephantina* Roxb., non Grah.; Elephant grass (E); Typhaceae; tall marshy reed. Plants are fed to elephants and also used for thatching, mats, wicker work and ropes; pulp is suitable for the manufacture of rayon. Rhizomes are astringent and diuretic, and are used in the treatment of dysentery. Fibre of ripe fruits is used for stuffing, and also as a binder in mortar.

Botal-brush – *see* Lal botal brush.

Bouli – *see* Kinkar.

Brahmadandi – *Tricholepis glaberrima* DC.; Compositae; herb. Plant is used as a nervine tonic, antiseptic and for treating skin ailments. Root bark is used in cough and urinary troubles.

Brahma-kamal – *Saussurea sacra* Edgew.; Sacred Saussurea (E), Yogiraj plant (E); Compositae; herb found in W. Himalayas. Roots are used in the indigenous system of medicine for nervous debility. Another species *S. obvallata* Wall ex C.B. Clarke is also known by the same Hindi name.

Brahma-kamal – *Saussurea obvallata* Wall. ex C.B. Clarke.; Compositae; herb. Roots are used in indigenous ointments to treat wounds and cuts.

Brahma manduki – *see* Brahmi.

Brahmi, Brahma-manduki; Mandukaparni (S) – *Centella asiatica* (L.) Urban; Asiatic pennywort (E); Hydrocotylaceae; prostrate herb rooting at nodes, and found in marshy locations. Stem and leaves act as a tonic and diuretic and are also used as a blood purifier and in treating leprosy. Asiaticoside, a glycoside is present, which is found to be specific for the treatment of leprosy. Another plant called Neer-brahmi is also known by the same Hindi name.

Brahmi – *see* Neer-brahmi.

Brihalloni (S) – *see* Kulfa.

Brinda – *see* Tulsi.

Buckripathi – *Dracaena angustifolia* Roxb.; Agavaceae; tall herb used as fodder for goats.

Budù, Baudala, Pudu; Gandhamadini (S), Jivantika (S) – *Viscum articulatum* Burm. f. Viscaceae; shrub. Paste of the plant is applied locally to cuts and wounds.

Bui, Kauraro – *Kochia indica* Wight; Chenopodiaceae; much branched herb. Plant is cultivated as an ornamental; also used as a cardiac stimulant. It is also used as fodder.

Buinowla, Panjuli; Krishna-kamboji (S) – *Kirganelia reticulata* (Poir.) Baill.; Euphorbiaceae; large straggling shrub. Cultivated as a hedge plant. Leaves are diuretic, and also used for diarrhoea in infants. Bark is astringent and diuretic, and also yields a dye.

Bukchi – *see* Babchi.

Burans – *Rhododendron arboreum* Sm.; Tree–Rhododendron (E); Ericaceae; small tree. Flower petals are used for making jams, jelly and cold drinks; also used to treat diarrhoea and dysentery. Wood is used for making plywood, boxes, tool handles and posts. Bark is used for preparing snuff. Tender leaves are edible.

Burhna, Haldwa – *Pulicaria crispa* (Cass.) Benth & Hook f.; Compositae; shrub. Decoction of the plant is considered to be a febrifuge and dried leaves are used for treating sores of bullocks.

Bussorah – *see* Fasli-gulab.

C

Cha – *see* Chai.

Chab, Chavi – *Piper retrofractum* Vahl; Java long pepper (E); Piperaceae; climber. Fruits are used as a spice, but are weaker in flavour than pepper. They act as a stimulant and carminative; also used for digestive ailments and haemorrhoids. Wood and roots yield a dye. Decoction of the roots is used for colic.

Chabeni, Gondni – *Grewia tenax* (Forsk.) Aschers & Schwt.; Tiliaceae; shrub. Fruits are edible, and wood is used for walking-sticks. Bark is the source of a mucilage reported to be used for tuberculosis. Leaves are lopped for fodder.

Chachinda – *Trichosanthes anguina* L.; Snake-gourd (E); Cucurbitaceae; trailing herb. Cultivated for its fruit which is used as vegetable. Roots and seeds are vermifuge and are used to combat diarrhoea and syphilis.

Chadua, Chato – *Rhamnus virgata* Roxb.; Indian buckthorn (E); Rhamnaceae; a shrub or small tree. Wood is used for fuel and for making implements. Leaves are lopped for fodder. Fruit is used in spleen disorders and also acts as a purgative.

Chagulputputi – *Euphorbia dracunculoides* Lam.; Euphorbiaceae; perennial herb. Seeds contain a drying oil. Capsules are used to treat warts.

Chai, Cha – *Camellia sinensis* (L.) O. Kuntze; Tea (E); Theaceae; evergreen cultivated shrub usually kept pruned as a hedge.

Cured leaves marketed as green tea or black tea (fermented) are used as a beverage. The stimulating effect is due to the presence of the alkaloids theine and caffeine. A small amount of theophylline is also present. Caffeine extracted from tea waste is used in medicine, and the tannins are used for preparing plywood adhesives. Fresh leaves yield a volatile oil. Brick tea, Oolong tea and Leppet are other well known forms of tea.

Chakotra, Sadaphal – *Citrus grandis* (L.) Osbeck.; Shaddock (E), Pummelo (E); Rutaceae; small tree. Fruit is consumed fresh and also made into marmalades. Naringin, a glucoside obtained from the fruit is used as a flavouring agent. Leaves are used to treat convulsive coughs and epilepsy.

Chaksu – *Cassia absus* L.; White sapota (E); Caesalpiniaceae; herb. Leaves act as an astringent and are used for getting rid of cough. Seeds are used for skin ailments and ophthalmia; they also yield a fatty oil.

Chakunda, Panevar; Dadamari (S) – *Cassia tora* L.; Sickle senna (E); Caesalpiniaceae; herb. Seeds are used as a mordant in dyeing. Paste of leaves and seeds is applied locally to cure eczema, ringworm and other skin ailments. Leaves are purgative.

Chakwat, Korake, Surake – *Atriplex hortensis* L.; Orache (E); Chenopodiaceae; bushy herb. Cultivated for its leaves and tender branches which are used as pot-herb. Leaves and seeds although rich in protein are diuretic. Alkaloids amaranthine and chenopodine are present. Prolonged consumption is not advised due to the presence of certain toxic substances in the seeds.

Chalta; Bharija (S) – *Dillenia indica* L.; Elephant apple (E); Dilleniaceae; medium-sized tree. Wood is used for construction work and for making tool handles and boats. Bark yields tannin. Fresh leaves are used as a feed for 'tusser' silkworms. Fleshy persistant sepals on the fruit, are made into jam and squashes, and are also used for flavouring.

Chambar-maya, Mored, Pabuna – *Ulmus wallichiana* Planch.; Himalayan elm (E); Ulmaceae; large tree. Wood is used for construction work and for making furniture; stem bark yields a strong fibre which is woven into sandals and also used for cordage.

Chameli; Chambeli (S) – *Jasminum grandiflorum* L.; Common jasmine (E); Oleaceae; straggling shrub. Grown as an ornamental for its intensely sweet-scented white flowers which are used in perfumery, and for scenting hair oils. Fresh leaves are chewed to treat ulceration of the mouth and fresh juice of leaves is applied on corns.

Cham-khirni – *Polyalthia suberosa* Thw.; Annonaceae; shrub or small tree. Wood is used for general carpentry. Fruit is edible. Root decoction is used as an abortifacient. Trees serve as a host to lac insect.

Champa – *see* Khair-champa; *see also* Champak.

Champak, Champa; Champaka (S) – *Michelia champaca* L.; Champak (E); Magnoliaceae; a large tree. Flowers are yellow in colour and highly scented. Essential oil from the flowers 'champa oil' is used in perfumery, and hair oils. Leaves also yield an essential oil similar to 'tulsi' or sacred basil oil. Wood is used for furniture, veneers, carving and ship-building; bark yields tannin and seeds contain a fatty oil.

Champaka (S) – *see* Champak.

Champa methi – *see* Kasuri methi.

Chamri-ki-bel – *see* Ramsar.

Chamror, Koda, Datranga – *Ehretia laevis* Roxb.; Ehretiaceae; small tree. Wood is used for making agricultural implements and match-sticks. Leaves are lopped for fodder.

Chamsur, Halim; Chandrashura (S) – *Lepidium sativum* L.; Garden cress (E); Cruciferae; herb. Plant is cultivated for its leaves which are used as salad and pot-herb. They are mildly diuretic and used in hepatic ailments. Seeds are tonic, diuretic, laxative and rubefacient; seed mucilage is used as gum-arabic. Seeds also yield a semi-drying oil which is used in soap industry.

Chana, Boot, Chanaka (S) – *Cicer arietinum* L.; Gram (E), Chickpea (E); Papilionaceae; much branched herb. Grown as an important pulse-crop; seeds are consumed either boiled, or parched or sprouted. Flour is used to prepare snacks and sweets. Soaked gram along with its husk is also fed to cattle and horses. Nutrient value of the grain is high.

Chanaka (S) – *see* Chana.

Chandal, Jasund – *Antiaris toxicaria* Lesch.; Upas tree (E); Moraceae; tree. Creamy white latex obtained from the bark contains antiarin a glycoside which is used in small doses as a mild cardiac stimulant. In large doses it acts as a poison and is used as an arrow poison. Bark also yields a fibre which is used for cordage and the wood is suitable for paper-pulp and match-boxes.

Chandan, Sandal; Chandana (S); Taliaparnam (S) – *Santalum album* L.; Sandalwood (E); Santalaceae; tree. Heartwood contains an essential oil termed sandalwood oil which is widely used in perfumery and toiletries. Wood is used mainly for distillation of the oil. Sandalwood is also highly esteemed for carving and is used for making exquisitely carved pieces of art. It is also used for religious ceremonies and sandalwood paste is applied to the forehead by the Hindus, and is considered to have a cooling effect. The oil and the wood are also used in medicine as a diuretic and diaphoretic. The tree is a partial root-parasite.

Chandana (S) – *see* Chandan.

Chandausi, Miana – *Medicago polymorpha* L.; Toothed bur clover (E); Papilionaceae; herb. The plant is used as a green manure and to check soil erosion. Leaves are a rich source of ascorbic acid.

Chandkal – *Macaranga peltata* (Roxb.) Muell.–Arg.; Euphorbiaceae; tree. Wood is suitable for paper pulp and match-sticks. Kino, a reddish gum obtained from the tree bark is used for sizing paper and for taking impressions for making casts. Bark and leaves contain tannin. Fruit is edible.

Chandni, Tagar; Tagara (S) – *Tabernaemontana divaricata* (L.) R. Br. ex Roem & Schult; Crape-jasmine (E); Apocynaceae; ornamental much branched shrub. Flowers are used for garlands. Red pulp around the seed is used as a dye.

Chandrabhaga – *see* Sarpagandha.

Chandrakanti (S) – *see* Dudhiakalmi.

Chandramallika (S) – *see* Guldaudi (chhoti).

Chandramula, Sidhoul; Chandramulika (S), Sugandhavacha (S) – *Kaempferia galanga* L.; Zingiberaceae; common ornamental herb. Rhizomes are used as a condiment, and in medicine as an expectorant, carminative and diuretic. They are also used in cosmetics.

Chandramulika (S) – *see* Chandramula.

Chandrashura (S) – *see* Chamsur.

Chandrika (S) – *see* Methi.

Chanhel – *Leptochloa chinensis* Nees.; Gramineae; annual slender grass. Plant is used as a fodder for cattle.

Chaplash – *Artocarpus chaplasha* Roxb.; Moraceae; tall tree. Wood is considered as a high class utility timber which is used for furniture, decorative panelling, carving, ship and house-building, turnery, general carpentry work and manufacture of plywood.

Chapra – *Myrsine africana* L.; Myrsinaceae; small shrub. Fruit is anthelmintic, and is used specifically for expelling the tapeworm; it is also a laxative and is used in ointments for treating ringworm and other skin diseases.

Chapri – *see* Matamar.

Char-koni Sem – *see* Chau-dhari phali.

Charangi, Kashshing – *Picrasma quassioides* (D. Don) Benn.; Simaroubaceae; tree. Stem bark and leaves are used as the source of an insecticide. Wood contains quassin and is used as a substitute for Jamaica quassia obtained from *P. excelsa* (Sw.) Planch. Fruit is edible, and the seeds yield a fatty oil.

Charas – *see* Bhang.

Charati (S) – *see* Ratanpurus.

Charoli – *see* Chironji.

Chatian, Satwin; Saptaparni (S) – *Alstonia scholaris* (L.) R. Br.; Devil's tree (E), Dita bark tree (E); Apocynaceae; evergreen tree. Grown as an ornamental avenue tree. Wood is used for the manufacture of pencils, match-sticks, veneers, plywood and paper pulp. Bark known in commerce as dita-bark is bitter, anthelmintic, febrifuge and astringent and is used to combat diarrhoea, dysentery, cardiac trouble and asthma. Echitamine is the chief alkaloid constituent of the bark. Flowers contain an essential oil and the alkaloid picrinine, which acts as a depressant for central nervous system. Latex from the plant is used for ulcers, sores and rheumatic inflammation.

Chato – *see* Chadua.

Chatri-matri – *see* Akra.

Chatroa, Kashmal – *Berberis vulgaris* L.; Common barberry (E); Berberidaceae; spiny shrub. Bark and the wood yield a yellow dye which is used for dyeing leather and wool. Fruit is edible.

Chau – *see* Peka.

Chau-dhari phali, Char-koni Sem – *Psophocarpus tetragonolobus* (L.) DC.; Goa bean (E); Papilionaceae; twining herb. Tender immature pods are used as vegetable. Seeds yield a fatty oil and the plant is also grown for fodder and green manure.

Chaulai, Sadanatya; Marisha (S) – *Amaranthus blitum* L. var. *oleracea* Duthie; Amaranth (E); Amaranthaceae; herb. Tender shoots are used as pot-herb; they are a rich source of iron and other minerals.

Chaulai-sag – *see* Lal-sag.

Chaulmogra, Dalmugri – *Hydnocarpus kurzii* (King) Warb.; Chaulmogra (E); Flacourtiaceae; tree. Seeds yield the real chaulmogra oil reported to be active against *Mycobacterium leprae* which causes leprosy. The oil is applied externally and has been in usage in India from very ancient times.

Chaulmoogra; Garudaphala (S), Tuvrak (S) – *Hydnocarpus laurifolia* (Dennst.) Sleumer; Flacourtiaceae; tree. Seeds yield hydnocarpous oil which is used in lepromatous leprosy. It is active against both *Mycobacterium leprae* and *M. tuberculosis*. The oil is also used externally for other chronic skin ailments, rheumatism and sprains.

Chaunkra, Jand, Khejri, Sami; Shami (S) – *Prosopis cineraria* (L.) Druce (syn. *P. spicigera* L.); Mimosaceae; tree. Wood is used for making tool handles and for fuel; it is also good for making charcoal. Gum from the tree is used as gum arabic. Young pods are edible and are also used as fodder.

Chaupatia, Uttanjan; Shikhi (S) – *Blepharis persica* (Burm. f.) Kuntze, Acanthaceae; undershrub. Seeds are diuretic and expectorant. Leaves are used in treating liver and spleen disorders, asthma, leucoderma and nasal haemorrhage. They are also lopped for fodder.

Chaval, Dhan; Syali (S), Tandula (S) – *Oryza sativa* L.; Rice (E); Gramineae; herb. Plant is cultivated throughout India for its grain and is one of the oldest and most important staple food crops. Unpolished rice and parboiled rice have higher nutritional value as compared to polished rice. Grain is consumed as boiled, puffed, or beaten rice and its flour is also used in various dishes. It is a source of starch and is also used for making an alcoholic beverage. Rice-bran oil is used for edible purposes and cosmetics. Rice husk is used as fuel, bedding material for poultry, and raw material for furfural. Rice bran is used as a stock-feed, and the rice straw is used for the manufacture of paper, mats and straw-boards.

Chavi – *see* Chab.

Chaya – *see* Gorakh boonti.

Cheen, Anu, Morha; Varaka (S) – *Panicum miliaceum* L.; Hog millet (E), Proso millet (E); Gramineae; tall herb. Cultivated since very ancient times for its grain which is edible. Straw is used as fodder.

Cheena narangi – *see* China orange.

Cheeniagulab – *see* Desi-gulab.

Chelwa – *Hibiscus tiliaceus* L.; Cuban bast (E), Yellow mallow (E); Malvaceae; large shrub or small tree. Grown as an ornamental. Bark yields a strong fibre which is used for ropes, sails, fishing nets, mats and cordage. Bark is also used for the manufacture of wrapping paper. Leaf decoction is used for treating ulcers, and is also used as a laxative. Mucilage from fresh bark is recommended in dysentery. Roots act as a diuretic and laxative, and the infusion of seeds is emetic.

Cherailu – *Rhododendron campanulatum* D. Don.; Ericaceae; Evergreen small tree. Leaves are used in combating syphilis, sciatica and rheumatism; they are also used as a snuff to cure colds when mixed with tobacco. Flowers yield an essential oil.

Cherana – *see* Bekkra.

Chetihola, Sicka – *Hovenia dulcis* Thunb.; Japanese raisin tree (E); Rhamnaceae; tree. Peduncles are edible and taste like pears.

Chhattri – *Polyporus officinalis* Fries.; Polyporaceae; saprophytic bracket fungus found on tree trunks. Plant is diuretic and contains agaricin which is used as a nervine tonic and to check excessive sweating.

Chhikika (S)–*see* Nak-chhikni.

Chhimber – *Eleusine flagellifera* Nees.; Gramineae; profusely tillered and branched grass creeping on the ground. Plant is used for forage and hay.

Chhirvel; Arkapushpi (S) – *Holostemma annularis* (Roxb.) K. Schum.; Asclepiadaceae; twining herb. Leaves, tender twigs with flowers and fruits are edible. Bark yields a fibre which is used for cordage. Root paste is applied to the eyes in ophthalmia. Root is used medicinally for treating gonorrhoea, diabetes, stomach ache and cough.

Chhota chand – *see* Sarpagandha.

Chhota-chirayeta – *Enicostema hyssopifolium* (Willd.) Verdoorn; Indian gentian (E); Gentianaceae; herb. Plant is used as a laxative, stomachic, blood purifier and bitter tonic. it also contains ophelic acid which is found in Chirayeta.

Chhota-gokhru – *see* Adhasisi.

Chhota-kanwal – *see* Bhenght.

Chhota-kulpha, Ratmandi; Surasa (S) – *Trichodesma indicum* R. Br.; Boraginaceae; herb. Plant usually used as pot-herb, is also considered as a diuretic. Roots are used in dysentery and are also applied locally to swollen joints.

Chhota-halkusa – *Leucas aspera* Spreng.; Labiatae; herb. Plant is used as an antipyretic. Flowers mixed with honey are given for curing cough and colds. Alcoholic extract of leaves is antibacterial. Leaf juice is used topically for treating inflammation, chronic skin eruption and psoriasis.

Chhota pilu, Jhak, Kharjal – *Salvadora persica* L.; Saltbush (E); Mustard tree (E); Salvadoraceae; evergreen small tree. The tree is cultivated for erecting shelter-belts and wind-breaks. Leaves are used as camel fodder. Fruits are edible. Leaf decoction is used for curing asthma and cough, and its poultice is used for piles. Root paste is used as a substitute for mustard plaster and its decoction is used for gonorrhoea.

Chhoti-dudhi; Laghududhika (S) – *Euphorbia thymifolia* L.; Euphorbiaceae; undershrub. Seeds and leaves act as an astringent, laxative and anthelmintic. Plant is used for the treatment of ringworm.

Chhoti-elaichi; Ela (S) – *Elettaria cardamomum* Maton; Lesser cardamom (E), Cardamom (E); Zingiberaceae; tall perennial herb. Fruits with seeds are used as a masticatory, spice and in medicine. Seeds are used in cordials, artificial fruit flavours, perfumery and as a carminative and diuretic. Seeds contain an essential oil called oleum cardamoni which is used in perfumery.

Chhoti-gulmohur – *see* Gulutora.

Chhoti-lani, Lonia, Lunak – *Suaeda fruticosa* (L.) Forsk. ex Gmel.; Seablite (E), Alkali seepweed (E); Chenopodiaceae; undershrub. Plant is used as fodder for camels and goats and dried plants are used as fuel. It is also useful in treating saline and water logged soils. Woolly outgrowth on the tip of branches is made into a paste and is mixed with oil to treat sores on the backs of camels.

Chhui mui – *see* Chui-mui.

Chian – *see* Gilla.

Chichoda – *Cyperus esculentus* L.; Chufa (E), Tiger nut (E); Cyperaceae; perennial sedge. Corms are edible. They are the source of a fatty oil termed chufa oil used for culinary purposes.

Chickora, Kala mewa; Vidari (S) – *Solanum erianthum* D. Don.; Potato tree (E); Solanaceae; small tree. Often cultivated in S. India for fruits used in curries. Root decoction is used for curing vertigo, urinary troubles and body ache. Leaf infusion is administered in vaginal discharge. Active principle present is a glyco-alkaloid called solasonine.

Chickua, Goria, Gurla – *Chrysopogon fulvus* (Spreng.) Chiov.; Gramineae; tall grass. Plants are densely tufted and are considered as good fodder when cut before flowering. Plant is also a good soil-binder.

Chidha (S) – *see* Chilgoza.

Chikrasi – *Chukrasia tabularis* A. Juss.; Indian redwood (E), White cedar (E); Meliaceae; tree. Wood is used for panelling, decorative work, high class furniture, and plywood. Leaves and bark yield tannin and a red gum exuded from the tree is used as an adhesive.

Chikri, Papri – *Buxus wallichiana* Baill.; Boxwood tree (E); Buxaceae; small tree. Wood is used for toys, carving, cabinet work, mathematical scales, boxes, and musical instruments. Leaves act as a purgative and are used in combating syphilis and rheumatism. Alkaloid buxine is present in the leaves and wood. Tincture of the bark is used as a febrifuge.

Chikti, Jhingharita (S) – *Triumfetta rhomboidea* Jacq.; Burbush (E), Burweed (E), Tiliaceae; herb. Stem is the source of a soft glossy fibre. Bark and leaves are used for controlling diarrhoea, and roots are used to treat dysentery and intestinal ulcers.

Chiku, Sapota – *Manilkara achras* (Mill.) Fosberg (syn. *Achras zapota* L.); Sapodilla (E); Sapotaceae; evergreen tree. Ripe fruits are sweet and edible. Milky latex is used for the manufacture of chewing gum and is called chickle.

Chil – *see* Kail.

Chila – *see* Birsa.

Chilauni, Makusal – *Schima wallichii* (DC.) Choisy; Needle wood (E); Theaceae; large tree. Wood provides valuable timber which is used for construction work, bridges, veneers, plywood, paper pulp, match boxes, pencils and fancy articles. Bark and leaves contain tannin. Bark is used in the tanning of leather and is also used to expel tapeworms.

Chilbil – *see* Kanju.

Chilgoza, Neoza; Chidha (S), Mukulaka (S) – *Pinus gerardiana* Wall.; Chilgoza pine (E); Pinaceae; tree. Seeds are edible, and are used as a dry fruit after roasting; they are also considered expectorant, carminative and stimulant. They are rich in a fatty oil. Plant is the source of an oleo-resin of good quality.

Chilla – *Casearia tomentosa* Roxb.; Flacourtiaceae; shrub or small tree. Bark contains tannin, and the powdered bark is used in the treatment of dropsy. Fruits are diuretic, and are also used as a fish-poison.

Chiluchi – *see* Shoti.

China orange, Cheena narangi – *Fortunella japonica* (Thunb.) Swingle (syn. *Citrus japonica* Thunb.); Kumquat (E); Rutaceae; shrub. Cultivated in the gardens as an ornamental shrub for its beautiful foliage and fragrant flowers forming perfect miniature fruits festooning the branches. Fruits are acidic and can be used for preparing marmalade.

Chingari karne – *Caryopteris odorata* (D. Don.) Robinson; Verbenaceae; shrub. Cultivated as an ornamental. Wood is used for making walking-sticks and has a pleasant cherry-wood fragrance.

Chinar – *Platanus orientalis* L.; Oriental plane (E); Platanaceae; tall beautiful tree with a dense crown. Cultivated for shade and as an ornamental. Wood is highly valued and is used for cabinet work, furniture, carving, lacquer work, and veneers. Bark is used for treating diarrhoea, dysentery and toothache. The tree is characteristic of the landscape of Kashmir valley.

Chipita (S) – *see* Kuchla.

Chir; Sarala (S) – *Pinus roxburghii* Sarg.; Chir Pine (E), Long-leaved pine (E); Pinaceae; coniferous tree. Wood yields timber which is much in demand for construction work, light furniture, packing cases and match industry. Resin from the stem is used in the preparation of paints and varnishes. Turpentine obtained from the oleo-resin is used as a solvent for paints and varnishes and also used in pharmaceuticals, perfumery industry, disinfectants, insecticides, denaturants, and as an important raw material for terpene chemicals used in many industries. Rosin or colopheny is used in cosmetics, paints, varnishes, polishes and also in the manufacture of linoleum, fireworks, explosives, sealing wax and several types of inks.

Chirabilva (S) – *see* Kanju.

Chirayeta, Kiryat-charayatah; Kirata-tikta (S) – *Swertia chirayita* (Roxb. ex Flem.) Karst.; Chiretta (E); Gentianaceae; herb. Dried plants are used as a remedy for treating anaemia, bronchial asthma, liver disorder, chronic fevers and also as a stomachic, tonic and laxative.

Chirchitta, Chirmethi – *Lycium barbarum* L.; Solanaceae; shrub. Leaves contain betaine, hydrocyanic acid and a mydriatic alkaloid in traces and are poisonous to livestock. Berries are considered as an aphrodisiac. Fresh flowering plant is used in homoeopathy as a diuretic.

Chire kutki – *Panicum psilopodium* Trin var. *psilopodium* and var. *coloratum* Hook. f.; Gramineae; herb. Plant is used as fodder. Grains are used for making an alcoholic beverage.

Chiriya bajra – *Phalaris minor* Retz.; Small canary-grass (E); Gramineae; small herb. Plant provides nutritive fodder for cattle. Grains are used as bird-feed.

Chiriya-ka-dana – *see* Tandlen.

Chirla – *Rhamnus pentapomica* Parker; Rhamnaceae; small tree. Fruit is edible and the wood is suitable for turnery. Bark yields a red dye. Leaves are lopped for fodder.

Chirmethi – *see* Chirchitta.

Chirmiti – *see* Ratti.

Chironji, Charoli; Tapasya-priya (S) – *Buchanania lanzan* Spreng.; Cuddapah almond (E); Anacardiaceae; small tree. Seeds are edible, nutritious, and used as a substitute for almonds. Seeds yield a fatty oil which is used in indigenous medicine and in confectionery. Wood is used for cheap furniture. Gum obtained from the stem is used for printing cloth, dyeing and tanning. Gum is also used for curing diarrhoea. Leaves are lopped for fodder.

Chirpoti, Patakona, Shana-sokha – *Zanonia indica* L.; Cucurbitaceae; climbing shrub. Fruit is used to treat cough and asthma. Fresh fruit juice is used as an antidote to gecko bites. Leaves are applied locally to reduce inflammation, and their decoction is used to reduce irritation due to boils.

Chirval, Saya – *Hedyotis umbellata* (L.) Lam. (syn. *Oldenlandia umbellata* L.); Chay-root (E); Rubiaceae; herb. Roots and leaves act as an expectorant, and are used in the treatment of bronchitis and asthma. Root bark yields chay-root dye.

Chitarak, Chitra; Chitraka (S) – *Plumbago zeylanica* L.; Plumbaginaceae; small shrub. Cultivated as an ornamental but occurs wild also. Root is used in remedies for curing diarrhoea, piles, dyspepsia and skin ailments. Root bark contains plumbagin which stimulates the secretion of bile and urine. Milky juice is used locally for scabies and ulcers.

Chiti – *see* Jiti.

Chitiphul – *Heliotropium strigosum* Willd.; Boraginaceae; herb. Plant is diuretic and laxative. Plant juice is applied locally to heal ulcers, gum-boils and sores.

Chitra – *see* Chitarak.

Chitrabeez – *see* Bilpat.

Chitraka (S) – *see* Chitarak.

Chob-chini – *Smilax china* L.; China root (E); Smilacaceae; climber. Root tubers are used to treat rheumatism, venereal diseases and chronic skin ailments. Roots contain steroidal saponin and tannin. *See also* Jangli-aushbah.

Chobehyat – *Guaiacum officinale* L.; Tree-of-life (E), Pockwood tree (E); Zygophyllaceae; small tree. Plant is the source of a wood called lignum vitae with self lubricating property, great compression strength and resistance to salt water; and hence put to very specific uses. It also yields a resin called guaiacum which is used in paints and varnishes, and used medicinally as a mild laxative and in lozenges for throat trouble.

Chokargond – *see* Lasora.

Choupultea, Pola, Pula – *Kydia calycina* Roxb.; Malvaceae; small tree. Wood is suitable for making match-sticks, packing boxes, plywood, veneers, turnery, news-print, paper-pulp, and agricultural implements. Leaves are lopped for fodder. Stem yields a fibre used for cordage and a kind of mucilage which is used for clarifying jaggery for the manufacture of sugar.

Chouri – *see* Jamrassi.

Chowli – *see* Lobhia.

Chucka; Bhutankusa (S) – *Croton oblongifolius* Roxb.; Euphorbiaceae; branched herb. Seeds yield an oil which is useful as a purgative, insecticide, and for stupefying fish.

Chui-mui, Chhui mui, Lajwanti; Lajja (S) – *Mimosa pudica* L.; Sensitive plant (E); Mimosaceae; herb. Decoction of the root is used for curing urinary disorders.

Chuk – *Rumex acetosella* L.; Sheep sorrel (E); Polygonaceae; herb. Young shoots are used as salad, and are a rich source of ascorbic acid. Fresh plant juice acts as a diuretic, diaphoretic and astringent. Seeds are used as poultry feed.

Chuka, Ambari palak – *Rumex vesicarius* L.; Bladder dock (E); Polygonaceae; herb. Tender shoots and leaves are used as a pot-herb, and in chutneys. Leaves contain oxalates and are harmful when taken raw by livestock in large quantity.

Chukandar – *Beta vulgaris* L.; Beet root (E); Garden beet (E); Chenopodiaceae; herb with spherical tuberous roots. Root is used raw or boiled in salads and soups. The white sugarbeet belongs to the variety *rapa* and is used for sugar manufacture.

Tops and the spent pulp are used as stock-feed. Leaves of some varieties are used as spinach. *See* Palak.

Chuka-tripatti – *see* Amrul.

Chuma – *see* Dhurchuk.

Chundrika (S) – *see* Sarpagandha.

Chupri-alu, Khamalu; Pindalu (S) – *Dioscorea alata* L.; Asiatic yam (E), Greater yam (E); Dioscoreaceae; climbing shrub. Cultivated for its tubers, which are rich in starch and used as vegetable.

Cinchona – *Cinchona calisaya* Wedd.; Quinine (E); Rubiaceae; tree. Bark is the source of quinine, which is used as a cure for malarial fever.

Cowa – *Garcinia cowa* Roxb. ex DC. Guttiferae; dioecious tree. Fruits are edible. Gum resin from the trunk and branches is used in the preparation of a varnish which is suitable for metallic surfaces. Leaves are used as vegetable. Sun-dried slices of fruit are prescribed in dysentery.

D

Dab; Darbha (S), Kusha (S) – *Desmostachya bipinnata* (L.) Stapf.; Gramineae; tall perennial grass. Culms are used for thatching, manufacture of writing and printing paper, rough ropes and brooms. Culms are also used in the treatment of dysentery.

Dabh, Siru, Ulu; Darbha (S) – *Imperata cylindrica* (L.) Beauv. var. *major* (Nees.) C.E. Hubb. ex Hubb. & Vaughan; Thatch grass (E), Cogon grass (E); Gramineae; perennial grass. Culms provide raw material for making paper and are also used for thatching. Plant is considered to be a good soil binder.

Dabiduba – *Xyris indica* L.; Xyridaceae; herb. Plant is used for leprosy, and for healing ringworm and other skin ailments accompanied by lot of itching.

Dabra; Prasniparni (S) – *Uraria picta* Desv.; Papilionaceae; herb. Extract of the plant has fracture-healing properties. Decoction of the roots is given in fevers and colds. Roots and pods are used for curing anus prolapse in infants. Root is used as one of the components of 'Dasamula' an Ayurvedic tonic preparation.

Dadamari (S) – *see* Chakunda.

Dadap, Mandara; Parijata (S) – *Erythrina indica* Lamk. var. *parcellii* Hort.; Indian coral tree (E); Papilionaceae; large tree. Cultivated as an ornamental for its beautiful coral red clusters of flowers. *See also* Raktamadar.

Dadia – *Lindera pulcherrima* (Nees.) Benth. ex Hook. f.; Lauraceae; small tree. Wood is suitable for construction purposes and for making tea boxes.

Dadima (S) – *see* Anar.

Dadmari – *Ammannia baccifera* L.; Blistering Ammannia (E); Lythraceae; herb growing in marshy areas. Fresh juice is used for curing ringworm and other skin diseases.

Dadmurdan – *Cassia alata* L.; Ringworm senna (E), Candalabara bush (E); Caesalpiniaceae; shrub. Cultivated as an ornamental. Juice or paste of fresh leaves mixed with lime juice is used topically for curing ringworm and other skin infections. Seeds act as a vermifuge.

Daduri, Katgularia, Kathumbar; Kakadumbura (S) – *Ficus hispida* L.f.; Moraceae; small tree. Mature fruits are edible and can be made into jam. Bark is the source of tannin, and leaves are lopped for fodder.

Dahana (S) – *see* Jangli-kalimirch.

Daheya, Siora; Shakhotaka (S) – *Streblus asper* Lour.; Siamese rough bush (E); Moraceae; tree. Plant serves as a host to lac insect. Fruits are edible. Tender twigs are chewed to cure pyorrhoea. Root poultice is used as a healer on inflammation, boils and ulcers. Bark yields fibre; seed paste is applied topically on leucoderma lesions. Leaves act as a galactagogue, and are also fed to cattle and elephants. Rough leaves are used for polishing ivory and horns.

Dahipalas, Dhaiman – *Cordia macleodii* Hook. f. & Thoms.; Ehretiaceae; tree. Wood is used for furniture, carving, yokes, carts and tools. Bark is used for treating jaundice.

Dailay, *see* Karer.

Dain, Kath-semul – *Schefflera venulosa* (Wight. & Arn.) Harms.; Araliaceae; a large straggling shrub. Roots mixed with rice are reported to cure dropsy.

Dak – *Ribes rubrum* L.; Red currant (E); Grossulariaceae; shrub. Fruits are very acidic and are used for making jams, and jellies. Seeds yield a drying oil.

Dalchini, Tamalapatra (S) – *Cinnamomum zeylanicum* Blume; Cinnamon (E); Lauraceae; an evergreen tree. Cultivated as a plantation crop in Kerala (India). Dried inner bark termed 'quills' is the cinnamon of commerce, and is used extensively as a spice and condiment. It is also used in medicine as an astringent, carminative and stimulant. The essential oil obtained from the bark is used in pharmaceuticals. According to recent studies, daily intake of even minute quantity of the spice helps in reducing blood sugar levels significantly in people with type II diabetes.

Dalme – *see* Bakarcha.

Dalmugri – *see* Chaulmogra.

Damahan, Dhamasa, Ustarkhar; Ajabhakshya (S) – *Fagonia cretica* L.; Khorasan thorn (E); Zygophyllaceae; small green spiny undershrub. Plant is an astringent, tonic, febrifuge, diuretic, and expectorant, and is considered to be useful in combating asthma, cough, general debility, diarrhoea and dysentery. Bark decoction is used in the treatment of scabies. Plant is used in the preparation of an Ayurvedic tonic called 'Kumari asava'.

Daman-papra, Parpata; Kshetraparpata (S) – *Hedyotis corymbosa* (L.) Lam.; Rubiaceae; herb. Decoction of the herb is prescribed in gastric trouble, and nervous depression caused by deranged bile and in other liver troubles.

Damar (S) – *see* Vilayati afsanthin.

Dampel, Tumul; Tapinijha (S) – *Garcinia xanthochymus* Hook. f.; Egg tree (E); Guttiferae; tree. Fruits are very acidic and are made into preserves and vinegar. Unripe mature fruits yield a gum resin which is used to make water colours.

Dandal, Katari – *Xylosma longifolium* Clos.; Flacourtiaceae; evergreen tree. Juice of tender leaves produces opium like effect. Wood is used as fuel and for making fences.

Dandotpala (S) – *see* Sankhaphuli.

Dangribet – *Calamus latifolius* Roxb.; East India cane (E); Palmae; climbing palm. Stems are used for wicker-work, walking-sticks and polo-sticks.

Cultivated as an ornamental. Flowers, leaves and bark are used for tanning. Flowers also yield red and yellow dyes. Dried buds, flowers and fruits are used in indigenous medicine for curing bowel complaints, haemorrhages and menorrhagia.

Daya – *Callicarpa macrophylla* Vahl.; Verbenaceae; shrub. Warmed leaves are applied locally to rheumatic joints. Oil from the roots is used in remedies for stomach disorders.

Debdari – *see* Ashoke.

Dela, Belkamu – *Porana paniculata* Roxb.; Bridal creeper (E); Convolvulaceae; climbing shrub. Cultivated as an ornamental. Twigs are employed for making coarse baskets. Flowers are highly esteemed in the preparation of bridal-bouquets for their lavender like fragrance.

Dendhu – *see* Bassant.

Deodar, Diar; Devadaru (S) – *Cedrus deodara* (Roxb.) Loud.; Himalayan cedar (E); Deodar (E); Pinaceae; evergreen tall tree. Wood is strong, and is used for railway sleepers, door and window frames, furniture, bridges and construction work. Roots and wood yield an oil and an oleo-resin. Oil is used in cosmetics, and skin ailments. Alcoholic extract of the stem yields sesquiterpenes which have spasmolitic activity.

Deodhan – *Sorghum vulgare* Pers. var. *saccharatum* Koern.; Sugar Sorghum (E), Sorgho (E); Gramineae; cultivated tall herb. Grains are consumed for food. Stem yields a sweet juice and leaves are used as fodder.

Deshi-badam – *see* Patee-badam.

Desi-gulab, Cheenia gulab – *Rosa bourboniana* Desportes; Bourbon rose (E); Rosaceae; shrub. Cultivated for its fragrant flowers. Flower petals are used for the manufacture of otto of roses and rose-water. Root marketed by the name of 'rajtarni' is used in eye troubles.

Deura – *see* Baunra.

Devadaru (S) – *see* Deodar.

Devadhupa (S) – *see* Guggul.

Devakili (S) – *see* Sabbajaya.

Devanala (S) – *see* Nala.

Devataruni (S) – *see* Gulab.

Dhai – *see* Dawi.

Dhaiman – *see* Dahipalas.

Dhaincha, Dhunchi; Jayanti (S) – *Sesbania cannabina* (Retz.) Pers.; Prickly sesban (E); Papilionaceae; tall herb. Cultivated as a green manure crop and for reclaiming saline and alkaline soils. Stems yield a strong fibre which is used for making sails, ropes, fishing-nets and fishing lines. Seeds yield a gum similar in uses to 'guar' gum.

Dhak, Tesu, Palas; Palasha (S) – *Butea monosperma* (Lamk.) Taubert (syn. *B. frondosa* Koenig ex Roxb.); Flame of the forest (E), Bengal kino (E); Papilionaceae; deciduous tree. Cultivated as an ornamental for its beautiful bloom. Tree yields a gum called Bengal kino which is used for controlling diarrhoea. Flowers yield an orange-yellow dye employed for dyeing clothes. Leaves are used for making disposable platters and cups. Root and bark yield a coarse fibre. Bark is astringent and used for treating piles and tumours. Wood is suitable for news-print paper. Tree serves as a host to lac insect. Seeds are anthelmintic and are the source of kino oil. Gum and bark are rich in kino-tannic acid and galic acid and the fresh seeds are rich in fat- and protein-digesting enzymes.

Dhakki- *see* Aamli.

Dhamasa – *see* Damahan.

Dhamasia – *see* Sarphonka.

Dhamni, Pharsa; Dhanuvriksha (S) – *Grewia tiliaefolia* Vahl.; Tiliaceae; tree. Fruits are edible. Wood is used for making bent-wood articles, bows and arrows, cricket stumps, tennis and badminton rackets, billiard cues, agricultural implements, and tool handles. Wood-pulp is considered to be suitable for manufacturing wrapping paper. Bark is used in remedies for curing dysentery.

Dhamsiria – *Hymenachne amplexicaulis* (Rudge) Nees.; Dal grass (E); Gramineae; floating aquatic grass. Plant is used as a stock-feed both in fresh and dried state and is high in protein content. It is reported to have a larvaecidal effect on mosquitoe larvae in stagnant pools. Pith is used for making garlands.

Dhan – *see* Chaval.

Dhania, Kustumburi (S) – *Coriandrum sativum* L.; Coriander (E); Umbelliferae; aromatic herb. Cultivated for its fruits and leaves which are a rich source of iron, magnesium and manganese and also reported to contain protective phytochemicals. They are used as a condiment for flavouring curries, soups, bakery products, tobacco products, and a wide variety of foods and liquor, specially gin. Fruits are diuretic, carminative and tonic, and yield an essential oil which is used as a flavouring agent for liqueurs and in cocoa and chocolate industry. Fatty oil from the seeds is used in the preparation of special soaps.

Dhanua, Marainda, Murchi – *Ischaemum rugosum* Salisb.; Gramineae; grass found on wet ground. Plant is used as fodder for cattle and horses; it is also used as hay.

Dhanuvriksha (S) – *see* Dhamni.

Dhao, Dhav – *Anogeissus pendula* Edgew.; Combretaceae; tree. Cultivated as an avenue tree. Wood is exceptionally strong, and is used for poles, carts, rafters and helves. Leaves are lopped for fodder.

Dharauli – *see* Dudhi.

Dharu – *Lavandula stoechas* L.; French lavender (E); Labiatae; fragrant herb. Flowers yield an essential oil which is used medicinally for colic, biliousness, chest infections and headache. It has a strong camphor-like odour. Flowers are used in the manufacture of perfumes, fumigating powders and medicated cushions.

Dhataki (S) – *see* Dawi.

Dhatri (S) – *see* Amla.

Dhattura (S) – *see* Dhatura.

Dhatura; Dhattura (S), Unmatta (S) – *Datura stramonium* L.; Thorn apple (E), Solanaceae; annual stout herb. The source of the drug stramonium (hyoscyamine as the chief alkaloid) are the leaves and flowering tops. The drug is used as a component of 'Kanaka asava' an Ayurvedic preparation used for the treatment of asthma and cough. It is an expectorant, demulcent, anodyne and antispasmodic. It also contains the alkaloid atropine.

Dhaula khejra – *Acacia polyacantha* Willd.; Mimosaceae; tree. Bark is the source of tannin and the heart-wood yields 'cutch'. Young branches along with the leaves are used as fodder.

Dhaula phindavri – *Nothosaerva brachiata* (L.) Wight; Amaranthaceae; annual herb. Tender shoots are used as pot-herb.

Dhaura, Seja, Sidi – *Lagerstroemia parviflora* Roxb.; Lythraceae; large tree. Wood is used for construction work, and for making boats, bridges, fences, carts, bent-wood furniture, agricultural implements and tool handles. Bark and leaves contain tannin. Tree yields an edible gum and the leaves are reported to serve as a feed for 'tusser' silkworm.

Dhar – *see* Dhao.

Dhawa, Dhawra; Vakavryksha (S) – *Anogeissus latifolia* (DC.) Wall. ex Bedd.; Axle wood (E), Gum ghatti (E); Combretaceae; deciduous tree. Stem yields a gum called ghati-gum which is considered to be a good substitute for gum-acacia. Wood is suitable for rayon-grade pulp, paper, bent-wood articles, wood charcoal and wood-alcohol. Gum-ghati is used extensively in calico-printing, in explosive industry as a desiccant, in petroleum industry as drilling mud conditioner, and in ceramics and paper manufacture as a sizing material.

Dhawra – *see* Dhawa.

Dhebri – *see* Jamrassi.

Dheniani – *Olax scandens* Roxb.; Olacaceae; shrub. Tender shoots along with leaves are used as pot-herb. Fruits are edible and are also preserved as squashes. Bark is used in medicine for anaemia.

Dhera – *see* Akola.

Dhey, Bhasma-kand – *Sauromatum venosum* (Ait.) Kunth.; Araceae; herb with large globose acrid tubers. Tubers are poisonous but are edible after thorough washing to remove the acrid principle. They are also used in stimulating poultices.

Dhiva (S) – *see* Tumru.

Dholasmudrika (S) – *see* Dholsamudra.

Dholdhak – *see* Pangra.

Dholphulio – *Eragrostis tremula* Hochst. ex Steud.; Gramineae; tufted annual herb. Plants are used for fodder.

Dholsamudra; Dholasmudrika (S) – *Leea macrophylla* Roxb.; Leeaceae; shrub. Mucilaginous root tubers are used to cure guinea worm and ringworm infection. Fruits are edible and leaves are used as vegetable.

Dhumra-patra – *see* Kiramar.

Dhunchi–*see* Dhaincha.

Dhup – *Juniperus macropoda* Bois.; India juniper (E); Cupressaceae; tree. Considered as the best wood for pencils. Twigs are burnt as a substitute for incense. Cedar-oil obtained from its wood shavings and sawdust is used for making linoleum. Fruiting bodies yield a volatile oil which is used as a substitute for juniper oil obtained from *J. communis.*

Dhurchuk, Chuma, Kalabis – *Hippophae rhamnoides* L.; Sea-buckthorn (E); Elaeagnaceae; shrub or small tree. Fruit is edible and is also made into preserve; syrup of the fruit is prescribed as a cure for respiratory complaints and its decoction is used in skin trouble. Fruit is rich in vitamin C, and the seeds yield a semi drying oil. Twigs and leaves contain tannin.

Dhurpi sag – *see* Goma.

Dhustura (S) – *see* Sadah-dhatura.

Diar – *see* Deodar.

Didhan, Laughauni, Phulan – *Aeschynomene indica* L.; Sola-pith (E); Papilionaceae; shrub found along canal banks. Soft wood is used for solar hats, but is not as good as *A. aspera*. Plant makes good fodder. Seeds yield a fatty oil.

Didhi – *Sonchus asper* Hill.; Spiny-leaved sow thistle (E); Compositae; herb. Plant is used as an emollient. Pounded herb paste is applied topically to wounds. Young shoots are used as pot-herb.

Dikamli; Pindava (S) – *Gardenia gummifera* L.f.; Gummy cape jasmine (E); Rubiaceae; shrub or small tree. Cumbi gum or 'dikamli' exuded from young shoots is used in remedies for nervous disorders, flatulent dyspepsia and diarrhoea in infants.

Din-ka-raja – *Cestrum diurnum* L.; Day jessamine (E); Solanaceae; shrub. Grown as an ornamental, for its sweet scented flowers.

Dipya (S) – *see* Khurasani-ajvayan.

Dirgha (S) – *see* Mari.

Dirghapatraka (S) – *see* Tendu.

Diva; Surna (S) – *Tacca leontopetaloides* (L.) O. Kuntze; Fiji arrowroot (E); Taccaceae; herb. Rhizomes are the source of starch which is used as a substitute for true arrowroot. It is used in many dishes and also as laundry starch. Split stems, scapes and petioles are braided to make hats.

Divana Babul – *see* Gandh babul.

Dodak – *Sonchus oleraceus* L.; Milk thistle (E); Compositae; herb. Leaves and roots act as a febrifuge and roots as vermifuge. Latex is boiled to form a gummy substance used for curing hydrothorax and ascites.

Dolsar, Moonj – *Erianthus ravennae* (L.) P. Beauv.; Ravenna grass (E); Gramineae; large tufted perennial herb. Culms are used for screens and are considered to be good raw material suitable for paper-pulp and rayon-grade pulp.

Dolu, Revand-chini; Revatchini (S), Gandhini (S) – *Rheum emodi* Wall. ex Meissn.; Indian rhubarb (E); Polygonaceae; herb. Dried rhizomes and root powder are used as a laxative and purgative. Powdered root mixed with madder and potash is used for dyeing cloth in red colour. Leaves and leaf stalks are consumed either boiled or cooked, or made into preserves. Flowers and leaves contain rutin.

Dom-sal, Gidar-rukh – *Miliusa velutina* Hook. f. & Thoms.; Annonaceae; tree. Wood is used for furniture, construction work, carts, tool handles and agricultural implements. Fruits are edible. Stem yields a fibre, and the bark is purgative.

Doob, Dubh; Durva (S) – *Cynodon dactylon* (L.) Pers.; Dhub grass (E), Bermuda grass (E); Gramineae; herb. Plant is highly valued as lawn grass or pasture grass, and also as a good soil binder. Rhizomes are used in urino-genital troubles.

Dopahariya; Arkavallabha (S) – *Pentapetes phoenicea* L.; Sterculiaceae; shrub. Decoction of the capsules is emollient; mucilage is used for bowel diseases. Roots are used for bilious flatulence and the leaves as tea substitute.

Dopattilata – *Ipomoea pes-caprae* (L.) Sweet.; Sea-side morning glory (E); Convolvulaceae; herb. Roots are edible. Seeds are used for stomach ache and cramps. Plant contains a volatile oil and leaves are used for external application in rheumatism; leaf juice is diuretic.

Dori – *Leptadenia reticulata* (Retz.) Wight & Arn.; Asclepiadaceae; twining shrub. Roots and leaves are used for skin ailments. Alcoholic extract of the roots and leaves shows anti-bacterial activity. Plant is reported to stimulate milk yield when fed to cattle and egg production when used as poultry feed. The plant is used by lactating mothers in some tribal communities and reportedly regularises female menstruation and enhances sperm count in males.

Draksha (S) – *see* Angoor.

Drek – *see* Bakain.

Dronapushpi (S) – *see* Goma.

Dubh – *see* Doob.

Dudhi, Dharauli – *Wrightia tomentosa* (Roxb.) Roem & Schult.; Apocynaceae; tree. Wood is used as a second class timber. Latex yields a yellow dye, used for dyeing fabrics. Tender shoots and leaves are used as pot-herb. Fruits yield a floss which is used for stuffing and seeds yield an oil which is used medicinally. Root bark and stem are reported to be useful against scorpion and snake-bites.

Dudhiakalmi; Chandrakanti (S) – *Ipomoea alba* L.; Moon flower (E); Convolvulaceae; herb. Cultivated as an ornamental for its fragrant nocturnal flowers. Root bark acts as a purgative. Fleshy calyx of flowers and young leaves are edible.

Dudhialata; Dugdhika (S) – *Oxystelma secamone* (L.) Karst.; Rosy milk-weed (E); Asclepiadaceae; climber. Plant is used as fodder. Herb is considered to be an antiseptic and galactogogue. Decoction is used as a gargle in sore-throat. Fresh roots are prescribed in jaundice.

Dugdhika (S) – *see* Dudhialata.

Dugdugia, Piaman – *Syzygium cerasoideum* (Roxb.) Raizada; Myrtaceae; tree. Bark of the tree is astringent, and is used in biliousness, bronchitis and dysentery. Concentrate of the root infusion is rubbed on painful joints. Fruits are prescribed in rheumatism. Wood is used for rafters, canoes and for building work.

Duhsparsha – *see* Barhanta.

Duku – *Peucedanum grande* C.B. Clarke; Umbelliferae; herb. Fruits are used as a condiment and in medicine as a carminative and diuretic for gastric and intestinal disorders.

Dulal – *see* Barau.

Durpa-tandar – *see* Kukar-makri.

Durva (S) – *see* Doob.

Dushpatrijati (S) – *see* Gulmehndi.

E

Ebans – *see* Abnus.

Ekadivi (S) – *see* Ekdania.

Ekdania, Khaja; Asana (S), Ekadivi (S) – *Bridelia retusa* Spreng.; Euphorbiaceae; tree. Fruits are edible, leaves are lopped for fodder. Wood is used for construction work, rafters, carts, and agricultural implements. Bark is used as a source of tannin.

Ela (S) – *see* Chhoti elaichi.

Elaichi – *see* Chhoti elaichi, Bari elaichi and Morang elaichi.

Errandi, Arandi; Uruvka (S) – *Ricinus communis* L.; Castor (E); Castor oil plant (E); Euphorbiaceae; sparsely branched shrub. Cultivated for its seeds which yield the castor-oil. The oil is used chiefly as a lubricant and purgative. The oil in crude form is used for dyeing cotton and for the manufacture of printing inks, imitation leathers, and many other industrial products such as resins for textile industry, disinfectants, hydraulic brake fluids and sebacic acid which is used in nylon manufacture. Castor-cake is used as manure. Although rich in protein and minerals the castor-cake is not used as a feed for livestock due to the presence of ricine which acts as a blood coagulant. Leaf poultice is applied to sores. Dried stems and seed hulls are used as fuel. 'Eri' silkworms are reared on castor leaves. The hydrogenated oil can substitute carnauba wax in the manufacture of candles, polishes, heat-sealing adhesives and insulating materials.

Etanayakam (S) – *Salacia reticulata* Wight; Hippocrateaceae; climbing shrub. Plant is accredited with mild antiseptic properties. Root bark is used to treat gonorrhoea and itch.

Eucalyptus, Safeda – *Eucalyptus citriodora* Hook. Lemon-scented Eucalyptus (E); Myrtaceae; tall tree successfully introduced into India from Australia both in the hills and the plains. Leaves are fragrant, and are the source of an essential oil which yields citronellal. Wood yields excellent heavy timber which is used for making bridges, shafts, underframing of the body of trucks and trolleys, and agricultural implements. Kino from the tree serves as a rich source of tannin. Many other species of *Eucalyptus* have been introduced in India under the same Hindi name.

F

Faridbuti – *Farsetia jacquemontii* Hook. f.; Cruciferae; herb. Tender twigs are made into chutney and are also used as a condiment. The plant is considered to be good and specific for the treatment of rheumatism.

Fasli-gulab, Bussorah; Shatapatri (S) – *Rosa damascena* Mill.; Damask rose (E); Rosaceae; bushy shrub. Flower petals are very fragrant and are used for the preparation of otto of roses and rose water. Petals are also made into a preserve called 'gulkand' which is used as a tonic and laxative and for soothing sore throat. Rose water is used as a refrigerant and a vehicle for medicines. Flower buds are astringent and used as a tonic.

Findak, Bindak – *Corylus avellana* L.; Hazel-nut (E), Filbert (E); Corylaceae; shrub or small tree. Cultivated as an ornamental in the hills. Kernels are edible, and yield a fatty oil which is used in soap manufacture.

Findora – *Lilium wallichianum* Schult. f.; Liliaceae; tall ornamental herb. Dried bulb scales are demulcent, and used in chest complaints.

Frash-bean, Rajmah, Vilayati sem – *Phaseolus vulgaris* L.; French bean (E), Haricot bean (E), Kidney bean (E); Papilionaceae; herb. Tender pods are used as vegetable. Dried beans are used as a pulse and have high protein content. Green pod shells are used as a diuretic in kidney and heart-trouble.

Frast – *Populus nigra* L. var. *italica* Koehne; Black poplar (E); Salicaceae; tree. Wood is used for the manufacture of packing cases, furniture, coaches, match-sticks, plywood and wood-pulp.

G

Gab, Kalatendu; Tinduka (S), Krishnasara (S) – *Diospyros peregrina* (Gaertn.) Gurke; Indian persimmon (E); Ebenaceae; small evergreen tree; Unripe fruits and bark contain tannin. Boiled and pulped fruits are used as a preservative for fishing nets. Infusion of fruit is used as a gargle for sore throat. Oil extracted from the seeds is used for treating diarrhoea and dysentery. Ripe fruits are edible.

Gadabani – *Trianthema decandra* L.; Aizoaceae; herb. Roots are prescribed for asthma and hepatitis.

Gadadhari (S) – *see* Kirmala.

Gadar-tambaku – *Verbascum coromandelianum* (Vahl.) Kuntze.; Scrophulariaceae; herb. Plant juice is used for healing eruptions of skin. Juice of leaves is sedative and is used to check diarrhoea and dysentery.

Gagandhul – *see* Keora.

Gagjadra – *see* Pakar.

Gair – *see* Barkau.

Gaithi – *see* Ratalu.

Gajapipal, Bari-pipli; Gaja-pippali (S) – *Scindapsus officinalis* (Roxb.) Schott.; Araceae; large epiphytic climber. Dried fruits are carminative, anthelmintic, stimulant and diaphoretic, and are used to treat diarrhoea. Decoction of fruit is used in asthma. Fruits yield a fatty oil and stems yield a fibre.

Gaja-pippali (S) – *see* Gajapipal.

Gajar; Shikha-mula (S) – *Daucus carota* L. var. *sativa* DC.; Carrot (E); Umbelliferae; herb. Fleshy tap roots are a rich source of carotene and are eaten raw or cooked, they are also preserved into jams and pickles. Seeds act as a carminative, stimulant and diuretic and are used in dropsy and kidney trouble. Essential oil from seeds is used in perfumery. Carrot tops are used as fodder. Purple-black carrots are used to prepare a beverage called 'kanji' in N. India, which is considered to be good as an appetizer.

Galgal – *see* Bara nibu.

Galion – *see* Banpalati.

Galwang – *Albizia lucida* Benth.; Mimosaceae; tree. Wood is used for rafters and posts. Tree serves as an important host to lac insect.

Gamathi pudina – see Vilayati pudina.

Gambhar, Kambhari; Kaasmari (S), Bhadraparni (S) – *Gmelina arborea* L.; Verbenaceae; tree. Wood yields timber used for bridges, ship-building, plywood, paper-pulp, match-sticks and a variety of articles *viz*.furniture, shafts, axles, musical instruments, artificial limbs, printing blocks and for carving. Root is used as one of the ingredients of 'Dasamula', an important Ayurvedic preparation.

Gambhira (S) – *see* Kali-tulsi.

Gandana, Biranjasif – *Achillea millefolium* L.; Milfoil (E), Yarrow (E); Compositae; herb. Flower-heads and leaves are considered to be tonic, astringent, diaphoretic, and carminative, and are used in colds and colic. Alkaloid achilline is present. Aromatic aerial parts are used for flavouring and as a substitute for hops in beer-preparation.

Gandana, Gundhun – *Allium ascalonicum* L.; Shallot (E); Alliaceae; herb. Cloves of bulbs (white or red) are used for flavouring and for making pickles. Green leaves are edible.

Gandhar – *see* Khas khas.

Gandh babul, Divana babul – *Acacia farnesiana* (L.) Willd.; Cassie (E); Sweet Acacia (E); Mimosaceae; small thorny tree. Flowers are golden yellow and fragrant; they yield cassie perfume. Pods and bark are used as tan. Bark is astringent and demulcent. Tree yields a gum used in confectionery, and serves as a host to lac insect. Seeds yield a fatty oil.

Gandhabiroza – *Ferula galbaniflua* Boiss. & Buhse.; Galbanum (E); Umbelliferae; perennial herb. Stem yields galbanum an oleo-gum resin, which is used in perfumery, and as a carminative, antispasmodic and expectorant in chronic bronchitis and asthma.

Gandhali, Somaraji; Prasarani (S) – *Paederia scandens* (Lour.) Merr; Rubiaceae; shrub. Roots are emetic. Juice of roots is used in piles and to treat pain in chest and liver. Leaf juice is administered for diarrhoea in children; leaves are considered to be tonic and astringent. Plant is considered to be specific for combating rheumatism.

Gandhamadini (S) – *see* Budu.

Gandhamalati (S) – see Maalati.

Gandharaj – *Gardenia jasminoides* Ellis; Cape-jasmine (E); Rubiaceae; shrub. Cultivated as an ornamental. Flowers yield an essential oil which is used in perfumery. Fruit pulp yields a yellow dye. Fruits are considered to be emetic and diuretic and are used in kidney and lung trouble. Roots are used in nervine disorders.

Gandhashati (S) – *see* Kapur-kachri.

Gandhata (S) – *see* Nakuli.

Gandh-bel – *see* Gandhej-ghas.

Gandhej ghas, Gandh-bel, Rohisha (S) – *Cymbopogon martinii* (Roxb.) Wats.; Rosha grass (E), Palma rosa (E); Gramineae; tall perennial grass. Leaves yield an essential oil. Oil obtained from the variety *motia* is referred to as palmarosa oil and that from the variety *sofia* as ginger-grass oil. Palmarosa oil is the source of commercial geraniol which is used in perfumery, soaps, cosmetics, flavouring of tobacco, and as an adulterant of otto of roses for its rose-like aroma. Palmarosa oil also known as rusa oil is used for the treatment of lumbago and painful stiff joints.

Gandhela – *see* Meetha neem.

Gandhi-buti; Bhissata (S), Okharadi (S) – *Mollugo lotoides* (L.) O. Kuntze; Molluginaceae; herb. Dried plant is used in abdominal disorders. Plant juice is used as a tonic.

Gandhini (S) – *see* Dolu.

Gandhpura – *Gaultheria fragrantissima* Wall.; Fragrant wintergreen (E); Ericaceae; shrub. Fruits are edible. Leaves yield a volatile oil which is used in perfumery, insecticidal preparations and medicine as a carminative and stimulant; it is also used for rheumatism and neuralgia.

Gandhuli – *see* Hulhul.

Gandhya – *see* Harmal.

Gangati – *see* Pindalu.

Gangtiya – *see* Latmahuria.

Gangwa – *Excoecaria agallocha* L.; Agallocha (E); Euphorbiaceae; tree. Wood is used for general carpentry work, toys, match-sticks, paper-pulp and incense. Latex acts as a strong purgative and also applied locally for rheumatism and paralysis. Bark is also purgative. Decoction of leaves is used to treat epilepsy.

Ganja – *see* Bhang.

Ganjini – *Cymbopogon nardus* (L.) Rendle; Citronella grass (E); Gramineae; tall perennial. Leaves are the source of an essential oil called citronella oil. Oil from the variety *'lenabatu'* is used for perfumery, toiletries and cosmetics and oil from the variety *'mahapengiri'* is used mainly in mosquito repellents and for preparing synthetic menthol. Citronella oil is the source of geraniol and citronellal.

Ganna, Paunda; Ikshu (S) – *Saccharum officinarum* L.; Sugarcane (E), Noble cane (E); Gramineae; tall perennial grass. Stems are juicy and are the source of crystalline sugar, jaggery and open pan-sugar known as 'khandsari'. By-products include molasses and bagasse or fibre. Molasses are used for the manufacture of industrial alcohol, synthetic rubber and rum. Bagasse is used for fuel and manufacture of cardboard, wrapping paper and other forms of paper. Molascuit a mixture of bagasse and molasses is used as fodder. Bagasse mixed with waste paper pulp is finding new use in the manufacture of light weight corrugated packing boxes. *See also* Ukh.

Ganna – *see* Ukh.

Ganth-gobhi – *Brassica oleracea* L. var. *gongylodes* L.; Kohlrabi (E), Knol-kohl (E); Cruciferae; herb. Aerial swollen stem is edible and also used as a stock-feed. Tender leaves are eaten raw or cooked.

Gaozaban, Shankhahuli – *Onosma bracteatum* Wall.; Boraginaceae; herb. Plant is considered to be tonic and, diuretic, and is used in syphilis, leprosy, rheumatism and irritation of bladder. The name Gaozaban has been used for several other plants also *viz.*, *Anchusa strigosa* Labill, *Anisomeles indica* Kuntze, *A. malabarica* R. Br., *Coccinea glauca* Savi, and *Macrotomia benthamii* DC.

Garari – *Cleistanthus collinus* (Roxb.) Benth. ex Hook. f.; Euphorbiaceae; small tree. Wood is used for construction work and paper-pulp. Bark, leaves and roots are used as fish poison. Leaves are considered to be abortifacient and leaves, bark and green fruits serve as the source of tannin.

Garbhada (S) – *see* Ram baigan.

Garbhaghatini (S) – *see* Kalihari.

Garbijaur, Medh – *Litsea glutinosa* (Lour.) C.B. Robins.; Lauraceae; aromatic small tree or shrub. Wood is used for furniture, agricultural implements and packing boxes. Fruits are edible. Seeds yield an aromatic fat used for making candles and soaps; the fat is source of lauric acid which is used for the manufacture of detergents. It is also used medicinally for rheumatism. Mucilaginous bark is used as a remedy for diarrhoea and dysentery. Leaves are used as fodder.

Gardha-bhanda (S) – *see* Paras-pipal.

Garmezu – *Astragalus strobiliferus* Royle; Papilionaceae; shrub. Plant is the source of a gum which is used as a substitute for gum-tragacanth. Gum which is collected by making incisions on the stem is of superior quality.

Garshuma – *see* Meda tumri.

Garsilug – *see* Meda tumri.

Garudaphala – *see* Chaulmoogra.

Gauj, Gonj – *Millettia extensa* Benth. ex Baker; Papilionaceae; woody straggling shrub. Powdered roots are used as a fish-poison, and to kill maggots in cattle wounds. Roots also possess insect-repellent properties and the infusion of roots is rubbed on cattle and horses to keep away the flies. Leaves are lopped for fodder. Bark yields a fibre used for making ropes.

Gauri – *Polyalthia fragrans* (Dalz.) Bedd.; Annonaceae; large tree. Wood yields timber which is used for light construction work, match-sticks, packing cases, picture frames, billiard cues, rackets and manufacture of plywood.

Gawar – *see* Guar.

Gazaria – *see* Kanta-alu.

Gehun, Kanak; Godhuma (S) – *Triticum aestivum* L. emend. Thell; Wheat (E); Gramineae; many tillered herb. Cultivated as an important staple food crop for its nutritious grains which also contain glutin, and are used for making leavened and unleavened bread, porridge, puffed wheat and various types of snacks and confectioneries. Straw and chaff are used as fodder. Straw-pulp is used for the manufacture of paper and strawboard. Wheat bran and germ are used for human consumption and also as stock feed.

Genda, Gultera, Sthalapushpa (S) – *Tagetes erecta* L.; African marigold (E), Aztec marigold (E); Compositae; herb. Cultivated for its beautiful bright yellow coloured flower-heads which are very popular and used either as such or made into garlands and used for worship and floral decorations in homes, temples, rituals, and ceremonial festivals as they remain fresh for a very long time. Root extract is laxative. Infusion of leaves and florets is carminative and diuretic; it is used for treating colds, cough, bronchitis and rheumatism. Florets yield a yellow dye and the xanthophyll fraction from petals on isolation, has the potential as poultry feed to improve the yellow colour of yolk in eggs. Seeds contain a fatty oil. Fresh plant is the source of an essential oil.

Ghabel – *see* Samandar-sokh.

Ghagra-bel – *see* Bindal.

Ghainchu, Tagarmul – *Limnanthemum cristatum* Griseb [syn. *Nymphoides indicum* (L.) Kuntze]; Gentianaceae; herb. Plant is used as a substitute of 'chirayeta' which is used in fevers and jaundice. Seeds are anthelmintic.

Ghant – *see* Moka.

Ghantarava – *see* Jhunjhunia.

Gharei kashmalu – *see* Tukhmalanga.

Ghechu; Kaangi (S) – *Aponogeton natans* (L.) Engl. & Krause; Aponogetonaceae; anchored aquatic herb. Tuberous starchy rootstocks are edible.

Ghee-kunvar, Guar-pattha; Ghrita-kumari (S) – *Aloe barbadensis* Mill. (syn. *Aloe vera* Tourn ex L.); Barbados aloe (E); Liliaceae; succulent shrub. Fresh mucilaginous leaf pulp is used internally to treat liver and spleen disorders and externally to alleviate the pain of burns and hasten their healing. It is considered the best remedy for sunburn and is used in innumerable cosmetics, moisturizers and skin creams. It is cultivated as an ornamental also. Leaf extract contains barbaloin, which inhibits the growth of *Mycobacterium tuberculosis*.

Ghia, Lauki, Kaddu; Alabu (S) – *Lagenaria siceraria* (Mol.) Standl; Bottle gourd (E); Calabash gourd (E); Cucurbitaceae; trailing or climbing herb. Plant is cultivated for its fruit which is used as vegetable and is rich in vitamins B and C. Seeds are anthelmintic and used in dropsy. Seed oil is used for curing headache. Dried fruit shells are very hard and are used for making blowing horns, musical instruments, water bottles and bowls.

Dansara, Dasni – *Rhus sinuata* Thunb.; Anacardiaceae; tree; Roasted fruits are edible. Stem bark is used for tanning and for imparting brown colour to leather. Leaves are also used for tanning. Wood is used for making fences and for small carpentry.

Danti; Jangli jamalgota – *Baliospermum montanum* (Willd.) Muell.–Arg.; Euphorbiaceae; an undershrub. Seeds act as a strong purgative. Oil from the seeds is also used as a strong cathartic. Roots are considered to be useful in treating jaundice. Seeds are sometimes substituted for the seeds of *Croton tiglium*, and therefore called Jangli jamalgota in Hindi.

Daradharsa (S) – *see* Taramira.

Darbha (S) – *see* Dabh, *see* also Dab.

Darhald – *see* Rasaut.

Darmar – *see* Timur; *see also* Tumru.

Daruharidra (S) – *see* Rasaut.

Darya-ka-naryal; Ubdie-narikaylum (S) – *Lodoicea maldivica* (Gmel) Pers.; Double coconut palm (E); Palmae; dioecious palm. Cultivated as an ornamental. Leaves are used for thatching and mats, and the mid-rib part is used for making brooms. Soft kernel and water in green fruits is antiacid and antibilious. Hard kernel (endosperm) yields vegetable ivory and the shells of large fruits are used as vessels for keeping water.

Dasni – *see* Dansara.

Datranga – *see* Chamror.

Daudotpala, Sadodi; Sahadevi (S) – *Vernonia cinerea* (L.) Less.; Purple fleabane (E), Ash-coloured fleabane (E); Compositae; herb. Infusion of the plant in combination with quinine is used to cure malaria. Decoction of the root is used to treat diarrhoea and stomach ache. Flowers are used for rheumatism and conjunctivitis. Seeds are anthelmintic, and are used in remedies for cough, flatulence, intestinal colic and leucoderma. Leaves are used for curing eczema and ringworm.

Dawi, Dhai; Agnijwala (S), Dhataki (S) – *Woodfordia fruticosa* (L.) Kurz.; Fire-flame bush (E), Shiranjitea (E); Lythraceae; shrub.

Ghiabati – *Ipomoea pes-tigridis* L.; Sea-side morning glory (E); Convolvulaceae; spreading annual herb. Plant is rich in calcium, phosphorus and proteins and forms nutritive fodder both in fresh and dried state. Roots contain resin and are used as a purgative. Leaf poultice is used on boils, sores and pimples.

Ghiabato, Boota; Nakhari (S) – *Ipomoea eriocarpa* R. Br.; Convolvulaceae; robust twining annual herb. Tender twigs and leaves are used as vegetable. Seeds are edible and provide a rich source of protein. Infusion of plant in oil is used topically for rheumatism, ulcers and leprosy. Plant is also used as fodder.

Ghiabel – *Merremia aegyptia* (L.) Urban (syn. *Ipomoea pentaphylla* Jacq.); Convolvulaceae; spreading annual herb. Seeds are nutritious and edible.

Ghiwain – *Elaeagnus latifolia* L.; Bastard oleaster (E); Elaeagnaceae; shrub or small tree. Ripe fruits are edible. Flowers are considered to be astringent.

Ghia tori – *see* Tori.

Ghogar, Kharpat, Toom – *Garuga pinnata* Roxb.; Burseraceae; tree. Fruits are edible. Plant provides useful timber considered to be good for making match-sticks, pencils, plywood and wrapping paper. Leaf galls are used for tanning. Leaves are lopped for fodder.

Ghrita-kumari (S) – *see* Ghee kunvar.

Ghuiyan – *see* Arvi.

Ghunghunian, Shanarghandika (S) – *Crotalaria retusa* L.; Golden yellow Crotalaria (E); Papilionaceae; shrub. Cultivated for the fibre obtained from its stem and used for cordage and canvas. Plant is used in scabies. Seed consumption by humans or cattle can cause cirrhosis of liver.

Ghurgia, Thanella – *Gardenia turgida* Roxb.; Rubiaceae; small tree. Wood is used for turnery, walking-sticks, and musical instruments. Fruits are edible after cooking.

Ghurush – *see* Sutri.

Gidar rukh – *see* Dom-sal.

Gidar tamaku – *see* Ban tambaku.

Gilas – *Prunus avium* L.; Sweet cherry (E); Mazard (E); Rosaceae; tree. Cultivated in the hilly regions for its juicy and fleshy delicious fruits which are used either fresh or canned.

Gilla, Barabi, Chian – *Entada phaseoloides* (L.) Merr. [syn. *E. scandens* (L.) Benth.]; Nicker bean (E); Mimosaceae; giant climbing shrub. Seeds, bark and fruit-pulp are used as fish poison. Stem fibre is used for fishing-nets and cordage. Seeds are considered to be emetic and anthelmintic. Stem and its bark are used as soap substitute. Seeds are used for crimping starched cottons and are also made into ornaments by tribals.

Giloe, Guduchi, Gulancha; Amrita (S) – *Tinospora cordifolia* (Willd.) Miers. ex Hook. f. & Thoms.; Menispermaceae; climbing shrub. Dry stems are a constituent of several Ayurvedic preparations which are used as tonic and to treat dyspepsia, urinary disorders and fevers. The drug has bitter principles present in the stems with intact bark. It acts as an analgesic, antispasmodic and anti-inflammatory. Leaf decoction is used as a remedy for gout and root decoction is used for obstruction in the viscera.

Ginighas – *Panicum maximum* Jacq.; Guinea grass (E); Gramineae; herb. Cultivated as a fodder plant and makes excellent hay and silage which is relished by cattle.

Gio, Jiban; Jivanti (S) – *Trema orientalis* (L.) Blume; Indian nettle tree (E); Charcoal tree (E); Ulmaceae; small tree. Stem bark yields fibre for cordage and also serves as the source of tannin. Fruits are edible. Wood is used for packing-cases, match-sticks, good quality paper and gunpowder charcoal. Decoction of roots is given to combat diarrhoea, and blood-cells discharge in urine. Leaves are lopped for fodder.

Girimalah – *see* Amaltas.

Girya – *see* Bhirra.

Gitoran – *see* Ardanda.

Goalilata; Godapadi (S); Suvaha (S) – *Cayratia pedata* (Wall.) Gagnep; Vitaceae; climber. Leaves are considered to be astringent and cooling. Leaf infusion is reported to check uterine reflexes.

Gobhi – *see* Samudulan.

Gobi – *see* Phool gobi.

Godapadi (S) – *see* Goali lata.

Godhuma (S) – *see* Gehun.

Goganda, Gogina – *Saurauia napaulensis* DC.; Saurauiaceae; tree. Fruits are edible. Leaves are lopped for fodder. Wood is used for packing cases and small carpentry.

Gogina – *see* Goganda.

Gogsa – *see* Phusera.

Gojihva (S) – *see* Samudulan.

Gokhru; Gokshura (S), Ikshugandha (S) – *Tribulus terrestris* L.; Land-caltrops (E); Zygophyllaceae; prostrate herb. Fruits are accredited with tonic and diuretic properties. Leaf paste is used for bladder stones. Herb yields saponins which on hydrolysis give steroidal sapogenins.

Gokhru-kalan – *Tribulus alatus* Delile; Zygophyllaceae; prostrate herb. Plants are used as fodder for camels, sheep and horses. Fruits are tonic and diuretic and are used in urinogenital disorders. Seeds act as an astringent and diuretic.

Gokshura (S) – *see* Gokhru.

Gokul-dhup – *Canarium sikkimense* King; Burseraceae; tall tree. Bark yields aromatic resin which is used as incense. Wood is suitable for tea-chests.

Gokurni – *see* Aparajit.

Gola – *see* Nariyal.

Gola-bet – *Daemonorops jenkinsianus* Mart; Palmae; tall palm. Long, soft stems are used for basketry.

Golainchi – *see* Khair-champa.

Golkandra – *see* Jangli karela.

Golmirch – *see* Kalimirch.

Golpatti pudina – *Mentha rotundifolia* (L.) Huds.; Apple mint (E); Labiatae; perennial herb. Cultivated for its fragrant leaves which are used for flavouring confectionery, curries and snacks.

Goma, Dhurpi sag; Dronapushpi (S) – *Leucas cephalotes* (Roth.) Spreng; Labiatae; herb. Flower syrup is used for treating cough and colds. Herb is considered to be diuretic, stimulant and anthelmintic.

Goncha – *see* Kiwach.

Gondi; Laghushlesh mataka (S) – *Cordia rothii* Roem. & Schult.; Ehretiaceae; small tree. Bark is astringent and used for sore throat as gargles; it also yields a fibre which is used for making ropes. Fruits are edible.

Gondni – *see* Chabeni.

Gonj – *Derris scandens* (Roxb.) Benth.; Papilionaceae; woody climber. Plant usually grows wild but is also cultivated as an ornamental for its dense foliage. Roots are used as fish poison but are not insecticidal. Stem is the source of a coarse fibre. *See* also 'Gauj'.

Gonj – *see* Gauj.

Gonte – *see* Baunra.

Gopabhadra (S) – *see* Badhara.

Gorakh-amli, Lichora – *Adansonia digitata* L.; Baobab (E); Monkey bread tree (E); Bombacaceae; tree. Fruit pulp is made into a fresh cooling drink. It is considered to be diaphoretic and is used in allergic dermatitis and stomach disorders. Seeds are edible and their oil is used for cooking. Inner bark yields a strong fibre and is also used for paper pulp. Wood pulp is suitable for the manufacture of paper.

Gorakh booti, Astmabayota (S) – *Aerva lanata* Juss. ex Schult.; Amaranthaceae; herb. Plant is used in sore-throat, cough and diabetes. Decoction of the herb is diuretic.

Gorakh-mundi – *see* Mundi.

Goran – *Ceriops tagal* (Perr.) C.B. Robins; Rhizophoraceae; small tree found in the Sundarbans and the Andaman islands. Bark and leaves are rich in tannin. Bark is used to check haemorrhages and malignant ulcers. Its extract is used to toughen fishing-nets and fishing-lines.

Gorani (S) – *see* Guar.

Goria – *see* Chickua.

Gorurna – *see* Amarkand.

Goth-ber – *see* Kat-ber.

Grahadruma (S) – *see* Patee-badam.

Grishma-sundaraka (S) – *see* Jima.

Gual, Lahichan, Punia – *Ehretia acuminata* R. Br. var. *serrata* (Roxb.) Johnston; Heliotrope tree (E); Ehretiaceae; tree. Fruits are edible, raw ones are pickled. Wood is used for agricultural implements; leaves are lopped for fodder.

Guar, Gawar, Khurti-ki-phali; Gorani (S) – *Cyamopsis tetragonoloba* (L.) Taub. [syn. *C. psoralioides* (Lamk.) DC.]; Cluster bean (E); Papilionaceae; robust bushy annual herb. The plant is cultivated for its mature seeds which yield the guar gum and its tender green pods which are used as a vegetable. It is also cultivated as a cover crop, forage crop and a green manure crop. The seed flour has very high viscosity due to the presence of a complex polysaccharide called galactomanan (guar gum) or mannogalacton, which has miscellaneous industrial uses. It is used as an emulsifier in salad dressings, thickener in food products, sizing agent in textile and paper industry, filter aid in mining industry and in the manufacture of cosmetics and pharmaceuticals. It is also used as a backing for postage stamps as it can form a very thin film on drying. The mature seeds are very rich in proteins and carbohydrates and are highly valued as a cattle-feed

Guar-pattha – *see* Ghee kunvar.

Guchha pushp, Mradupatra (S) – *Malva verticillata* L.; Malvaceae; herb. Leaves are used as pot-herb. Ash of dried leaves is used in scabies. Roots are used for curing whooping cough.

Gudhapatra – *see* Karer.

Guduchi – *see* Giloe.

Guggul; Devadhupa (S), Koushikaha (S) – *Commiphora wightii* (Arnott) Bhandari; Indian bdellium tree (E); Burseraceae; small tree. Bark yields a fragrant gum resin known as gum-guggul or Indian myrrh, which is used as a fixative in perfumery and as incense. Fragrant oleo-resin is also used in Ayurvedic medicine as an expectorant, carminative, diuretic and pain killer for muscular rheumatism. It is also reported to lower down the cholestrol level of blood. 'Bol', 'rasagaduhi' or myrrh is the gum resin obtained from *Commiphora myrrha* Nees.

Guggul dhup – *Ailanthus triphysa* (Dennst.) Alston.; Simaroubaceae; tree. Bark yields a fragrant resin which is used as an incense. Bark juice is used for curing bronchitis, asthma and dysentery. Leaves yield a black dye. Wood is suitable for match-sticks, plywood, veneers and paper pulp. Fruits contain a fatty oil.

Gujur – *Pastinaca sativa* L. [syn. *Peucedanum sativum* (L.) Hook. f.]; Parsnip (E); Umbelliferae; herb. Roots are fleshy and used as salad or vegetable, they are also used for soups. Herb acts as a carminative and diuretic. Fruits are used for stomach and bladder disorders, and contain a fatty oil. All parts of the herb contain an essential oil.

Gulab; Devataruni (S) – *Rosa centifolia* L.; Cabbage rose (E), Provence rose (E); Rosaceae; small shrub. Cultivated for its fragrant flowers. Petals yield rose water and an essential oil known as otto of roses. Decoction of flowers is used in ulceration of the intestines. Floral wax a by-product of rose perfume is used in soap industry. Fruit is a rich source of vitamin C.

Gulabash, Gul-abbas, Krishnakeli (S) – *Mirabilis jalapa* L.; Four o'clock plant (E); Nyctaginaceae; herb. Cultivated as an ornamental for its beautiful flowers which also yield a crimson dye. Leaf extract is used for bruises, sores, boils and abscesses. Leaves are also edible; powdered seeds are used in cosmetics.

Gul-abbas – *see* Gulabash.

Gulab jaman – *Syzygium jambos* (L.) Alston.; Rose-apple (E); Myrtaceae; tree. Cultivated as an avenue tree. Fruits are edible. Leaves yield an essential oil.

Gulati – *Crotalaria medicaginea* Lamk. var. *luxurians* (Benth.) Baker; Papilionaceae; perennial herb. Plants are used as fodder for camels. Seeds are also used as fodder for cattle.

Gulancha – *see* Giloe.

Gular, Umar, Udumbara (S) – *Ficus glomerata* Roxb.; Cluster fig (E); Moraceae; deciduous tree. Cultivated as a road-side tree. Fruits are edible. Leaves are lopped for fodder. Latex is used in diarrhoea and piles. Roots are used in controlling diarrhoea and diabetes. Leaves are prescribed in bile disorders. Fruits are considered carminative and stomachic. Bark yields tannin. Wood is used for cheap furniture. The tree serves as a host to summer brood of lac insect.

Gulcheri – *see* Rajnigandha.

Guldaudi (chhoti), Gulechini; Chandramallika (S) – *Chrysanthemum coronarium* L.; Garland Chrysanthemum (E), Crown daisy (E); Compositae; annual herb. Cultivated as an ornamental, and the flowers-heads are used as a substitute for chamomile for stimulating digestion. *See also* Guldaudi; Sevanti (S).

Guldaudi; Sevanti (S) – *Chrysanthemum indicum* L. (syn. *C. japonicum* Thunb.); Japanese Chrysanthemum (E); Compositae; herb. Cultivated as an ornamental for its beautiful flowers which remain fresh for a very long time and are very popular for floral decorations. Leaves are prescribed for migraine.

Gulechini – *see* Guldaudi (chhoti).

Gulga – *Nipa fruticans* Thunb.; Palmae; tall palm. Plant is the source of toddy. Leaves are used for thatching, mats and basketry. Leaf paste is used topically for treating ulcers and bites of centipedes. Immature fruits are made into preserves.

Guliajaib – *see* Shalapara.

Gulkhair, Kunzi, Vilayati-kangai – *Malva sylvestris* L.; Malvaceae; perennial herb. Tender shoots with young fruits are used as pot-herb. All parts contain mucilage, carotene and calcium. Plant is used for treating urinary infection and whooping cough and also used externally on inflammation and abscesses.

Gul-khera – *Althaea rosea* (L.) Cav.; Hollyhock (E); Malvaceae; tall herb. Cultivated as an ornamental. Flowers yield a red dye which is used as an indicator in measuring acidity and alkalinity. It is also used medicinally in chest infections.

Gulmehndi; Dushpatrijati (S) – *Impatiens balsamina* L.; Garden balsam (E); Balsaminaceae; annual herb. Cultivated as an ornamental for its beautiful flowers. Alcoholic extract of the flowers is reported to be fungicidal and bactericidal. Seeds yield a fatty oil. Flowers are mucilaginous, and are used for lumbago, and to improve circulation.

Gul mohar – *Delonix regia* (Boj.) Raf.; Gold mohur (E); Caesalpiniaceae; tree. Cultivated as an avenue tree for its beautiful foliage and flowers.

Gulsakari – *Sida spinosa* L.; Prickly Sida (E); Malvaceae; undershrub. Roots are tonic and diaphoretic and are used in fevers, debility, irritability of bladder and gonorrhoea.

Gul-shabbo – *see* Rajnigandha.

Gulsham – *Eranthemum roseum* (Vahl.) R. Br.; Acanthaceae; shrub. Tuberous roots boiled in milk are used for combating leucorrhoea.

Gultera – *see* Genda.

Gulu, Kulu – *Sterculia urens* Roxb.; Karaya-gum Sterculia (E); Sterculiaceae; tall tree. Stem yields gum-karaya which is used similar to tragacanth-gum obtained from *Astragalus gummifer* Labill. It finds uses in pharmaceutical, medicinal and cosmetic preparations such as emulsions, lotions, pastes, lozenges, laxatives and sprays. Its usage extends to food, baking and dairy as dressings and spreads, as a thickener in printing pastes for textiles, and as a pulp-binder in paper industry. Seeds are edible after roasting and seed protein yields an adhesive used in plywood industry. Wood is used for making toys, guitars and packing cases; stem bark yields a fibre used for making ropes.

Gulutora, Chhoti-gulmohur, Ratnagandhi (S) – *Caesalpinia pulcherrima* (L.) Sw.; Peacock flower (E), Barbados pride (E);

Caesalpiniaceae; shrub. Cultivated as an ornamental for its beautiful flowers. Pods and leaves are used as a substitute for senna. Flowers yield a dye. Bark is abortifacient, leaves are purgative and infusion of flowers is used for curing bronchitis and asthma.

Guma – *see* Halkusa.

Gunara, Bansi–*Panicum antidotale* Retz.; Blue Panicum (E); Gramineae; tall grass. Plant is used as fodder when young and tender, and is considered to be a good soil binder and wind-break.

Gunchi – *see* Ratti.

Gundhun – *see* Gandana.

Gundra (S) – *see* Bora.

Gunja (S) – *see* Ratti.

Gunkar – *Themeda quadrivalvis* (L.) Kuntze; Kangaroo grass (E); Gramineae; tall grass. Young tender plants are used as cattle feed. Culms are considered to be good for thatching and paper pulp. Plant is also a good soil binder.

Gurgu – *Pistacia khinjuk* Stocks; Chian turpentine tree (E), East Indian mastiche (E); Pistaciaceae; tree. Plant is the source of an ornamental mottled wood which is also used for carving. Galls and bark are used for dyeing and tanning. Leaves are lopped for fodder.

Gurhal, Jasum, Javakusum; Rudra pushpam (S) – *Hibiscus rosa-sinensis* L.; Shoe-flower (E), China-rose (E); Malvaceae; bushy evergreen shrub. Cultivated as an ornamental. Flowers are used for worship, they also yield a dark-purplish dye employed in preparing hair-dyeing oils and shoe-polishes. Flower-decoction is prescribed in bronchial catarrh and root-decoction in venereal diseases. Leaves are used medicinally as an anodyne and laxative.

Gurla – *see* Chickua.

Gurlu – *see* Sankru.

Gur-mar – *see* Merasingi.

Guthari – *see* Madana-ghanti.

Gwaladarim, Kura – *Gymnosporia royleana* M. Laws.; Celastraceae; tree. Wood is used as a substitute for box-wood which is used for carving and engraving; it is also used for walking-sticks.

Gwalam – *see* Jangli seb.

H

Hab-el-ghar – *Laurus nobilis* L.; True laurel (E), Sweet bay (E); Lauraceae; shrub or small tree. Leaves contain an essential oil and are used as a condiment. Seeds are the source of an aromatic fat which is used for diarrhoea, dropsy and local application in sprains; it is also used in perfumery and soap manufacture. Wood is used for cabinet work.

Habulas – *see* Murad.

Hadjora, Harshankari; Asthisanhara (S) – *Cissus quadrangularis* L.; Edible-stemmed vine (E); Vitaceae; succulent twiner. Plant acts as an anthelmintic, carminative and blood purifier. Stem juice and powdered roots are reported to be used for setting fractured bones. Juice is also prescribed in scurvy. Stems and roots yield a strong fibre.

Haiza, Rungru, Tatra – *Kalanchoe integra* (Medic.) Kuntze; Crassulaceae; succulent perennial herb. Leaves are considered to be antiseptic and insecticidal, and leaf juice is purgative. Leaf-ash is applied to abscesses.

Hakna, Sakena – *Indigofera pulchella* Roxb.; Papilionaceae; herb. Decoction of the herb is used for curing cough.

Hakshardana – *Euphorbia hypericifolia* L.; Euphorbiaceae; herb. Infusion of the herb is astringent and is used for treating diarrhoea, dysentery and leucorrhoea.

Haldi; Haridra (S) – *Curcuma domestica* Valeton; Turmeric (E); Zingiberaceae; perennial herb. Cultivated for its rhizomes which are used as a condiment, seasoning for food, tonic, antiseptic, blood purifier, and in ointments for skin, in cosmetics and for wounds and sprains. The yellow pigment curcumin which is a powerful antioxidant and an active principle present in turmeric is used in pharmacy, home-remedies, confectionery, foods, textiles and paint industry. Rhizomes are also used as an offering in certain rituals of the Hindus.

Haldu – *Adina cordifolia* (Roxb.) Hook f. ex Brandis; Yellow teak (E); Naucleaceae; tree. Wood is fairly strong and considered very good for bobbins, flooring and panelling of railway carriages, plywood and paper manufacture. Bark is the source of tannin, and the spent bark is used for the manufacture of boards.

Haldwa – *see* Burhna.

Halganne – *Palaquium ellipticum* (Dalz.) Engl.; Indian gutta-percha (E); Sapotaceae; tall tree. Wood is used for building purposes, veneers, plywood and bent wood furniture. Seeds are the source of a fatty oil used for soap manufacture while the tree is the source of pala-gum an inferior kind of gutta-percha.

Halim – *see* Chamsur.

Halis – *Podocarpus neriifolius* D. Don; Mounteak (E), Thitmin (E); Podocarpaceae; tree. Plant is the source of high class timber used for furniture, oars, paddles, masts, tea boxes and ladders; it is also used for making pencils after proper treatment. Fleshy receptacles of fruiting bodies are edible.

Halkusa, Guma – *Leucas lavandulaefolia* Rees; Labiatae; herb or undershrub. Leaves are used as a febrifuge and leaf juice is used for healing psoriasis, painful swellings and skin eruptions. Flowers mixed with honey are used to treat cough and colds.

Halsi – *Aegiceras corniculatum* (L.) Blanco; Goat's horn mangrove (E); Myrsinaceae; tree found in swamps. Bark contains tannin and saponin, and is used for tanning and fish poisoning.

Halwa-tendu – *Diospyros kaki* L.f.; Japanese persimmon (E), Kaki (E); Ebenaceae; small tree. Wood is used for ornamental work and mosaics. Fully ripe fruits are edible. Tannin from unripe fruits is used for dyeing and as a preservative for wood.

Halyun, Seet-muli – *Asparagus officinalis* L.; Garden Asparagus (E); Liliaceae; perennial herb. Young succulent shoots called spears are used as vegetable and marketed either fresh, frozen or canned. Herb contains asparagine which is used as a diuretic and for combating chronic gout.

Hamsagar – *Kalanchoe laciniata* (L.) DC.; Crassulaceae; herb with succulent leaves. Leaves antiseptic and astringent, and are applied to sores and wounds. Leaf juice is prescribed in diarrhoea and dysentery.

Hans-lata – *Aristolochia grandiflora* Sw.; Pelican-flower (E); Aristolochiaceae; climbing shrub. The plant is cultivated as an ornamental for its beautiful flowers and foliage.

Hansraj, Mubaraka – *Adiantum capillus-veneris* L.; Maiden-hair fern (E); Adiantaceae, herb. The whole plant is used as a pectoral, demulcent, tonic, expectorant and febrifuge; herb boiled in wine is used for hard tumours of spleen, and also contains an essential oil.

Hanuman phala, Lakshmanphal – *Annona cherimolia* Mill.; Cherimoya (E); Annonaceae; small tree. Cultivated for its edible fruit, eaten raw as a dessert fruit or made into squashes and milk shakes. Seeds are emetic and cathartic.

Hapusa (S) – *see* Mundi.

Harachampaka (S) – *see* Hari-champa.

Haranpadi, Hiranpadi, Prasarna; Bhadrabala (S) – *Convolvulus arvensis* L.; Deer's foot (E); Convolvulaceae; herb. Seeds contain a fixed oil. Roots are cathartic.

Harfarauri – *Cicca acida* (L.) Merr. [syn. *Phyllanthus acidus* (L.) Skeels.]; Stargoose-berry (E); Euphorbiaceae; small tree. Plant is cultivated for its edible fruits and leaves. Bark is the source of tannin. Roots and seeds are cathartic.

Hargoza – *see* Harkuch kanta.

Hari-champa; Harchampaka (S) – *Artabotrys uncinatus* (Lam.) Merr.; Climbing ylang-ylang (E); Annonaceae; scandent shrub. Flowers contain an essential oil which is used in perfumery; they are also used for the preparation of a tea-like stimulating beverage. Leaves reportedly possess contraceptive properties.

Haridra (S) – *see* Haldi.

Harin-harra; Rohituka (S) – *Aphanamixis polystachya* (Wall.) Parker; Sohaga (E); Meliaceae; tree. Wood is used for construction work, furniture, canoes, and cabinet work. Seeds are laxative and anthelmintic. Bark paste is used in rheumatism. Bark is reported to act as an immuno-suppressive drug with anti-cancer activity; it is also used as a remedy for liver and spleen disorders and tumours.

Haripriya (S) – *see* Peeli Kaner.

Harira – *Terminalia citrina* Roxb. ex Flem.; Combretaceae; tree found in the foothills of East India. Fruits are a rich source of tannin and are used in the same way as 'harra' or chebulic myrobalan. Bark is diuretic and cardiotonic; it also serves as the source of a dark blue dye. Wood is used for construction work.

Harita-manjari (S) – *see* Khokali.

Harjori – *see* Akanadi.

Harkuch; Hilamochi – *Enhydra fluctuans* Lour.; Compositae; herb. Leaves contain an essential oil, and are consumed as vegetable and salad. Leaves are considered to be antibilious, demulcent and laxative and are used in nervous and cutaneous disorders.

Harkuch kanta, Hargoza; Harkusa (S) – *Acanthus ilicifolius* L.; Sea holly (E); Acanthaceae; spinous herb. Leaves are used as an expectorant and for fomentation in neuralgia. Roots are used in asthma, leucorrhoea and paralysis.

Harkusa (S) – *see* Harkuch kanta.

Harmal, Gandhya, Lahouri-hurmul – *Peganum harmala* L.; Wild rue (E); Foreign henna (E); Zygophyllaceae; herb. Dried seeds contain several alkaloids and possess narcotic, antispasmodic, emetic and hypnotic properties; they are used to treat rheumatism, hysteria, gall-stones, colic and menstrual pain and fever. Seeds yield a red dye. Powdered roots mixed with oil are used to kill human lice. Recent reports indicate that the seeds act as protozoicidal and coronary dilators. Leaves are anthelmintic; their decoction is given in rheumatism.

Harra – *Terminalia chebula* Retz.; Chebulic myrobalan (E), Yellow myrobalan (E); Combretaceae; tree. Dried fruits are a rich source of tannin, other parts also contain tannin. They are used as stomachic, tonic and laxative and form an important constituent of an Ayurvedic preparation called 'Triphala'. Fruit pulp is used in dentifrices. Wood is used for construction work, carts and tool handles and the tree yields a gum. Fruit extract is used in oil-drilling preparations.

Harsankari – *see* Hadjora.

Harsinghar; Sephalika (S) – *Nyctanthes arbor-tristis* L.; Tree of sorrow (E); Coral jasmine (E); Nyctanthaceae; small tree. Flower pedicels yield an orange coloured dye which has been used for colouring silks and cotton since very ancient times in India. Flowers are also used to make garlands for worship and hair adornments. They yield an essential oil similar to jasmine. Seeds yield a fixed oil. Bark is a rich source of tannin. Leaves are used in the treatment of rheumatism and their decoction is used in sciatica; leaf-juice is anthelmintic and diuretic.

Hartho – *see* Ainta.

Hathajori, Bichu – *Martynia annua* L.; Tiger claw (E), Devil's claw (E); Martyniaceae; herb. Leaf juice is used as a gargle for sore-throat. Leaves are used in epilepsy. Fruits are used for reducing inflammation. Plant is used as a remedy against the sting of scorpions, and seeds yield a semi-drying oil.

Hathhathoria – *see* Nag-phani.

Hathhazori – *Blechnum orientale* L.; Blechnaceae; herb. Rhizomes are edible and are applied to boils in poultice form; they are also reported to be anthelmintic and are used for urinary disorders.

Hathichak, Hathichoke – *Cynara scolymus* L.; Burr artichoke (E), Globe artichoke (E); Compositae; perennial herb. Fleshy flower-head receptacles are a rich source of insulin, and considered to be useful in the diet of diabetics. Flower-heads are consumed as vegetable. Leaves are bitter, and are used in remedies for rheumatism and dropsy.

Hathichoke – *see* Hathichak, *see also* Hathichuk.

Hathichuk, Hathichoke – *Helianthus tuberosus* L.; Jerusalem artichoke (E); Compositae; undershrub. Cultivated for its edible, subterranean stem tubers. Tubers form the commercial source of laevulose, which is used as a sweetening agent for diabetics. They are consumed raw, boiled or made into flour; they are also preserved as chips and pickles. Crushed tubers are used for the manufacture of industrial alcohol. Stalks are pulped for the manufacture of paper. Green aerial parts are used as stock feed.

Hathi denkiya – *Pothos cathcarti* Schott.; Araceae; epiphytic climber on tree trunks. Leaves are consumed after frying in butter to get relief from body pain.

Hati-sunda – *see* Hati-sura.

Hati-sura, Hati-sunda; Bhurundi (S), Sri-hastini (S) – *Heliotropium indicum* L.; Boraginaceae; herb or undershrub. Leaves are applied locally to gum-boils, ulcers, and wounds. Leaf decoction is used in urticaria, and root decoction is administered in cough and fever. Leaves yield a dye.

Hattian – *see* Safed semul.

Haubera – *see* Abhal.

Haulia – *Phoebe lanceolata* (Nees) Nees; Lauraceae; tree. Wood is used for canoes. Leaves are lopped for fodder. Ash of berries is used for healing sores.

Hazar mani – *Phyllanthus urinaria* L.; Euphorbiaceae; herb. Plant is diuretic and is used in urino-genital disorders. Juice of leaves with coconut milk is used as an appetizer. Herb is often used as a substitute of 'jaramla' (*P. fraternus* Webster).

Hejurchei – *Leonotis nepetaefolia* (L.) Ait.; Labiatae; herb. Flower-head ashes are applied to burns, ringworm and itchy skin conditions. Leaves are used for rheumatism. Seeds are considered antimalarial, and are the source of a fatty oil.

Hemakanda – *Maerua oblongifolia* (Forsk) A Rich; Capparidaceae; large woody straggling shrub. Roots possess tonic and stimulant properties. Unripe fruits are consumed after boiling.

Henna – *see* Mehndi.

Hetenuria; Jhingi (S) – *Trichodesma zeylanicum* R. Br.; Boraginaceae; herb. Leaves are considered to be diuretic, and demulcent and are used for the preparation of a type of beer. Pulverized root is used as an analgesic on sores and wounds. Flowers are used in medicines to cure chest infections.

Hijjal, Ingar – *Barringtonia acutangula* Gaertn.; Barringtoniaceae; small tree. Seeds, bark and roots are used as fish poison. Powdered seeds are expectorant. Bark contains tannin. Tree is grown for its ornamental flowers. Fruit is astringent and is used in nasal catarrh; leaf juice is used for controlling diarrhoea. Wood is used for boats and cabinet work.

Hikka gadi – *see* Bamna.

Hila – *Garcinia cambogia* Desr. var. *cambogia*; Gamboge tree (E); Guttiferae; tree. Fruits very acidic, edible, and are also pickled. Dried rind of fruit is used as a condiment and its decoction is used in bowel disorders. Seeds yield an edible fat. Wood is good for match-stick industry. Bark yields a gum-resin which is used for varnish and in miniature paintings and water colours.

Himalcheri – *Antidesma bunius* (L.) Spreng.; Chinese laurel (E); Stilaginaceae; small tree. Fruits are edible, they are also made into preserves and wine. Leaves are also edible, and considered to be diaphoretic. Wood pulp is used for making cardboard and bark fibre for ropes.

Him champa – *see* Anda champa.

Himu, Kimu – *Morus serrata* Roxb.; Himalayan mulberry (E); Moraceae; tree. Fruit is edible. Wood is suitable for sports goods, toys, furniture, panelling and carving. Leaves are used for fodder; they are also used for feeding silkworms.

Hindichobchini – *Smilax lanceifolia* Roxb.; Smilacaceae; climber. The strained juice of tuberous root is given in rheumatic pain and the leftover residue is used on painful joints in the form of poultice.

Hindi-sana, Sena, Senai; Bhumiari (S) – *Cassia angustifolia* Vahl.; Indian senna (E); Caesalpiniaceae; small shrub. Fruits and leaves are used as purgative, laxative and vermifuge..

Hing; Hingu (S), Balhika (S) – *Ferula assafoetida* L.; Asafetida (E); Umbelliferae; perennial herb. Tap roots exude a gum-resin when incised which is used for flavouring food. It is considered to be antispasmodic, laxative and expectorant and is used in medicine for flatulent colic, whooping cough, bronchitis in children and asthma. Gum-resin is also the source of an essential oil called oleum asae-foetidae. Another species *F. narthex* also yields an oleo-gum-resin with similar uses and is known by the same Hindi name.

Hingan, Hingot; Ingudi (S) – *Balanites aegyptiaca* (L.) Delile; Balanites (E); Balanitaceae; small spiny tree. Ripe fruits are used for treating skin troubles and whooping cough. Seeds are rich in a fixed oil and protein, and are used in colic and whooping cough; seed extract is hypotensive. Seeds serve as raw material for steroid industry; and the steroid sapogenine is used in oral contraceptives and steroid drugs.

Hingot – *see* Hingan.

Hingu – *see* Hing.

Hinsalu – *see* Anchhu.

Hiradukhi – *see* Aprang.

Hirankhuri – *Emilia sonchifolia* (L.) DC.; Compositae; herb. Leaves are edible; their decoction is used in bowel disorders. Juice of leaves is used for giving relief to sore-eyes.

Hiranpadi – *see* Haranpadi.

Hirantutiya, Surinjan; Hiranyatutha (S) – *Colchicum luteum* Baker; Golden collyrium (E); Liliaceae; perennial herb. Corms are used in rheumatism, gout, and liver- and spleen disorders. Dried corms contain a high content of colchicine.

Hiranyatutha (S) – *see* Hirantutiya.

Hirik – *Sterculia guttata* Roxb.; Sterculiaceae; tree. Seed is edible in roasted form. Bark fibre is used for cordage. Gum exuded from the plant is used similar to gum-tragacanth.

Hirruseeah, Mahabi – *Euphorbia helioscopia* L.; Sun spurge (E); Euphorbiaceae; herb. Roots are anthelmintic. Juice of plant is prescribed to treat rheumatism, neuralgia, and warts, while the latex is used as a fish poison. Seeds are used in cholera, they also yield a drying oil, which is used as a purgative.

Hisalu – *Rubus lanatus* Wall.; Rosaceae; shrub. Fruits are of inferior quality but are edible.

Hol – *see* Vilayati gawuth.

Hribera – *see* Sugandha-bala.

Hukakanda – *Platanthera susannae* (L.) Lindl; Orchidaceae; herb. Tubers are used as a cure for bullae or blebs occurring on palms.

Holak – *Terminalia myriocarpa* Heurck & Muell.-Arg.; Hollock (E); Combretaceae; tree found in E. Himalayas. Wood is used for construction work, furniture, packing boxes, trucks and heavy vehicle bodies and the wood pulp is used for paper manufacture. Wood is also used for the manufacture of plywood and match boxes. Bark yields tannin and is used medicinally as a diuretic and cardiac stimulant.

Hulhul, Hurhur; Adityabhakta (S), Arkakanta (S) – *Cleome viscosa* L.; Sticky Cleome (E); Capparidaceae; pubescent herb. Seeds are anthelmintic and carminative, they are also used as a condiment; poultice of the seeds is used on painful joints.

Hulul, Gandhuli; Arkapushpika (S) – *Gynandropsis gynandra* (L.) Brig.; Capparidaceae; pubescent glandular herb. Leaves are used for flavouring curries and sauces. Bruised leaves are used on rheumatic joints and for headache and other localized pains. Seeds are anthelmintic and yield a semi-drying oil; they are also used as a fish poison.

Hunraj – *see* Bannalia.

Hurhur – *see* Hulhul.

Hurna – *Sapium indicum* Willd.; Euphorbiaceae; evergreen tree. Leaves are the source of a greenish yellow dye used for dyeing fabrics. Root-bark decoction is emetic; it is also used in insanity and hydrophobia. Fruits possess a toxic principle called aesculetin which is used as a fish poison.

Hyamaraka (S) – *see* Indrajau.

I

Ijjul; Samudraphala (S) – *Barringtonia racemosa* (L.) Spreng.; Barringtoniaceae; small tree. Fruits are used in cough and asthma and kernels are given with milk for treating jaundice and bile disorders. Bark is the source of tannin and is also used as a fish-poison.

Ikshu (S) – *see* Ganna.

Ikshugandha (S) – *see* Gokhru.

Illarbillar – *see* Parwatti.

Imli, Amli; Amlika (S) – *Tamarindus indica* L.; Tamarind tree (E); Caesalpiniaceae; tree. Cultivated as an avenue tree. Fruit pulp is used extensively in chutneys, curries and sauces. It contains large amounts of tartaric acid along with some citric- and lactic acids and finds use in foods, pharmaceutical industry, dyeing, tanning and polishing of metal-ware. Fruit-pulp and infusion of leaves is used in indigenous medicine as a carminative, laxative and in bilious disorders. Tamarind kernel powder is the source of jellose, which is used as a substitute for fruit pectins in the preservation of fruits in the form of marmalades and jellies. Its usage extends to textile industry as a sizing agent and in rubber industry as a creaming agent for concentration of the latex. Wood is used for turnery, tool handles, tent-pegs, furniture, panelling and printing blocks.

Idhana (S) – *see* Vilayati afsanthin.

Indrajau, Mitha-indrajau; Hyamaraka (S) – *Wrightia tinctoria* R. Br.; Sweet indrajao (E), Pala indigo plant (E); Apocynaceae; tree. Wood is used for turnery, carving, match-stick industry, printing blocks, toys, bobbins and stained-wood inlay-work. Wood pulp is good for the manufacture of wrapping paper. Flowers and fruits are the source of a blue dye. Seeds and bark are used in bilious disorders and flatulence. Fresh raw fruit juice and fresh latex are proteolytic and are used to curdle milk. Seeds yield a semi-drying oil. Tender leaves, flowers and young fruits are eaten.

Indrayan, Makal; Mahendravaruni (S) – *Citrullus colocynthis* (L.) Kuntz.; Bitter apple (E), Cucurbitaceae; perennial trailing herb. Fruits are used as a purgative; fruit pulp is reported to be bactericidal. Roots are used as a remedy for jaundice, urinary disorders, and rheumatism. Seeds yield a fixed oil.

Ingar – *see* Hijjal.

Ingudi (S) – *see* Hingan.

Irsia – *see* Sosun.

Isfanaj – *see* Palak.

Ishadgola (S) – *see* Isubgol.

Isharmul; Ishvarimul (S) – *Aristolochia indica* L.; Indian birthwort (E); Aristolochiaceae; shrubby twiner. Dried roots and stems contain the drug which is used in low concentration as a gastric stimulant and tonic; they are also used for menstrual regulation and for curing fever. The drug is reported to contain aristolochic acid as the active principle. Leaf juice is expectorant, and used for getting rid of cough. Seeds are used for biliousness and inflammation.

Ishvarimul (S) – *see* Isharmul.

Isubgol; Ishadgola (S) – *Plantago ovata* Forsk.; Blonde psyllium (E); Plantaginaceae; herb. Cultivated for its seeds and seed husk. Seeds are used in the preparation of medicines used for kidney, bladder and urethra disorders. Crushed seed poultice is used for rheumatism and glandular swellings. Seed-husk is highly esteemed and a rich source of mucilage and fibre, which is used in chronic constipation, diarrhoea, dysentery and inflammatory conditions of intestines and urinary tract. Seed mucilage is used in the preparation of cosmetics, ice-creams and chocolates. Husk is also used as a binder in compressed tablets.

Iswara (S) – *see* Kotagandhal.

J

Jadwar, Nirbisi; Apavish (S) – *Delphinium denudatum* Wall.; Ranunculaceae; herb. Roots are used as a tonic, in toothaches and to adulterate aconite. Seeds are the source of many alkaloids; they are also used in the treatment of itch and skin eruptions and for making insecticidal preparations.

Jafran – *see* Kesar.

Jahrphali – *see* Khewnau.

Jaie, Javi – *Avena sativa* L.; Oat (E); Gramineae; herb. Cultivated to a limited extent only. Grain is rich in protein, but lacks gluten and fat. Oatmeal is used for the preparation of breakfast foods, biscuits and cakes. Grain hulls serve as a rich source of furfural, an industrial solvent.

Jainti, Balmota; Jayantika (S) – *Sesbania sesban* (L.) Merr.; Egyptian rattle pod (E); Papilionaceae; large shrub or small tree. The plant is cultivated as a live support and wind-break for pepper, betel and grape vines and to provide shade to turmeric, coffee, tea, sweet orange and cotton plantations. Tender shoots are lopped for fodder. Wood is used for making toys; bark is source of a fibre for ropes. Seeds are used in ointments for skin ailments and for treating diarrhoea and spleen enlargement.

Jaiphal, Javitri; Jatiphala (S) – *Myristica fragrans* Houtt.; Nutmeg tree (E); Myristicaceae; tree. Fruit is the source of two important spices viz., nutmeg and mace. Kernel is the 'jaiphal' or nutmeg of commerce and its dried fibrous aril constitutes the 'javitri' or mace. Both contain an essential oil and are used for flavouring foods, cosmetics and soaps. Fat from the kernel is used as a stimulant in various ointments for rheumatism, paralysis and sprains. Pericarp is used for making jellies and pickles; nutmeg oil is carminative, stimulant and astringent and is used for stomach ache, vomiting, and dysentery. Leaves also yield an essential oil which is used for flavouring essences and in the preparation of chewing-gum.

Jaitoon – *see* Zaitoon.

Jalapapili – *Phyla nodiflora* (L.) Greene; (syn. *Lippia nodiflora* Rich.); Verbenaceae; herb. The plant is used as a febrifuge and diuretic. Fresh plant paste is used for curing swollen cervical glands, ulcers, erysiphales infections and boils.

Jalaphala – *see* Singhara.

Jalapippali (S) – *see* Jalpipari.

Jaldhania; Kandir (S) – *Ranunculus sceleratus* L.; Blister butter cup (E); Celery-leaved crowfoot (E); Ranunculaceae; herb. Leaf-juice is used in asthma, gripe, pneumonia, rheumatism and sciatica. Seeds are used in kidney trouble. Protonemonin present in the plant is responsible for causing blisters.

Jalkhumbi, Takapana; Kumbhika (S) – *Pistia stratiotes* L. var. *cuneata* Engl.; Water lettuce (E); Tropical duckweed (E); Araceae; herb. Plant is aquatic, and forms an excellent source of fish-food. Leaves are rich in vitamins A, B and C. Ash is rich in potash and plants are used as manure. Leaves are used to treat eczema, skin ailments, ulcers, leprosy and piles, and the plant ash for curing ringworm.

Jallil, Sawala, Syala – *Vallisneria spiralis* L.; Eel grass (E), Hydrocharitaceae; herb. Aquatic submerged plant considered to be a good oxygenator for fish. It is also considered to be stomachic, demulcent and cooling and is used to treat leucorrhoea.

Jallur – *see* Maljhan.

Jalnimba – *see* Neer-brahmi.

Jalpai – *Elaeocarpus serratus* L.; Çeylon olive (E); Elaeocarpaceae; tree. Fruits are either eaten in curries or pickled. Wood is suitable for match-boxes. Fruits are used in diarrhoea and dysentery. Leaves are used as an antidote to poisoning and in combating rheumatism.

Jalpipari, Jalapippali (S) – *Commelina salicifolia* Roxb. Commelinaceae; herb. The plant is used as a remedy for dysentery; it is also used as a cattle-feed.

Jalsamoka (S) – *see* Samak.

Jamalgota; Jayaphala (S) – *Croton tiglium* L.; Purging croton (E); Euphorbiaceae; shrub or small tree. Seeds and seed oil act as a strong purgative and vesicant. Seeds are also used to stupefy fish.

Jaman, Jamun – *Syzygium cumini* (L.) Skeels; Jambolan (E), Java plum (E); Myrtaceae; large tree. Ripe fruits edible, they are also made into preserves, vinegar and wine. Wood is used for construction work, packing boxes, agricultural implements, tool handles, and various other purposes. Leaves are lopped for fodder, and are also used to feed 'tassar' silkworms. Bark is used for tanning and its decoction is used for gargles and mouthwash. Infusion of seed powder and bark is administered in diabetes.

Jambira – *see* Bara-nibu.

Jambu, Suria; Kanakakuli (S) – *Xylia xylocarpa* (Roxb.) Taub.; Pyinkado (E); Mimosaceae; tree. Wood yields valuable timber and is considered to be a good substitute for 'sal' and teak. Wood pulp is suitable for wrapping paper. Wood yields good quality charcoal. Decoction of bark is vermifuge, and is used to check vomiting and diarrhoea. Fruits are the source of a fatty oil. Ripe fruits and seeds are edible.

Jamoah – *Eugenia cuspidata* Berg.; Myrtaceae; tree. Cultivated as an avenue tree.

Jamphal – *see* Amrud.

Jamrassi, Chouri, Dhebri – *Elaeodendron glaucum* Pers.; Celastraceae; tree. Cultivated as an ornamental. Wood is used for cabinet work. Tree yields a gum called 'jamrassi'. Bark and leaves are rich in tannin. Powdered roots are used as a fumigatory.

Jamrul, Amrool – *Syzygium samarangense* (Bl.) Merr. & Perry; Samarang rose-apple (E); Myrtaceae; tree. Wood is used for building huts and fruits are edible.

Jamti-ki-bel; Patalagarudi – *Cocculus hirsutus* (L.) Diels.; Menispermaceae; climbing shrub. Roots are demulcent and laxative, and are used in bilious dyspepsia, venereal diseases and chronic rheumatism. Extract of roots and stems is spasmolytic and is used as a sedative, cardiotonic and hypotensive. Mucilaginous juice of leaves is applied topically to treat eczema.

Jamun – *see* Jaman.

Jand – *see* Chaunkra.

Jangal jalebi, Vilayati imli – *Pithecellobium dulce* (Roxb.) Benth.; (syn. *Inga dulcis* Willd.); Manila tamarind (E); Mimosaceae; tree. Cultivated for prickly hedges, and for fuel as it is a quick-growing plant. Seeds are edible with a sweet aril. Mature seeds yield a fatty oil which is used in soap manufacture and for edible purposes. Oil cake is used as a stock-feed. Leaves and pods are used as fodder.

Jangli adrak, Banada; Vanardraka (S) – *Zingiber cassumunar* Roxb.; Cassumunar ginger; Zingiberaceae; perennial herb. Rhizomes act as a carminative and stimulant and are used in colic and diarrhoea; they are the source of an essential oil which is used in the preparation of artificial pepper, rose and geranium oils and flavours.

Jangli akhrot; Aksota (S) – *Aleurites moluccana* (L.) Willd.; Candle nut tree (E); Euphorbiaceae; evergreen tree. Seeds yield a drying oil which makes a water-proof hard film highly resistant to acids and alkalies, and is much in demand for paints, varnishes and soap manufacture. Wood pulp is considered to be good for the manufacture of paper and the wood for match-sticks. Seed-oil is purgative. Bark is the source of tannin.

Jangli am – *see* Amara.

Jangli amli – *see* Jaramla.

Jangli angoor – *Ampelocissus arnottiana* (Wight & Arn) Planch; Vitidaceae; climbing shrub. Juice of roots is diuretic and depurative, and is used for eye trouble and ulcers.

Jangli arand – *see* Bagbherenda.

Jangli aushbah, Ram-dataun – *Smilax zeylanica* L.; Smilacaceae; shrub. Roots are used to combat dysentery, urinary disorders and rheumatism; they are also used as a substitute for 'anantamul' or Indian sarsaparilla (*Hemidesmus indicus*). Tender shoots are used as vegetable.

Jangli badam – *Sterculia foetida* L.; Wild almond (E); Sterculiaceae; tree. Seeds called Java olives are edible after roasting; they are the source of a fatty oil which is used as a laxative, illuminant and for soap manufacture.

Jangli bhendi, Bankapas – *Azanza lampas* (Cav.) Alef.; Malvaceae; small shrub. Young stems are the source of a fibre used for ropes, cordage and fishing-nets. Flowers yield a dye, and floral parts are used for skin ailments. Seeds are rich in a fatty oil. Roots are used for the treatment of syphilis and gonorrhoea.

Jangli chachinda, Rambel; Kasht-bhanjan (S) - *Trichosanthes cucumerina* L.; Cucurbitaceae; trailing herb. Cultivated for its fruits used as vegetable. Seeds are anti-febrile and anthelmintic. Roots are used in bronchitis and also applied locally for boils. Leaf juice is prescribed for hair regrowth on bald patches, and in biliousness.

Jangli chaulai; Tanduliya (S), Vishagna (S) – *Amaranthus viridis* L.; Wild amaranth (E); Amaranthaceae; herb. Tender shoots and leaves are used as pot-herb. Plant is used as fodder for cattle.

Janglidal; Aranya-dhanya (S) – *Hygroryza aristata* (Retz.) Nees ex Wight & Arn.; Gramineae; floating grass in slow-moving streams or lakes. Plants make good fodder. Grains are sweet, digestible, and used in biliousness.

Jangli dalchini – *Cinnamomum iners* Reinw.; Lauraceae; tree. Bark contains an essential oil which is used for cough and dysentery in children. Wood is used for furniture.

Jangli dhan – *Leersia hexandra* Sw.; Rice grass (E). Gramineae; aquatic perennial grass. Plant is used as fodder, both fresh and as hay.

Jangli dungy – *Tetrameles nudiflora* R. Br.; Baing tree (E), Maina tree (E); Tetramelaceae; large buttressed tree. Wood is coarse but soft and is used for canoes, packing cases, match-sticks and plywood. Decoction of bark is reported to be used as a remedy for jaundice, dropsy and rheumatism.

Jangli-erandi – *see* Undarbibi.

Jangli frast – *see* Safed frast.

Jangli haldi; Vana-haridra (S) – *Curcuma aromatica* Salisb.; Wild turmeric (E), Yellow zedoary (E); Zingiberaceae; perennial herb. Cultivated for its rhizomes which are rich in an essential oil with camphor-like odour and are used medicinally as a tonic, carminative and in ointments for sprains. They are also used in cosmetics and as a dye.

Jangli jamalgota – *see* Danti.

Jangli jhan – *see* Jangli saru.

Jangli kalimirch, Kanj; Dahana (S) – *Toddalia asiatica* (L.) Lam; Wild orange-tree (E); Forest-pepper (E); Rutaceae; shrub. Fruits edible, acrid, and are also pickled; fresh root bark infusion acts as a tonic and carminative and is used for controlling diarrhoea. Root bark also yields a yellow dye. Fresh leaves contain an essential oil and are prescribed for bowel-pain.

Jangli karela, Golkandra; Vahisi (S) – *Momordica dioica* Roxb. ex Willd.; Small bitter-gourd (E); Cucurbitaceae; spreading or climbing shrub. Fruits are used as vegetable. Semi-drying oil obtained from the kernels is used in paints and varnishes. Snuff of powdered dry fruits stimulates copious flow of mucous discharge from nostrils. Roots are used for treating urinary disorders, and bleeding piles.

Jangli khajur, Khajeria, Thakal – *Phoenix acaulis* Roxb. ex Buch.-Ham.; Palmae; Stemless palm. Terminal leaf buds are used as vegetable. Fruits and young peduncles are edible. Pith yields starch for sago. Leaves are used for thatching, and for making mats, ropes and brooms.

Jangli madan-mast-ka-phul; Varaguna (S) – *Cycas circinalis* L.; Fern palm (E); Cycadaceae; palm-like short tree. Cultivated in gardens as an ornamental for its beautiful evergreen foliage. Pith and cortex yield starch for sago. Seeds also yield an edible starch, which can be used only after removal of the toxic principles.

Jangli matar – *Lathyrus aphaca* L.; Yellow vetchling (E); Papilionaceae; trailing herb. Plant is used as fodder. Ripe seeds are narcotic in effect.

Jangli methi – *Indigofera trifoliata* L.; Papilionaceae; herb. Seeds are astringent and aphrodisiac, and are used for combating leucorrhoea and rheumatism.

Jangli nimbu; Atavi jambira (S) – *Atalantia malabarica* (Rafin) Tanaka (syn. *A. monophylla* Correa); Wild lime (E); Rutaceae; small spinous ornamental tree. Wood is used for cabinet work. Fruits yield a medicinal oil which is applied topically to painful rheumatic joints.

Jangli palak – *see* Ambavah.

Jangli pikvam – *see* Antamul.

Jangli piyaz – *see* Ban piyazi.

Jangli pudina – *Mentha longifolia* (L.) Huds.; Horsemint (E); Labiatae; perennial herb. Leaves are consumed in the form of chutney or dry powder for flavouring. They are a rich source of an essential oil which is considered as a stimulant, carminative and antiseptic. *M. longifolia* (L.) Huds. var. *incana* Willd. is considered to be an astringent, and is used for treating rheumatic pain.

Jangli sarson – *see* Khubkalan.

Jangli saru, Jangli jhau – *Casuarina equisetifolia* L.; Beefwood (E), Casuarina (E); Casuarinaceae; tree. Cultivated for fuel and for other purposes. Growth of the plant is rapid. Tree yields a resin and its bark is astringent and used in diarrhoea and dysentery; it is also used for tanning and dyeing. Leaf decoction is used in colic and the thin needle leaves are used for making activated carbon.

Jangli sawuk, Sawank – *Echinochloa colona* (L.) Link.; Shama millet (E); Gramineae; herb. Cultivated for fodder. Grains are edible.

Jangli seb, Gwalam, Patol – *Malus baccata* (L.) Borkh.; Siberian crab apple (E); Rosaceae; small tree. Cultivated for the supply of rooted cuttings to serve as a hardy stock for grafting superior apple varieties. Fruits are used as vegetable or as a preserve.

Jangli selai – *Licuala spinosa* Wurmb.; Palmae; densely tufted palm. Cultivated as an ornamental. Leaves are used for thatching, and the bark for treating tuberculosis.

Jangli toot – *Broussonetia papyrifera* Vent.; Paper mulberry (E); Moraceae; small tree. Bark yields a strong lustrous fibre which is used for making paper lanterns, writing paper, tapa-cloth and umbrellas. Wood is good for rayon-grade pulp, writing paper and news-print paper.

Japani pudina – *Mentha arvensis* L. var. *piperascens* Holmes; Japanese pepper mint (E); Labiatae; perennial herb. Cultivated for its leaves rich in an essential oil which is the chief source of menthol, used for treating colds. The oil is used as a substitute for true peppermint oil obtained from Vilayati pudina (*M. piperita*).

Jaramla, Jangli amli; Bhumyamalaki (S) – *Phyllanthus fraternus* Webster; Euphorbiaceae; herb. Plant acts as an astringent, diuretic and febrifuge and is used for diarrhoea, dysentery, colic, indigestion, dropsy and urinogenital complaints. Fresh roots are used in jaundice. Decoction of stems and leaves yields a black dye used for dyeing cotton cloth.

Jarayupriya (S), Makshikavisha (S) – *Erigeron canadensis* L.; Canada fleabane (E); Compositae; herb. Plant is an astringent, diuretic and stimulant and is used in diarrhoea, dysentery, kidney trouble, dropsy, uterine haemorrhage, ringworm and eczema. Dry plants on steam distillation yield the oil of fleabane which is used in medicine.

Jargadi (S) – *see* Sankru.

Jargi – *Chloris inflata* Link.; Gramineae; herb. The plant is regarded as one of the drought resistant alkali tolerant grasses. It makes good fodder before flowering.

Jari; Kaninika (S) – *Ficus tsiela* Roxb.; Moraceae; tree. Wood is used for making furniture. Leaves are lopped for fodder. Bark is used as a remedy for colic.

Jarul – *Lagerstroemia speciosa* Pers.; Queen crape-myrtle (E); Lythraceae; tree. Cultivated as an ornamental avenue tree. It is the source of 'jarul', a timber of commercial importance which is used for bridges, ships, boats, railway carriages, sleepers, and interior fittings. Wood-pulp yields good quality paper. Fruits and leaves are a rich source of tannin.

Jasum – *see* Gurhal.

Jasund – *see* Chandal.

Jatamansi, Bal-chir; Maamsi (S), Lomasaa (S) – *Nardostachys jatamansi* (D. Don) DC.; Spikenard (E); Valerianaceae; perennial herb. Rhizomes yield an essential oil known as spikenard oil, which acts as an hypotensive and depressant to central nervous system in moderate doses. Infusion of rhizomes is used in hysteria, palpitation of heart, and leprosy. Tincture of rhizomes is prescribed in epilepsy and convulsions. Spikenard oil is also used to improve hair-growth and darken the colour of hair.

Jatiphala (S) – *see* Jaiphal.

Jau, Jav; Java (S), Yava (S) – *Hordeum vulgare* (L.) emend. Bowden.; Barley (E); Gramineae; annual herb. Cultivated for its grain which is used like wheat for flour, parched grains, and for malting and brewing industry specially for the preparation of beer. Malt is also used for making malted milk, infant foods, candy and some pharmaceutical preparations. Barley water is used as a diuretic. The culms are used for fodder.

Jav – *see* Jau.

Java (S) – *see* Jau.

Java kusum – *see* Gurhal.

Java-ki-rani – *Cassia javanica* L.; Java Cassia (E); Caesalpiniaceae; small tree. Cultivated as an ornamental tree for its beautiful pink flowers.

Javi – *see* Jaie.

Javitri – *see* Jaiphal.

Jawasa, Bharbharra – *Alhagi pseudalhagi* (Bieb.) Desv.; Camel thorn (E), Persian manna plant (E); Papilionaceae; spiny shrub. Plant is expectorant, antibilious, diuretic, antiseptic and laxative. The decoction of twigs is used for cough and root decoction for inflammation and abscesses. A sugary exudation from it called 'taranjabin' is used as a laxative, expectorant and anti-emetic. Oil from the leaves is used for painful rheumatic joints. Leaves and shoots are used as camel fodder.

Jayanti (S) – *see* Dhaincha.

Jayantika (S) – *see* Jainti.

Jayaphala (S) – *see* Jamalgota.

Jhak – *see* Chhota pilu.

Jhal – *see* Bara pilu.

Jhamo, Khip – *Crotalaria burhia* Buch-Ham. ex Benth.; Papilionaceae; xerophytic undershrub. Stem is the source of a fibre used for ropes. Plant is used as fodder for camels.

Jhangi – *see* Kureli.

Jharberi, Bhukamtaka (S), Sukshamaphala (S) – *Ziziphus nummularia* (Burm. f.) Wight & Arn.; Wild jujube (E); Rhamnaceae; spiny shrub. Fruits are edible. Plants are cultivated for shelter belts and wind-breaks. Bark is used for tanning and leaves for curing scabies. Root bark contains nummularine alkaloids. Wood is used for making high quality charcoal.

Jhari-haldi; Daru haridra (S) – *Coscinium fenestratum* (Gaertn.) Colebr.; False calumba (E), Tree turmeric (E); Menispermaceae; climbing shrub. Stems yield a yellow dye called false calumba and are used as a substitute for 'kalam-ki-jar' or calumba a drug obtained from the roots of *Jateorhiza palmata*. The dye is used medicinally for dressing ulcers and wounds, and the stems are used for treating indigestion and general debility.

Jhar fanoos – *Kigelia pinnata* DC.; Sausage tree (E); Bignoniaceae; large tree with dense spreading crown. Cultivated as a shade tree on road sides and in parks. Fruits are woody, brown and hang down from long and sturdy cord-like stalks. Bark is used in indigenous medicine for treating venereal diseases, dysentery and rheumatism.

Jhau, Jhav; Jhavuka (S); Shavaka (S) – *Tamarix troupii* Hole; French tamarisk (E); Tamaricaceae; bushy shrub to small tree. Cultivated as an ornamental. Galls formed on the branches called 'bari-main' are considered astringent, and are used for diarrhoea, dysentery, gargles for sore throat, and piles. Galls are also used for tanning and give a nice yellow colour. Wood is suitable for agricultural implements. *Tamarix ericoides* a shrub occurring in riverbeds of S. India and *T. dioica*, a small tree distributed throughout India in river-beds and sea-coasts are also known by the same Hindi name.

Jhav – *see* Jhau.

Jhavuka (S) – *see* Jhau.

Jhingan, Kaimil, Mohin – *Lannea coromandelica* (Houtt.) Merr; Anacardiaceae; tree. Wood is used for multipurposes, it is also used for carving, bobbins, pencils and plywood. Wood pulp is used for paper. Stem is tapped for 'jhingan' gum which is used in confectionery, sizing of cloth, calico printing and ink manufacture. Bark is astringent and is used for dyeing and printing cloth.

Jhinga Tori – *see* Kali tori.

Jhingi (S) – *see* Hetenuria.

Jhinjharita (S) – *see* Chikti.

Jhinti, Katsareya; Karunta (S) – *Barleria prionitis* L.; Acanthaceae; shrub. Roots are febrifuge, and root paste is used to cure boils and glandular swellings. Leaves are chewed to relieve toothache, and leaf juice mixed with honey is used for catarrhal disorders.

Juhighas – *Alysicarpus monilifer* DC.; Papilionaceae; prostrate herb. Plant is used as fodder.

Jhumko lata – *Passiflora edulis* Sims; Passion fruit (E), Purple granadilla (E); Passifloraceae; shrubby climber. Fruits are edible and made into cordials, syrups, squashes, jellies, juice concentrates and powders. Peels are rich in pectin. Seeds yield a semi-drying oil which is used in paints and varnishes. Seed cake is used both as a manure and stock-feed.

Jhunjhunia – *Crotalaria spectabilis* Roth; Papilionaceae; undershrub. Cultivated for green manure. Stems are the source of a fibre. Plant is used in scabies.

Jhunjhuni-ankari – *see* Mumuna.

Jhusa – *Eragrostis plumosa* Link.; Gramineae; small grass. The plants are used for fodder.

Jiaputa – *see* Putranjiva.

Jiban – *see* Gio.

Jilpai – *see* Kotagandhal.

Jima; Phanija (S), Grishma-sundaraka (S) – *Mollugo oppositifolia* L.; Molluginaceae; herb. Plant is considered to be antiseptic and stomachic. It is used for skin ailments and mixed with castor oil, for curing earache.

Jira, Zeera, Jiraka (S) – *Cuminum cyminum* L.; Cumin (E); Umbelliferae; herb. Cultivated for its aromatic fruits and used as a condiment either alone or mixed with other spices. Essential oil from the fruits is used in perfumery and for flavouring beverages. Fruits are used in medicine for combating diarrhoea and indigestion.

Jiraka (S) – *see* Jira.

Jiti, Chiti, Tongus – *Marsdenia tenacissima* (Roxb.) Moon; Rajmahal hemp (E); Asclepiadaceae; climbing shrub. Stems yield a very strong fibre used for making fishing lines and bowstrings. Roots yield the drug 'safed nisoth' or white turpeth which is used as a purgative in indigenous medicine. The latex mixed with latex of other plants is used to produce rubber.

Jivanti (S) – *see* Gio.

Jivantika (S) – *see* Budu.

Joar, Jowar – *Sorghum vulgare* Pers.; Sorghum (E); Gramineae; tall herb. Cultivated for its grain used as food and the culms used as fodder. Grain is the source of starch and malt which are used in malting and fermentation industry for the production of industrial alcohol and acetone.

Jonkhmari – *Anagallis arvensis* L.; Scarlet pimpernel (E); Primulaceae; herb. Plant is diaphoretic, expectorant and stimulant and is used for the treatment of dropsy, leprosy and some cerebral disorders. It is also used to expel leeches from the nostrils of cattle, and intoxicate fish.

Jowar – *see* Joar.

Jub-palum – *Rumex maritimus* L.; Golden dock (E); Polygonaceae; herb. Roots and leaves are cathartic, and are also applied to burns. Plant is used as pot-herb.

Juhi, Jui; Juthika (S), Mugdhee (S) – *Jasminum auriculatum* Vahl; Oleaceae; Bushy climbing shrub. Cultivated for its very delicate, beautiful and aromatic flowers which are rich in an essential oil and are used in perfumery.

Jui – *see* Juhi.

Jukutam (S) – *see* Baigan.

Jungi – *Millettia racemosa* Benth.; Papilionaceae; small tree. Roots are used to kill maggots in cattle wounds, and are also used as a fish-poison. Leaves are lopped for fodder.

Juthika (S) – *see* Juhi.

Jutuk, Utran, Sadovani; Uttaravaruni (S) – *Pergularia daemia* (Forsk.) Chiov.; Asclepiadaceae; twiner. Leaves and flowers are eaten. Leaf-juice is administered for infantile diarrhoea and mixed with lime is used for inflamed rheumatic joints. Leaf-decoction is used for asthma. Plant extract is used for curing menstrual and uterine disorders.

Juvashur – *Opopanax chironium* Koch.; Opopanax (E). Umbelliferae; herb. Gum-resin called 'javashur' or opopanax, obtained from the dried milky-juice exuded after roots are incised is used in perfumery. It is also accredited with stimulant, antiseptic and antispasmodic properties.

Jyotishka – *see* Bhadradanti.

Jyotishmati – *see* Malkangni.

K

Kaangi (S) – *see* Ghenchu.

Kaasmari (S) – *see* Gambhar.

Kabab-chini, Sheetal-chini – *Piper cubeba* L.f.; Cubeb (E), Tailed pepper (E); Piperaceae; climbing shrub. Fruits called cubebs, are used as a spice, condiment, and in perfumery. They are also considered as diuretic, carminative, stimulant and sedative, and are used for bronchial troubles, gonorrhoea and rheumatism. Oil of cubebs is used as a condiment, as a flavouring for lozenges and in urinary disorders.

Kabra – *Capparis spinosa* L.; Caper-bush (E); Capparidaceae; small prostrate shrub. Flower buds known as capers, are used for treating scurvy. Bark is used for combating rheumatism, paralysis and tubercular glands; it is also considered to be a tonic and diuretic. Seeds yield a fatty oil.

Kachalu – *see* Arvi.

Kachha-shimbi – *Menyanthes trifoliata* L.; Buck bean (E), Bog bean (E); Menyanthaceae; perennial aquatic herb. Plant is considered as emetic, cathartic, tonic and diaphoretic; it is used medicinally in remedies for gout, rheumatism, dropsy and skin ailments. Leaves contain ascorbic acid and an alkaloid gentianine.

Kachlora; Aragvadha (S) – *Pithecellobium monadelphum* Kosterm.; Mimosaceae; tree. Decoction of leaves is used for treating leprosy and for promoting hair growth. Seeds contain pithecolobine and their decoction is prescribed in diabetes mellitus; wood is suitable for match-industry.

Kachnal, Ashta; Svetkanchagna (S) – *Bauhinia racemosa* Lamk.; Caesalpiniaceae; small tree. Bark is astringent, and is used in dysentery; it also yields strong cordage fibre. Flower buds are edible. Leaves are anthelmintic, and are used for treating diarrhoea.

Kachnar – *Bauhinia variegata* L.; Variegated Bauhinia (E), Mountain ebony (E); Caesalpiniaceae; small tree. Cultivated as an ornamental for its beautiful flowers. Flower-buds are used as vegetable. Roots are carminative. Bark is used for dyeing and tanning; it also yields a fibre. It is used medicinally for curing sore throat, bad breath, cutaneous ailments, boils and ulcers.

Kachri, Phoont – *Cucumis melo* L. var. *momordica* Duth. & Full.; Snap melon (E); Cucurbitaceae; trailing herb. Cultivated for its edible fruits, which are consumed fresh when ripe.

Kachu (S) – *see* Arvi.

Kachur, Kasis – *Cornus macrophylla* Wall.; Cornaceae; tree. Wood is used for bobbins, pulleys, shuttles and for gunpowder charcoal. Fruits are edible.

Kachura; Sati (S), Karchura (S) – *Curcuma zedoaria* (Berg.) Rose; Zedoary (E); Zingiberaceae; perennial herb. Cultivated for its bitter rhizomes which are used as a stimulant, carminative and stomachic, and serve as the source of an essential oil which is used in cosmetics and perfumery. Rhizomes are also the source of 'shoti' starch and zedoary which is used as a condiment.

Kadali (S) – *see* Kela.

Kadamb; Kadamba (S) – *Anthocephalus cadamba* (Roxb.) Miq.; Kadam (E); Naucleaceae; moderate sized deciduous tree. Cultivated as an ornamental for its beautiful foliage and fragrant globose flower-heads, used for making garlands. Flowers yield an essential oil, and flower receptacle is edible. Wood is used for packing-cases and light construction work. Wood-pulp is suitable for making cheap-quality paper.

Kadamba (S) – *see* Kadamb.

Kadavanchi – *Momordica tuberosa* (Roxb.) Cogn.; Cucurbitaceae; trailing herb. Tender fruits are used as vegetable. Roots are considered to be abortifacient.

Kaddu, Kansiphal, Sitaphal, Lal kumra – *Cucurbita maxima* Duch.; Red-pumpkin (E), Winter squash (E); Cucurbitaceae; trailing annual herb. Cultivated for its fruit used as vegetable. Tender shoots with flowers are used as pot-herb. Fruit pulp poultice is used on inflammation and burns. Seeds are tonic, diuretic and vermicidal; they are also used as taeniacide.

Kaddu – *see also* Ghia.

Kadhera, Nilkattai – *Heliotropium ellipticum* Ledebour; Boraginaceae; tomentose herb. Leaves are used for treating earache, ulcers and warts.

Kadna banjam – *Ardisia umbellata* Baker; Myrsinaceae; shrub. Cultivated as an ornamental for its beautiful pink flowers borne in corymbs.

Kadua-gokhru – *see* Bara Gokhru.

Kafi, Kahva – *Coffea arabica* L.; Arabian coffee (E); Rubiaceae, evergreen small tree or shrub. Cultivated for its dried beans which on roasting develop the fine aroma, typical of brewed coffee; it is used as a stimulating beverage. An alkaloid caffeine is present. It is also used medicinally as a diuretic, nervine and stimulant.

Kafurkapat – *Meriandra benghalensis* Benth.; Bengal sage (E); Labiatae; herb. Cultivated for its aromatic leaves which are used as a condiment. Herb is the source of meriandra oil which on cooling yields 'kapoor' or camphor. Plant is considered to be astringent, antiseptic, and carminative. Infusion of leaves is used as a gargle for sore-throat.

Kaghzi-bans – *Dendrocalamus hamiltonii* Nees & Arn. ex Munro; Gramineae; tall tufted bamboo. Young culms are edible. Stems with long hollow internodes and big lumen are used as water conduits. Plant is used chiefly for paper manufacture.

Kagzi nimbu, Nimbu – *Citrus aurantifolia* (Christm.) Sw.; Lime (E) Rutaceae; shrub. Cultivated for its fruits used extensively for culinary purposes. Fruit is an appetizer and good source of vitamin C, used either fresh or preserved as pickle, jam, jelly and marmalade.

Kahimal, Keol, Plaksha (S) – *Ficus lucescens* Blume.; Moraceae; tree with dense crown. Cultivated on roadsides for shade. Ripe fruits are edible. Wood is used for making paper pulp and bark for gargles. Leaves are used for fodder.

Kahu – *see* Arjun.

Kahva – *see* Kafi.

Kaiger – *see* Son-khair.

Kail, Chil – *Pinus wallichiana* A.B. Jackson; Blue pine (E); Pinaceae; tall tree. Wood yields timber which is used for construction work, furniture, railway sleepers, pencils and match boxes. Plant is the source of good quality turpentine and rosin; the latter is used in the manufacture of inks, oil cloth, sealing wax, soaps and for sizing paper.

Kaim – *see* Kalmi kadassa.

Kaimil – *see* Jhingan.

Kaiphal, Katphal – *Myrica esculenta* Buch.-Ham. ex D. Don.; Box myrtle (E), Bay berry (E); Myricaceae; evergreen small tree. Bark is the source of tannin and a yellow dye. Bark decoction is used in diarrhoea, lung and bronchial disorders, asthma, and to wash and clean open rotting sores. Bark is chewed to relieve toothache and also used as a fish-poison. Fruits are edible and wax on the pericarp is used for making candles.

Kaith – *see* Kavitha.

Kaju; Kajutaka (S) – *Anacardium occidentale* L.; Cashew nut tree (E); Anacardiaceae; evergreen small tree. Cultivated for its nutritious kernels which are used raw, roasted and fried or made into sweetmeats. Fleshy peduncle called cashew-apple is edible and used for making jams and wines. The fruit pericarp yields cashew-shell oil which is used for termite proofing, water proofing, and as a high class lubricant. It is also used in the manufacture of inks, gums, oil cloth, laminating resins, varnishes, acid and alkali resistant cement, insulation coatings, adhesives, metal anticorrosives, and lacquers. Being rich source of phenol it is further used in the manufacture of certain plastics and synthetic resins which are used for the treatment of water in boilers, ice plants, air-conditioning units and textile industries. India is the chief producer of cashewnuts and cashew-shell oil.

Kajutaka (S) – *see* Kaju.

Kakadumbura (S) – *see* Daduri.

Kakajangha – *Leea aequata* L.; Leeaceae; shrub. Leaves are antiseptic and used as poultice for wounds. Essential oil obtained from the leaves and stems inhibits the growth of *Mycobacterium tuberculosis* bacteria.

Kakamachi (S) – *see* Makoi.

Kakamari (S) – *see* Kakmari.

Kakandan, Madama – *Bruguiera cylindrica* Wight & Arn.; Rhizophoraceae; tree found in tidal forests. Bark is the source of tannin.

Kakaria – *Bergia odorata* Edgew.; Elatinaceae; undershrub. Leaf-poultice is used for fractures and sores.

Kakaronda – *Blumea balsamifera* (L.) DC.; Ngai camphor (E); Compositae; aromatic herb found in the hills. Leaves are rich in an essential oil and are the source of blumea-camphor. Leaves are used as fish-poison and leaf extract is used for insomnia.

Kakarundah – *see* Kukurbicha.

Kakatundi, Kaura-dodi – *Asclepias curassavica* L.; Curassavian swallow-wort (E), False ipecac (E); Asclepiadaceae; small shrub. Cultivated as an ornamental. Leaf juice is anthelmintic, and is used for treating dysentery. Latex is used for treating corns and warts. Roots are used for treating gonorrhoea and piles and also as an adulterant of ipecac.

Kakki – *see* Kath bewal.

Kakmari; Kakamari (S) – *Anamirta cocculus* (L.) Wight & Arn.; Fish berries (E), Levant nut (E); Menispermaceae; trailing shrub. Fruits are used to stupefy fish. They are also used locally for curing ringworm and chronic skin ailments.

Kakoli (S) – *see* Sugandh kokila.

Kakra – *Pistacia integerrima* Stewart ex Brandis; Pistaciaceae, small tree. Wood is beautifully mottled, and is used for ornamentation inlay-work, panelling and carving. Galls on the leaves called 'kakra-singi' are used for asthma, respiratory infections and dysentery. Essential oil from the galls is considered carminative. Bark and leaves contain tannin.

Kakrai – *Abutilon glaucum* Sweet.; Malvaceae; undershrub. Leaves are rich in mucilage and are used for treating piles. Stem yields fibre. Plant is used as fodder.

Kakranda; Kukuradru (S) – *Blumea lacera* DC.; Compositae; aromatic herb. Leaf-juice is anthelmintic, specifically used for threadworms. Herb is stimulant, diuretic and febrifuge. Essential oil present in the herb yields blumea-camphor.

Kakrasingi; Kakratshringi (S) – *Rhus succedanea* L.; Japanese wax tree (E), Wild varnish tree (E); Anacardiaceae; small tree or shrub. Mesocarp of the fruit yields a wax which is used for the manufacture of wax-matches, candles, crayons, pencils, leather and textile finishes, pharmaceuticals, furniture polish, special soaps, packing of foods, pomades, lipsticks and as a substitute for bee-wax. Kernels yield a fatty oil. Alcoholic extract of the leaves is anti-viral and anti-cancerous. Latex from the stem is used in varnishes and lacquer work. Galls on the twigs and branches called 'kakra singhi' are considered tonic, expectorant and astringent, and are used in diarrhoea and dysentery. *See also* Kakra–*Pistacia integerrima.*

Kakri; Bahukanda (S) – *Cucumis melo* L. var. *utilissimus* Duth. & Full.; Snake cucumber (E); Cucurbitaceae; herb. Cultivated for its long, tender and nutritious fruits used raw for salad. Mature seeds are considered to be cooling and diuretic.

Kakrol, Bhat kerela; Karkataka (S) – *Momordica cochinchinensis* Spreng.; Cucurbitaceae; trailing herb. Young leafy shoots and tender fruits are eaten as vegetable. Fruits and leaves are also used in ointments used for local applications for fractures, ulceration and lumbago. Seeds are the source of a fatty oil which is used in paints and varnishes.

Kala anchhu – *see* Kala hisalu.

Kala bhangra – *Anisomeles indica* (L.) Kuntze (syn. *Nepeta indica* L.); Labiatae; undershrub. Plant acts as an astringent and carminative and is used as a condiment. Essential oil has camphor like odour and is used medicinally in uterine disorders.

Kalabis – *see* Dhurchuk.

Kala chakma – *Lithocarpus fenestratus* (Roxb.) Rehd.; Fagaceae; tree. Wood is used for timber, building purposes and agricultural implements. Bark is rich in tannin and is used for tanning of leather in light colour.

Kala damar – *Shorea tumbuggaia* Roxb.; Dipterocarpaceae; large tree. Plant is the source of resin which is used as incense and as a substitute of pitch in marine yards. Wood is used for beams, posts, planking, implements and turnery.

Kala-dammar – *Canarium strictum* Roxb.; Black damar (E); Burseraceae; large deciduous tree. Wood is used for making packing cases and tea-chests. Stem bark is tapped for resin which is used as a substitute of Burgundy pitch in medical plasters; it is also used in varnishes.

Kala dana – *see* Nilkalmi.

Kala dhatura – *see* Sadah-dhatura.

Kala hinsalu, Kali anchhi – *Rubus niveus* Thunb.; Mysore raspberry (E), Mahabaleshwar raspberry (E); Rosaceae; shrub. Fruits are eaten either fresh or preserved as jam and jelly.

Kala hisalu, Kala anchhu – *Rubus paniculatus* Sm.; Ceylon raspberry (E); Rosaceae; shrub. Fruits are eaten as dessert or made into preserves.

Kala isabgol – *Plantago psyllium* L.; Black psyllium (E); Plantaginaceae; herb. Dry seeds are used as laxative, demulcent and expectorant. Fatty oil from the seeds is used in varnishes and the oil-cake is used as a stock feed. Psyllium mucilage is also used in sizing of silk and paper manufacture.

Kala jira – *see* Kalonji.

Kala kantala (S) – *see* Bans keora.

Kala kiryat – *see* Kastula.

Kalaklitaka (S) – *see* Surmainil.

Kala matar – *see* Bakla.

Kalamb-ki-jar – *Jateorhiza palmata* (Lamk.) Miers. (syn. *Cocculus palmatus* DC.); Menispermaceae; scandent undershrub. Cultivated for its roots known commercially as 'kalam ki jar' or *radix columba*. They are used for treating dyspepsia, diarrhoea, dysentery and morning sickness in pregnant women. Powdered roots are antiseptic and applied to open sores. Chief alkaloids present in the roots are jateorhizine, columbine, and palmatine.

Kalameshika (S) – *see* Manjit.

Kala mewa – *see* Chichora.

Kalamnor – *Ficus asperrima* roxb.; Moraceae; tree. Bark is used for tanning.

Kalamucha – *see* Baru.

Kalasaka (S) – *see* Pat.

Kala-shisham; Shishapa (S) – *Dalbergia latifolia* Roxb.; Indian rosewood (E); Papilionaceae; large tree. Wood is considered as one of the best for furniture, cabinet work, carving, veneers and plyboard. It is also used for other miscellaneous purposes such as calico-printing blocks, picture frames, shuttles, boats, agricultural implements, bent wood articles and keys of violin.

Kala siras – *Albizia odoratissima* (L.f.) Benth. (syn. *Mimosa odoratissima* L.f.); Fragrant Albizia (E); Mimosaceae; tree. Cultivated as an avenue tree. Wood is used for construction work, railway sleepers, bridges, panelling, furniture and implements. Tree yields a gum similar to gum arabic, and serves as a host to lac insect. Leaves are lopped for fodder.

Kala tendu – *see* Gab.

Kala til, Ram til, Surguja – *Guizotia abyssinica* Cass.; Niger seed (E); Compositae; herb. Cultivated for its seeds which are the source of an oil used for cooking, and manufacture of soaps, paints and varnishes. Seed-oil cake is used as a stock-feed and manure.

Kala-zira, Shah-zirah – *Bunium persicum* (Boiss.) Fedts.; Earth nut (E), Black caraway (E); Umbelliferae; perennial herb. Cultivated for its aromatic fruits which are used as a condiment, and the starchy tubers which are consumed as vegetable.

Kali anchhi – *see* Kala hinsalu.

Kaliar, Lal kachnar – *Bauhinia purpurea* L.; Camel's foot tree (E); Pink Bauhinia (E); Caesalpiniaceae; tree. Cultivated as an ornamental. Flower buds and young fruits are used as vegetable. Bark is a rich source of tannin and is used for tanning and dyeing. Leaves are lopped for fodder.

Kalidudhi, Siamlata; Paravalli (S) – *Ichnocarpus frutescens* R. Br.; Black creeper (E); Apocynaceae; climbing shrub. Cultivated as an ornamental. Roots are considered to be tonic, diuretic and demulcent and are used in powdered form for treating diabetes and bladder-stones.

Kali haldi, Nar-kachura – *Curcuma caesia* Roxb.; Black zedoary (E); Zingiberaceae; herb. Cultivated for its aromatic rhizomes which are used as a cosmetic and for the treatment of sprains and bruises. Essential oil contains camphor.

Kalihari; Agnimukhi (S), Agnishikha (S),. Garbhagatini (S) – *Gloriosa suberba* L.; Tiger's claws (E). Glory-lily (E); Liliaceae; perennial herb. Cultivated as an ornamental. Tubers are anthelmintic, stomachic and tonic, but are highly poisonous in large doses. They are also used for promoting labour pains and as an abortifacient and applied externally for skin troubles. Leaf juice is used to kill hair lice. Chief alkaloid present is colchicine along with many others.

Kalijhant – *Adiantum philippense* L. (syn. *A. lunulatum* Burm.); Walking maiden-hair fern (E); Adiantaceae; perennial herb. Rhizomes are used in epileptic fits and in fever due to elephantiasis. Fronds burnt in boiling hot oil are used for itchy skin ailments.

Kalijiri, Somraj; Somraji (S) – *Centratherum anthelminticum* (L.) Kuntze; Compositae; herb. Achenes are anthelmintic and are used specifically against threadworms; they also contain a fixed oil.

Kalikatbhi, Kumbi; Kumbhi (S) – *Careya arborea* Roxb.; Patana oak (E); Barringtoniaceae; large tree. Wood is used for construction work, gun-stocks and cabinets. Bark is used for tanning and dyeing; it is also source of a fibre used for cordage. Leaves are used as beedi-wrapper. Seeds are edible.

Kali khatai – *see* Aamli.

Kali mirch, Golmirch; Maricha (S) – *Piper nigrum* L.; Black pepper (E); Piperaceae; trailing perennial shrub. Cultivated extensively for its dried ripe fruits which are used as a spice and condiment. Pepper contains alkaloids piperidine and piperine, an oleoresin chavicine responsible for the pungent taste, and an essential oil called pepper-oil which is responsible for the aroma and used as an adjunct in flavouring foods, sauces and beverages. Pepper is used externally as a rubefacient for piles, cutaneous ailments and for sore throat.

Kali musli, Musali-kand; Mushali (S) – *Curculigo orchioides* Gaertn.; Hypoxidaceae; perennial herb found in the hills. Black tuberous roots are tonic and diuretic and are used for curing diarrhoea, piles, asthma, jaundice and skin ailment. Roots are also edible.

Kalinga – *see* Kutaja.

Kali rai – *see* Banarasi rai.

Kali sarson, Maghi, Toriva – *Brassica napus* L. var. *napus;* Rape (E); Cruciferae; herb. Cultivated as an important oil-seed crop. Seeds yield an edible oil which is also used for soap manufacture and as a lubricant. Leaves are used as salad and for stock-feed.

Kali tori, Jhinga tori; Koshataki (S) – *Luffa acutangula* (L.) Roxb.; Ribbed gourd (E); Cucurbitaceae; trailing herb. Cultivated for its tender fruits which are used as vegetable. Fibrous dried ripe fruits are used as bath sponge. Leaf juice is used for treating conjunctivitis and leaf poultice for leprosy and haemorrhoids. Ripe seeds are emetic and purgative, they also yield a fatty-oil. Oil cake is toxic, and is used as manure.

Kali tulsi, Mamri; Gambhira (S) – *Ocimum americanum* L.; Hoary basil (E); Labiatae; aromatic herb. Leaves yield an essential oil used in cosmetics and soaps. They are also used as a condiment. Tender shoots are used as pot-herb. Decoction of leaves is used as mouth-wash and for treating cough and dysentery. Seeds are mucilaginous, and considered to be tonic and diuretic; they also yield a semi-drying fatty oil.

Kallai – *see* Aggai.

Kalmegh – *see* Kirayat.

Kalmi kadassa, Kaim – *Mitragyna parvifolia* (Roxb.) Korth.; Rubiaceae; tree. Wood is used for construction purposes, furniture, carving, match-industry, and calico-printing blocks. Wood pulp is used for making wrapping paper. Bark and roots are used in colic, as a febrifuge and in tribal medicine for the treatment of rabies. Bark is rich in tannin and fibre which is used for cordage.

Kalmisag, Patuasag, Sarnali – *Ipomoea reptans* (L.) Poir.; Water spinach (E), Swamp cabbage (E); Convolvulaceae; semi-aquatic trailing herb. Tender shoots are rich in vitamins and minerals and are used as vegetable. Plant is used for fodder. Root-juice is emetic and is used for the treatment of opium- and arsenic-poisoning.

Kalo bilauni – *Antidesma acuminatum* Wall.; Stilaginaceae; tree. Fruits are edible.

Kalonji, Kala jira, Mugrela – *Nigella sativa* L.; Black cumin (E), Small fennel (E); Ranunculaceae; herb. Cultivated for its seeds which are used as a spice and condiment; they are also used medicinally as a stimulant, carminative and diuretic and applied locally for skin ailments. Ripe seeds are also used for curing inflammation of the mucous membrane of intestines. Seed extract shows antibacterial activity.

Kamal, Kanwal; Padma (S), Pankaj (S) – *Nelumbo nucifera* Gaertn.; Lotus (E), Sacred lotus (E); Nelumbonaceae; aquatic perennial herb. Starchy rhizomes called 'kamal-kakri' or 'bhein' are used as vegetable. They are the source of a kind of arrowroot. Fruiting torus called 'kamal-gutta' contains numerous oblong carpels. The mature seeds are eaten raw or roasted. Alkaloid nelumbine is present in the petioles, pedicels and bitter embryos. Flowers are considered sacred and as a symbol of purity and divinity by the Hindus.

Kamalata – *Ipomoea quamoclit* L.; Cypress wine (E), Indian pink (E); Convolvulaceae; twining shrub. Cultivated as an ornamental. Leaves are used as vegetable. Leaf paste is used for treating carbuncles and haemorrhoids.

Kamalgatta – *see* Kamal.

Kamal-kakri – *see* Kamal.

Kambhari – *see* Gambhar.

Kamela, Sindur, Rohini – *Mallotus philippensis* (Lamk.) Muell-Arg.; Monkey face tree (E), Kamala tree (E); Euphorbiaceae; tree. Glandular hair on fruit pericarp are the source of Kamela dye which is used for dyeing silk and wool. It is also used as an anthelmintic and anti-oxidant for vegetable oils, and externally for skin ailments. Seeds yield an oil used in hair-fixers and ointments; oil cake is used as manure and for making insulating-boards. Wood is suitable for match-boxes and bark yields tannin. Leaves are lopped for fodder.

Kamini, Bisar – *Murraya paniculata* (L.) Jack (syn. *M. exotica* L.); Orange jessamine (E); Rutaceae; shrub. Cultivated usually as a hedge plant. Root bark and leaves are used in medicine for combating rheumatism, hysteria and cough; leaves contain an essential oil. Flowers contain murrayin and are used in cosmetics. Wood is used for pen and brush holders, tool-handles and walking-sticks.

Kampti – *see* Madhavilata.

Kamrakh, Karmal – *Averrhoa carambola* L.; Carambola (E); Averrhoaceae; tree. Cultivated for its fleshy fruits which are either eaten raw or cooked and made into preserves. Fruit is rich in vitamin B and C and iron. Some varieties bear acidic fruit, the others bear sweet and sour.

Kamrup, Chilkan; Kuni (S) – *Ficus microcarpa* L.f., [syn. *F. retusa* auct. (non L.)] Moraceae; tree. Wood is suitable for furniture. Bark is used for liver ailments and root bark, boiled in oil is used for wounds. Leaves are used as fodder.

Kanak – *see* Gehun.

Kanakakuli (S) – *see* Jambu.

Kanak-champa, Kaniar, Muchkand; Karnikara (S) – *Pterospermum acerifolium* Willd.; Sterculiaceae; tree. Wood is used for construction work, panelling, bridges, boats, veneers, plywood, match industry, toys and miscellaneous articles. Leaves are used for making disposable plates, as packing material for tobacco and for thatching. Flowers are considered antiseptic and are used as a remedy for inflammation and ulcers; they are also edible. *See also* Khambar.

Kanakchampa (S) – *see* Khambar.

Kananaeranda – *see* Bagbherenda.

Kananashigru (S) – *see* Ban sigru.

Kanchara, Kancowa; Kanchata (S) – *Commelina benghalensis* L.; Commelinaceae; straggling herb. Plant is used as fodder. Leaves are used as pot herb. They are also considered to be laxative and demulcent.

Kanchari, Nadarang – *Alternanthera amoena* Voss; Amaranthaceae; herb. Cultivated for its tender young shoots which are used as vegetable.

Kanchata (S) – *see* Kanchara.

Kancowa – *see* Kanchara; *see also* Kankauwa.

Kandalu (S) – *see* Pitmari.

Kander – *Ischaemum aristatum* L.; Gramineae; perennial herb. Plant is relished by cattle but imparts an undesirable odour to the milk.

Kandir (S) – *see* Jaldhania.

Kandla, Semla – *Bauhinia retusa* Buch-Ham.; Caesalpiniaceae; small tree. The plant yields a gum known as 'semla gond' which is used for sizing paper and cloth and as a binder in charcoal briquettes. Wood is suitable for rafters.

Kanduri – *see* Kundru.

Kaner – *Nerium oleander* L.; Oleander (E); Apocynaceae; evergreen shrub. Cultivated as an ornamental for its beautiful pink flowers which are not fragrant but showy. Stem bark, leaves and flowers are cardiotonic and diuretic. Seeds contain a fatty oil and numerous glycosides. Leaf-juice is used for skin eruptions. *See also* Kaner; Karavira (S).

Kaner; Karavira (S) – *Nerium indicum* Mill.; Indian oleander (E); Apocynaceae; evergreen shrub with aromatic flowers. Root bark is a carminative, diaphoretic, attenuant and anthelmintic, and possesses active principles *viz.*, nerioderin and karabin, with digitoxin-like activity. Leaves also contain oleandrin which is a cardiotonic. Root paste and oil from the root bark are used externally for treating skin ailments, swellings and leprosy. The plant is usually cultivated as an ornamental.

Kanghi; Atibala (S) – *Abutilon indicum* (L.) Sweet; Indian Abutilon (E). Country mallow (E); Malvaceae; hairy undershrub. Stem yields a fibre used for cordage. Seeds called 'balbeej' are mucilaginous, and used as a laxative and demulcent. Seeds also yield a semi-drying oil. Bark is astringent and diuretic. Roots called 'atibala' are antipyretic and used as a nervine tonic, and for treating piles; they are also mixed with chaulmogra oil for the treatment of leucoderma.

Kangiabel, Khaji – *Bridelia stipularis* Blume; Euphorbiaceae; tree. Fruit is edible. Seeds possess haemagglutinating property, and also yield a fatty oil. Leaves are used for treating jaundice and twigs for making baskets. Decoction of bark is hypotensive and is used as a remedy for fever, cough and asthma.

Kangni, Kangu; Kangunika (S) – *Setaria italica* (L.) Beauv.; Fox-tail millet (E), Italian millet (E); Gramineae; herb. Cultivated for both fodder and grain; Grains are malted and mixed with barley for the preparation of beer to make it more strong. Grains are diuretic and astringent, and are used for combating rheumatism and relieving pain after childbirth. Straw is used for thatching and fodder.

Kangu – *see* Kangni.

Kangunika (S) – *see* Kangni.

Kaniar – *see* Kanak champa.

Kaninika – *see* Jari.

Kanj – *see* Jangli kalimirch.

Kanjanbura, Mudunirbisha – *Kaempferia angustifolia* Rosc.; Zingiberaceae; perennial herb. Rhizomes are used as a masticatory and for treating cough.

Kanju, Banchilla, Chilbil; Chirabilva (S) – *Holoptelea integrifolia* (Roxb.) Planch.; Ulmaceae; tree. Timber is used for furniture, decorative panelling, carving, cabinet work, yokes, ploughs, carts, bobbins, match-sticks, plywood and paper-pulp. Bark is used for making insulation-boards.

Kanjuna – *Commelina paludosa* Bl.; Commelinaceae; herb. Tender shoots are used as vegetable. Roots considered to be laxative are used in bilious disorder.

Kanka-jariya – *Digitaria longiflora* (Retz.) Pers.; Gramineae; herb. Plants are used as fodder.

Kankauwa, Kancowa – *Commelina forskalii* Vahl.; Commelinaceae; prostrate straggling herb. Tender shoots are used as vegetable. Plant is used as fodder.

Kankhura – *Boehmeria nivea* (L.) Gaud.; Ramie (E), Rhea (E); Urticaceae; undershrub. Cultivated for fibre obtained from the inner bark of its stem. Fibre called rhea or ramie is exceptionally strong, durable, silky and lustrous. It is generally blended with cotton, silk and wool to produce non-creasable fabrics. It is also used for ropes, fishing-nets, fishing-lines, motor-tyre fabrics, gas mantles, thread for leather goods and as a binding material.

Kankra – *Bruguiera gymnorrhiza* (L.) Lamk.; Rhizophoraceae; tree. Bark serves as a rich source of tannin. Wooden poles after harvesting the bark are used for rafters.

Kanocha, Bazarmani, Ranavali – *Phyllanthus maderaspatensis* L.; Euphorbiaceae; herb. Leaf-infusion is used for curing headaches. Seeds act as a carminative, diuretic and laxative; they are also rich in a fatty oil.

Kanor – *see* Bankhor.

Kanphuti; Karnasphota (S) – *Cardiospermum halicacabum* L.; Balloon vine (E); Sapindaceae; climbing herb. Roots are diaphoretic, emetic, diuretic and laxative and are used for curing stiffness of joints and nervous disorders. Leaf-juice is used for earache and leaf poultice for rheumatism.

Kans; Kas, Kasa (S) – *Saccharum spontaneum* L.; Thatch grass (E); Gramineae; perennial tall and robust wild grass. Culms are used for thatching, plant is a very good soil binder. It is considered very valuable in breeding work for incorporating the quality of disease resistance in cultivated sugarcanes by hybridization technique. Pulp is suitable for paper manufacture.

Kansa – *see* Luchra.

Kanshurra; Koshapushpi – *Commelina nudiflora* L.; Commelinaceae; herb. Plant is used as pot-herb and for fodder. Crushed leaves are applied topically to burns and itches, and leaf poultice is used for sores.

Kansiphal – *see* Kaddu. *See also* Mitha kaddu.

Kanta-alu, Bhusa, Gazaria – *Dioscorea pentaphylla* L.; Dioscoreaceae; climbing shrub. Tubers are consumed after boiling and washing. They are also used for curing inflammation. Flowers are used as vegetable.

Kantagur-kamai; Kundali (S) – *Azima tetracantha* Lamk.; Salvadoraceae; rambling shrub with axillary spines. The plant is considered good for hedges. Berries are edible. Bark is expectorant. The juice of leaves is used in cough and asthma. Plant is reported to be an effective remedy in tribal medicine of S. India for the treatment of rheumatic arthritis and paralysis.

Kantakari – *see* Kanteri.

Kantala – *Agave cantala* Roxb.; Manila maguey (E), Cantala (E), Bombay aloe (E); Agavaceae; hardy perennial. It is cultivated as a soil binder and for fencing because of its xerophytic nature and long narrow, spine-tipped leaves on a reduced stem. Leaves yield a pure white fibre used for twines, ropes and cordage. Pulp left after harvesting fibre is used for the extraction of hecogenin which is employed in the manufacture of steroid hormones.

Kantalu – *see* Utkanta.

Kanteri, Kateli, Bhatkatiya; Kantakari (S) – *Solanum surattense* Burm. f.; Yellow-berried nightshade (E); Solanaceae; spiny herb. Root serves as one of the ingredients of an Ayurvedic preparation called 'Dasamula'. Roots are expectorant and are used in cough, chest pain, and asthma. Leaf-juice mixed with pepper is used for rheumatism. Aqueous and alcoholic extract of the plant is hypotensive. Herb is used in the preparation of several other indigenous medicines used for curing fever due to chest infections, bronchitis and bronchial asthma. Fruits are used in curries. Seeds yield a semi-drying oil.

Kanthapunkha – *Tephrosia uniflora* Pers. ssp. *petrosa* (Blatt & Halb) Gill & Ali; Papilionaceae; herb. Leaf decoction is used in syphilis. Roots and seeds are insecticidal and piscicidal. Root decoction is used for treating asthma, rheumatism, dyspepsia and urinary infections. Extract of the herb is considered to be useful in liver cirrhosis.

Kanthari – *Capparis sepiaria* L.; India caper (E); Capparidaceae; thorny spreading or climbing shrub. Plant is considered to be a tonic and febrifuge and is also useful in skin troubles.

Kantiari, Kateri – *Carthamus oxyacantha* M. Bieb.; Wild safflower (E); Compositae; spiny herb. Cultivated as an oil seed crop. Oil extracted by cold expression method is called poli-oil which is used for preparing macassar hair oil and for water proofing tarpaulins. Oil derived by hot dry process is called roghum-oil and is employed in the manufacture of 'afridi' wax-cloth and for greasing well-ropes and leather buckles. Oil is also used for itch and foul ulcers.

Kanujera, Siran – *Albizia chinensis* (Osbeck) Merr.; Mimosaceae; tree. Cultivated as a shade tree in tea and coffee plantations. Wood is used for tea-chests and small turnery. Tree is the source of a gum used for sizing paper. Wood-pulp is considered to be good for paper-manufacture. Tender-shoots are used as fodder.

Kanukpa – *Euodia fraxinifolia* Hook. f.; American beach (E); Rutaceae; tree. Fruits are edible and are used in chutneys; they are also used in the treatment of dysentery. Wood is used for match-industry, tea-chests and posts.

Kant-swarniyas – *Meconopsis aculeata* Royle; Blue poppy (E); Papaveraceae; perennial herb. Roots are poisonous, they are also considered to be narcotic.

Kanwal – *see* Kamal.

Kao – *see* Kau.

Kapas, Rui – *Gossypium arboreum* L.; Tree cotton (E); Malvaceae; shrub. Cultivated as a fibre plant. Staple or lint fibre obtained from the surface of seeds, is utilized extensively in the manufacture of cotton textiles and rubber-tyre fabrics. Short fibre known as fuzz or linters are the source of high grade cellulose and are used in the manufacture of viscose rayons, cellulose ethers, esters and nitrocellulose lacquers; they are also used for stuffing purposes. Cotton-seeds yield a semi-drying oil which is used in toilet preparations, leather industry, lubricants, paints and varnishes. Refined oil is used for the manufacture of cooking oil, shortening and margarine. Seed-cake is used as fertilizer and as a stock-feed after removal of gossypol, a toxic principle. Seed-hull is used as cattle-feed, soil conditioner, fertilizer and in the manufacture of insulating materials, Cotton-rag fibre and cotton combers are used in the manufacture of fine quality paper. *See* Kapas for other cultivated species.

Kapas, Rui – *Gossypium herbaceum* L.; Asiatic cotton (E), Levant cotton (E), Malvaceae; cultivated shrub. Uses are similar to *G. arboreum*.

Kapas, Rui – *Gossypium hirsutum* L.; Upland cotton (E); Malvaceae; cultivated shrub densely covered with woolly hair. Uses are similar to *G. arboreum*.

Kapas, Rui – *Gossypium barbadense* L.; Egyptian cotton (E), Sea-island cotton (E); Malvaceae; shrub. Cultivated to a limited extent only. Uses are similar to *G. arboreum*.

Kapittha – *see* Kavitha.

Kapni – *Holmskioldia sanguinea* Retz.; Chinese hat-plat (E), Parasol flower (E); Verbenaceae; shrub. Cultivated as an ornamental for its orange red flowers arranged in cymes. Plant is also used as fodder for sheep and goats.

Kapur, Mushkapur; Karpur (S) – *Cinnamomum camphora* (L.) T. Nees & Eberm.; Camphor tree (E); Lauraceae; evergreen tree. Chipped wood on distillation yields camphor and safrole which is used in the manufacture of delicate perfumes. Camphor is extensively used externally for sprains, inflammations and rheumatic pain, and internally as a cardiac stimulant and for treating diarrhoea. It is also used as a soothing agent in hysteria and nervousness. Leaves yield a volatile oil and seeds are the source of an aromatic fat with high laurin content.

Kapuri – *see* Anantamul.

Kapur-kachri, Sitruti; Gandhashati (S) – *Hedychium spicatum* Buch-Ham. ex Smith; Spiked ginger-lily (E); Zingiberaceae; Tall perennial herb. Rhizomes are aromatic and are used as carminative, stomachic, tonic and as a flavouring agent for perfuming tobacco. Rhizomes are also the source of an essential oil used in perfumery and considered to be active against fungi and gram positive bacteria.

Kapur tulsi – *Ocimum kilimandscharicum* Guerke; Camphor basil (E); Labiatae; undershrub. Cultivated for its leaves which yield camphor which is used medicinally in ointments and balms for sprains and pain.

Karamadika (S) – *see* Karanda.

Karamarda (S) – *see* Karaunda.

Karambha (S) – *see* Ardanda.

Karamkalla – *see* Patta-gobi.

Karamsag – *Brassica oleracea* L. var. *acephala* DC.; Tall kale (E), Borecole (E); Cruciferae; herb. Cultivated for its tender shoots and leaves which are used for vegetable, soups and salads.

Karanda; Karamadika (S) – *Carissa spinarum* L. Apocynaceae; evergreen shrub. Cultivated for hedges and for its fragrant flowers. Fruits are edible. Roots act as a purgative and leaves are rich in tannin.

Karanj; Karanja (S) – *Pongamia pinnata* L.; Pierre.; Indian beech (E); Pongam (E); Papilionaceae; small tree with dense crown. Cultivated for its seeds which are the source of pongam oil used in the manufacture of washing soaps, candles, tanning industry and as a lubricant of heavy engines, lathes and chains. 'Karanj' oil or pongam oil is also used for illumination and shows potential as a petro-fuel. Oil is used medicinally for herpes, scabies, leucoderma and other skin ailments. Active principle present is karanjine. Oil is used internally as a remedy in sluggish liver and dyspepsia. Wood is used for small carpentry. Leaf-juice is used in cough, diarrhoea, dyspepsia, gonorrhoea and leprosy. Leaves and roots are used as fish-poison. Fresh bark is given for treating piles. Bark is also the source of fibre used for cordage. Leaves are lopped for fodder.

Karanja (S) – *see* Karanj.

Karanju, Kat-karanja; Putikaranja (S) – *Caesalpinia crista* L.; Molucca bean (E), Bonduc nut (E); Caesalpiniaceae; scandent prickly shrub. Often cultivated as a hedge plant. Seeds are tonic and antipyretic and are used for treating colic and intermittent fevers; seed-oil is used in cosmetics to treat freckles on the face and check discharge from the ear.

Karanta – *Cryptolepis buchanani* R. & S.; Periplocaceae; twining shrub. Plant is the source of floss, a fibre of local importance which is used for cordage and a special type of cloth.

Karas – *see* Salaree.

Karaunda, Karonda; Karamarda (S), Avighna (S) – *Carissa carandas* L.; Karanda (E); Apocynaceae; evergreen spiny shrub. Cultivated for fencing and hedges. Fruit is acidic and is made into jams, chutney and pickles. Ripe fruits are sweet and used in tarts and jellies. Root is anthelmintic and stomachic.

Karavira (S) – *see* Kaner.

Karbuia – *Bergia suffruticosa* (Del.) Fenzl.; Elatinaceae; undershrub found in the states of Gujarat and Rajasthan. Tender stem-cuttings are used for brushing and cleaning the teeth.

Karchura (S) – *see* Kachura.

Kardi – *see* Kasumbh.

Karela – *Momordica charantia* L.; Bitter gourd (E); Cucurbitaceae; trailing herb. Cultivated for its fruits which are used as vegetable. Tender shoots with leaves are also used as vegetable. Fruits are tonic, stomachic, and carminative and are used for combating diabetes, rheumatism, gout, and diseases of spleen and liver. Roots are considered to be good for haemorrhoids and leaf juice for biliousness.

Karer, Tantee; Karira (S), Gudhapatra (S) – *Capparis decidua* (Forsk.) Edgew.; Capparidaceae; evergreen leafless spinous shrub. Young green fruits commonly known as 'tantee' or 'dailay' are pickled; they are considered to be good for biliousness and heart-trouble. Flower buds are used as vegetable. Tender shoot-poultice is used for inflammation. Bark of the stem is used as a remedy for asthma and cough, and root-bark for intermittent fevers. Plant is xerophytic, and is cultivated for shelter-belts and wind-breaks.

Kari, Kirua – *Miliusa tomentosa* (Roxb.) J. Sinclair; Annonaceae; tree. Wood is used for cabinet work, shutters, billiard cues, bobbins and carving. Tree is the source of 'kari gum' which is used as a substitute for gum tragacanth. Fruits are edible, and leaves are lopped for fodder.

Karira (S) – *see* Karer.

Kariyartharani – *Stachytarpheta jamaicensis* Vahl.; Verbenaceae; herb. Occasionally cultivated in gardens for its beautiful deep blue flowers arranged in terminal spikes. Fresh leaves are used as vegetable. Dried leaves are marketed as Brazilian tea. Herb decoction is used as an abortifacient and leaf decoction for nose ulcers. Herb is used for treating stomach disorders, intestinal worms, ulcers, venereal diseases, and erysiphales infection. Leaf-juice is used for cataract.

Karkataka (S) – *see* Kakrol.

Karkhandu (S) – *see* Mokoh.

Karmal – *see* Kamrakh.

Karnasphota (S) – *see* Kanphuti.

Karnikara (S) – *see* Kanak champa.

Karonda – *see* Karaunda.

Karpur (S) – *see* Kapur.

Karpura haridra (S) – *see* Am haldi.

Karrah – *see* Kusumbh.

Karshu, Barchar – *Quercus semecarpifolia* Smith; Brown oak of Himalayas (E), Kharshu oak (E); Fagaceae; large tree. Wood is used for construction work, ploughs and furniture; it also yields good charcoal. Wood pulp is used for the manufacture of wrapping-paper. Leaves and bark contain tannin and the leaves are lopped for fodder.

Kartah, Khel – *Dichanthium caricosum* (L.) A. Camus; Gramineae; herb. Plant is used as fodder.

Karu, Kutki – *Gentiana kurroo* Royle; Indian gentian root (E), Himalayan gentian (E); Gentianaceae; perennial herb. Rhizomes (entire or split) together with roots constitute the drug 'traymana' or Indian gentian which is rich in gentiopicrin and gentianic acid. Rhizomes are considered to be tonic, stomachic, febrifuge, anthelmintic and digestive, and are used in hepatic, digestive and urinary disorders.

Karu dhak – *Ribes glaciale* Wall.; Grossulariaceae; shrub found in the Himalayas. Fruits are edible.

Karukand – *Dioscorea hispida* Dennst.; Dioscoreaceae; perennial herbaceous climber with tuberous roots. Tubers are poisonous and can be used only after thorough washing in times of scarcity.

Karunta (S) – *see* Jhinti.

Karvi tori; Katukoshataki (S) – *Luffa acutangula* (L.) Roxb. var. *amara* (Roxb.) C.B. Clarke; Cucurbitaceae; annual climbing herb. Plant is used in spleen enlargement, asthma and skin trouble. Seeds act as an emetic and expectorant.

Karwa-inderjau – *see* Kutaja.

Karwanth – *see* Bega.

Kas – *see* Kans.

Kasa (S) – *see* Kans.

Kasa alu – *Dioscorea puber* Blume.; Dioscoreaceae; perennial herbaceous climber with tuberous root. Tubers are edible, some varieties emit offensive odour.

Kasamarda (S) – *see* Kasondi.

Kasaunda – *Cassia sophera* L.; Sophera senna (E); Caesalpiniaceae; undershrub. Leaves, bark and seeds are laxative. Leaf juice is used for curing ringworm.

Kasbeeze-mradupatra – *see* Panirak.

Kaseru; Kaseruka (S) – *Scirpus grossus* L.f.; Cyperaceae; large perennial herb. Tubers are edible, and are considered to be tonic, diuretic and laxative; they are used to stop vomiting and diarrhoea. Culms are used as fodder; they are also used for thatching and basketry.

Kaseruka (S) – *see* Kaseru.

Kashini – *see* Kasni.

Kashmal – *see* Chatroa.

Kashshing – *see* Charangi.

Kasht-bhanjan (S) – *see* Jangli chachinda.

Kasini – *Cichorium endivia* L.; Garden endive (E), Endive (E); Compositae; herb. Broad-leaved varieties are used as vegetable. Achenes (fruits) are used in biliousness. Roots are considered to be tonic and demulcent.

Kasis – *see* Kachur.

Kasmol – *see* Ban-bakar.

Kasni, Kashini – *Cichorium intybus* L.; Chicory (E); Compositae; hispid herb. Leaves are used as vegetable, they are also used as fodder. Dried roots are diuretic, stomachic and tonic. Dried, roasted and powdered roots are blended with coffee.

Kasondi; Kasmarda (S) – *Cassia occidentalis* L.; Negro coffee (E); Caesalpiniaceae; herb. Leaves and seeds act as a purgative. Seed powder and paste are applied externally for skin-ailments. Seeds are used to adulterate coffee.

Kaspat, Kathu, Phaphra – *Fagopyrum tataricum* (L.) Gaertn.; Tartary buckwheat (E), Duck-wheat (E); Polygonaceae; herb. Cultivated for its grains used as poultry feed, and as a substitute for cereals. Rutin, flavonol glucoside is present in the leaves and flowers, and is used for treating capillary fragility. Leaves are used as pot-herb.

Kastula, Kala Kirayat – *Haplanthus verticillatus* (Roxb.) Nees.; Acanthaceae; herb. Plant is used as a febrifuge.

Kasturi dana, Mushk dana; Latakasturikam (S) – *Abelmoschus moschatus* (L.) Medic.; Muskmallow (E), Ambrette seed (E); Malvaceae; shrub. Musk-scented seeds are the source of an essential oil called ambrette-seed oil which is used in very expensive perfumes with musk-odour, they also contain a fatty oil. Seeds are also used as a flavouring agent, carminative, and stimulant. Flowers are used for flavouring tobacco. Root-mucilage is used for sizing paper. Tender shoots and leaves are used in soups.

Kasuri methi, Champa methi; Malya (S) – *Trigonella corniculata* L.; Papilionaceae; herb. Leaves are used as pot-herb. Fruits are bitter and considered to be astringent. Diosgenin is present.

Kataili chaulai, Tanduliya (S) – *Amaranthus spinosus* L.; Amaranth (prickly) (E); Amaranthaceae; spinous undershrub. Leaves are used as pot-herb. Infusion of shoots is used for eczema, and the leaves are also used as an emollient.

Kataka – *see* Neimal.

Kataphal, Latkua – *Baccaurea sapida* (Roxb.) Muel.-Arg. (syn. *Pierardia sapida* Roxb.); Euphorbiaceae; tree. Fruits, flowers and leaves are edible. Fruit is also made into wine. Bark and leaves are used for dyeing.

Katari – *see* Dandal.

Katathohar; Patrasnuhi (S) – *Euphorbia nivulia* Buch.-Ham.; Euphorbiaceae; small tree. Root-bark is used in dropsy; latex of the plant is used for curing wounds. Juice is purgative and diuretic. Plant is used for rheumatism and earache. Bark is suitable for making composite cork-board when blended with *Hevea* latex as a binder.

Kat-ber, Goth-ber – *Ziziphus xylopyra* Willd.; Rhamnaceae; tree. Plant is used as an important host to lac insect. Fruits are rich in catechol tannin; bark is also used for tanning. Wood is used for agricultural implements, inlay-work, panelling and other ornamental purposes. Leaves are lopped for fodder.

Kateli – *see* Kanteri, *see also* Bharband.

Kateri – *see* Kantiari.

Kateri indrayan – *Ecballium elaterium* A. Rich.; Squirting cucumber (E); Cucurbitaceae; trailing herb. Dried immature fruits are marketed as the source of the drug called elatarium. Active principle present is elatarin, a powerful hydragogue cathartic.

Katgularia – *see* Daduri.

Kathachampa, Papari; Papata (S) – *Pavetta indica* L.; White pavetta (E); Rubiaceae; small tree. Roots contain an essential oil. They are considered as a purgative and diuretic and are used for urinary disorders, headache, jaundice and visceral obstructions. Decoction of leaves is used for treating haemorrhoids and ulcerated nose. Flower infusion is used as a cosmetic. Fruits and flowers are edible.

Kathal; Panas; Panasa (S) – *Artocarpus heterophyllus* Lamk.; Jack fruit (E); Moraceae; tall evergreen tree. Unripe fruits are used as vegetable, ripe ones are eaten raw or preserved. Wood is rated as high-grade timber and used for furniture, inlay work, musical instruments, toys, and carving. Wood is also the source of a yellow dye. Leaves are lopped for fodder.

Kath-bewal, Kakki – *Grewia glabra* Blume.; Tiliaceae; tree. Wood is used for turnery. Bark is the source of fibre which is used for cordage. Leaves are used as fodder.

Kaththa – *see* Khair.

Kath-kuththa – *Uncaria gambier* (Hunt.) Roxb.; White cutch (E); Pale catechu (E); Rubiaceae; climbing shrub. Young branches and leaves are the source of a resinous substance which is used for tanning of leather and medicinally as a powerful astringent. It is also used as a masticatory and as a dye stuff.

Kath-semul – *see* Dain.

Kathsola – *Sesbania roxburghii* Merr.; Papilionaceae; herb. Soft wood is used for making mats and toys. Leaves are used in poultices; they are also used as pot-herb and fodder. Seeds are stimulant. Plant is cultivated for fencing the boundaries.

Kathu – *see* Kaspat.

Kathumbar – *see* Daduri.

Katira gond – *see* Peeli kapas.

Katiragabina-gond – *Astragalus heratensis* Bunge; Indian tragacanth (E); Papilionaceae; large shrub. Stem yields a gum called 'katira gabina' which is used for glazing.

Kat-karanja – *see* Karanju.

Katki, Kutki, Kuru; Katuka (S) – *Picrorhiza kurroa* Royle ex. Benth.; Scrophulariaceae; trailing herb. Dried rhizomes and roots constitute the drug 'katki' or picrorhiza which is used as a substitute of 'karu' or 'traymana' or Indian gentian. Drug from the rhizomes and roots is used to improve appetite and tone up digestion. It is a strong cathartic in large doses, and is also effective in dropsy. Active principles present include picrorhizin and kutkin.

Katmarra – *see* Meda.

Katphal – *see* Kaiphal.

Katsareya – *see* Jhinti.

Katsol – *Rubus moluccanus* L.; Black cherry (E); Rosaceae; shrub. Fruits are edible. Root-juice is used for treating fistula.

Katuka (S) – *see* Katki.

Katukoshataki (S) – *see* Karvi tori.

Katul, Panar, Pindalu – *Randia uliginosa* DC.; Rubiaceae; tree. Fruits are edible after they are boiled or roasted. Mature but unripe fruit pulp is astringent, and is used in diarrhoea, dysentery, dyeing, intensifying colour and as a fish poison. Roots are used in biliousness. Flowers are the source of an essential oil. Leaves are lopped for fodder. Wood is used for turnery.

Kau, Kao – *Olea ferruginea* Royle; Indian olive (E); Oleaceae; tree. Wood is used for turnery articles, carving, toys, walking-sticks, ploughs, boats, ginning machines, printing blocks, engraving, panelling, cabinet work and veneers. Fruits are edible, they are also the source of a fatty oil. Leaves are used to cure gonorrhoea. Leaves and bark are used as a febrifuge and in tonics for general debility.

Kauathodi – *Pentatropis spiralis* (Forsk.) Decne. Asclepiadaceae; slender twining undershrub. Roots are astringent and are used in gonorrhoea. Tubers are sweet and edible.

Kaura-dodi – *see* Kakatundi.

Kauraj – *Ampelocissus araneosa* (M. Laws.) Planch.; Vitidaceaee; climbing shrub. Root tubers are sliced and dried, and marketed as 'chamar-musli'; they are considered to be refrigerant and astringent. Young twigs make good fodder for horses.

Kaura-ro – *see* Bui.

Kavitha, Kaith, Bilin; Kapittha (S) – *Feronia limonia* (L.) Sw. (syn. *Limonia acidissima* L.; *Feronia elephantum* Correa); Elephant apple (E); Rutaceae; tree. Fruits are edible, they are also preserved as cordials, and considered to be good as a tonic. Leaves are aromatic and yield an essential oil. Wood is used for walking-sticks, agricultural implements and carving. Trunk of the tree exudes a gum which is used for similar purposes as gum arabic.

Kawala – *Machilus odoratissima* Nees.; Lauraceae; tree. Wood is used for construction work, furniture and plywood. Seeds yield a semi-drying oil, and leaves are used for feeding 'muga' silkworms.

Kawanch, Alkusi – *Mucuna pruriens* (L.) DC.; Horse-eye bean (E); Papilionaceae; twiner. Fruits are used as vegetable.

Kayaputi – *Melaleuca leucadendron* L.; Cajeput tree (E); Myrtaceae; tree. Cultivated as an ornamental, often for hedges. Tender shoots and leaves are the source of cajeput oil which is used as an expectorant, carminative, anthelmintic against roundworms, mosquito repellent and insecticide. Wood is very strong and is used for railway sleepers and ship building.

Keetavasa (S) – *see* Majuphal.

Kela; Kadali (S), Rambha (S) – *Musa paradisiaca* L. (syn. *M. sapientum* L.); Banana (E); Musaceae; large tree-like herb. Cultivated for its highly nutritious fruits which are used as a widely popular dessert fruit when ripe, and vegetable when green and raw. Ripe fruits are considered to be useful in diarrhoea, dysentery, nephritis, uraemia, diabetes, gout, hypertension and heart diseases. Ripe fruits are a rich source of sugars, minerals and vitamins. The core of pseudo-stem and young flowers are used as vegetable; the starch obtained from pseudo-stem is used for sizing cloth. Fresh leaves are used as disposable platters and they are also considered to be auspicious and used for decoration in many Hindu rituals. The plant includes all the diploid and tetraploid clones, chiefly hybrids of *M. acuminata* Colla, and *M. balbisiana* Colla. The latter also has edible fruits (syn. *M. sapientum* var. *pruinosa* King ex. Cowan & Cowan).

Keli – *see* Sabbajaya.

Kemuka (S) – *see* Keu.

Kendu, Temru – *Diospyros exsculpta* Buch-Ham.; Nepal ebony persimmon (E); Ebenaceae; small tree. Leaves are used as 'beedi' wrappers. Fruits are edible. Wood is traded as black ebony and is used for cabinet work, picture frames, caskets and carving.

Kendwa – *see* Khirun.

Keol – *see* Kahimal.

Keora, Gagandhul; Ketaki (S) – *Pandanus odoratissimus* L.f.; Screw-pine (E); Pandanaceae; shrub. Male inflorescence is the source of 'kewra attar', a highly esteemed and popular perfume, used for scenting syrups, hair oils, incense, soaps and cosmetics. It is also used for flavouring Indian sweetmeats, foods and soft drinks. Seeds, tender floral spathes and terminal bud are edible. Leaves are used for mats, baskets, hats, thatching and as a source of fibre which is good for paper manufacture and sacks. Leaves are used medicinally for brain and heart diseases and externally for treating scabies and leprosy.

Keora-ka-mul; Padma-pushkara (S) – *Iris germanica* L.; German iris (E), Orris (E); Iridaceae; perennial herb. Rhizomes are the source of orris oil used in perfumery. They are also used for liver disorder, dropsy and bronchitis. All parts are rich in ascorbic acid. Leaf extract is rich in vitamin P and ascorbic acid and is used for curing injury to frozen feet caused by frostbite.

Keri – *see* Banpatara.

Kesar, Jafran, Zafran; Keshara (S) – *Crocus sativus* L.; Saffron crocus (E); Iridaceae; bulbous herb. Flower part called stigmas is collected, dried, and marketed as saffron of commerce, and considered to be stomachic, stimulant and sedative, but is used chiefly as a food-flavouring and colouring agent for confectionery, culinary and bakery products. Stigmas are rich in crocin a yellow glycoside and picrocrocin a colourless one, along with some volatile oils.

Kesaraja (S) – *see* Bhangra and Peela bhangra.

Kesari – *see* Khesari.

Keshara (S) – *see* Kesar.

Ketaki (S) – *see* Keora.

Keu; Kemuka (S) – *Costus speciosus* (Koen. Ex Retz.) Sm.; Costaceae; herb. Cultivated as an ornamental. Rhizomes are edible after cooking, and are considered to be a tonic and purgative. Roots are anthelmintic. Rhizomes are commercially important as they are a rich source of diosgenin, a precursor of steroids.

Khadira (S) – *see* Khair.

Khair, Kaththa; Khadira (S) – *Acacia catechu* (L.f.) Willd.; Black cutch (E), Catechu (E); Mimosaceae; tree. 'Kaththa' or catechu is obtained from the heartwood, and is extensively consumed as an important ingredient of betel leaf chewed as a masticatory in the Indian subcontinent. Cutch which is also extracted from the heartwood is used for dyeing canvas, ropes, fishing nets and in plywood adhesives. 'Kheersal', another product which is found in some of the older trees, is used for curing cough and sore-throat in indigenous systems of medicine. Gum exuded by the tree called 'khair' gum is used as a substitute for gum-arabic. Wood is used for tools and implements and is considered excellent for wheel-spokes and wheel-hubs.

Khair champa, Son champa, Golainchi; Kshira champa (S) – *Plumeria rubra* forma *acuminata* Sant. & Irani ex Shah.; Pagoda tree (E), Temple tree (E), Frangipani (E); Apocynaceae; small dichotomously branched tree. Cultivated as an ornamental tree for its beautiful and fragrant creamy white flowers with yellow centre. Latex of the plant contains alkaloids and is used in ointments for itch, gum troubles and rheumatism. Bark decoction is used in venereal diseases and is also considered to be antiherpatic. Wood is termite free and is used for some musical instruments. Roots are cathartic. Recent studies show that the tree can withstand drought, salt sprays and very adverse conditions. It is popular for landscaping besides people's preference to plant it near religious places.

Khaja – *see* Ekdania.

Khajeria – *see* Jangli khajur.

Khajur, Pind khajur – *Phoenix dactylifera* L.; Date palm (E); Palmae; tall unbranched tree with terminal crown. Cultivated for its edible fruits. Ripe fruits are highly nutritious and rich in sugars and minerals, they are consumed both fresh and preserved. They are considered to be expectorant, laxative and demulcent, and also fermented to prepare good quality brandy. Softened seeds are used as feed for goats, camels and horses and are rich in oxalic acid. Tree is tapped for its sweet sap which is used for preparing date-palm sugar and jaggery. Leaves are used for basketry and thatching. Gum obtained from the tree is used for diarrhoea.

Khajuri, Khajur – *Phoenix sylvestris* (L.) Roxb.; Wild date-palm (E), Date-sugar palm (E); Palmae; tall palm. Cultivated for its sweet fruits, which are eaten fresh and preserved as dry fruit or as jams and jellies. Sap obtained from tapped trees known as 'nira' provides a refreshing drink rich in vitamin B and C and it is also fermented to prepare toddy. It can also be concentrated to give highly nutritive date-sugar and date-jaggery. Leaves are used for basketry, mats, brooms, fishing-nets and thatching. Roots are chewed to relieve toothache.

Khakan – *see* Bara pilu.

Khamalu – *see* Chupri alu.

Khamara – *see* Bhillaura.

Khambar; Kanakchampa (S) – *Ochna jabotapita* L.; Ochnaceae; small tree. Cultivated as an ornamental. Wood is considered to be good for carving, inlay-work and walking-sticks. Root decoction is used in menstrual disorders and asthma. Bark is used as a tonic. Leaves are lopped for fodder.

Khantodi – *Ceropegia hirsuta* Wight & Arn.; Asclepiadaceae; twining herb. Root tubers are edible. Another species *C. oculata* Hook. is also known by the same Hindi name and also bears edible root tubers.

Khapparkadu – *Ceropegia bulbosa* Roxb.; Asclepiadaceae; herb. Root tubers and the succulent acidic leaves are edible.

Kharbuja; Madhupaka (S) – *Cucumis melo* L.; Muskmelon (E); Cucurbitaceae; creeping annual herb. Cultivated for its delicious fruits eaten as dessert. Seed kernels are edible, rich in a fatty oil, and considered to be cooling and diuretic. Roasted seed kernels are used in confectionery and snacks. Seed pulp is used for treating chronic eczema.

Khardol – *see* Banharria.

Kharenta – *see* Bariara.

Kharenti – *see* Kungyi.

Khari-lani – *Suaeda maritima* (L.) Dum.; Common Indian saltwort (E); Chenopodiaceae; herb characteristic of moist saline soils. Plant is considered to be a good sand-binder on sea shores and for reclaiming saline soils. Leaves are edible after cooking.

Kharindroyan – *Cucumis prophetarum* L.; Wild cucumber (E); Cucurbitaceae; herb. Plant is considered to be highly toxic, emetic and purgative.

Kharjal – *see* Chhota pilu.

Kharmor – *Rungia repens* (L.) Nees.; Acanthaceae; herb. Dried and pulverized plants are used for cough and fever, and are also considered to be diuretic and vermifuge. Fresh leaf juice mixed with castor oil is used for curing the scaly infection of scalp, caused by *Tinea capititis*.

Kharnub – *Ceratonia siliqua* (L.); Locust bean (E), Carob tree (E); Caesalpiniaceae; tree. Fruits and seeds are rich in proteins and sugar and are used as a stock feed; they are also considered good for preparing syrups. Seed endosperm is the source of a gum called carob gum which is used as a thickner in calico-printing, colour pastes and sauces. It is also used in sizing of paper, tanning, cosmetics, pharmaceuticals, paints, adhesives, polishes and ceramics. St John's bread considered to be a delicacy, is the sweet mucilaginous pulp from the beans. Seeds are used as a substitute of coffee and also yield a fatty oil besides the gum. Pods are used for cough.

Kharpat – *see* Ghogar.

Kharpudi – *Ceropegia lawii* Hook.; Asclepiadaceae; succulent herb. Root tubers are edible.

Khartua – *Chenopodium murale* L.; Chenopodiaceae; herb. Plants make good fodder.

Khas – *see* Afim.

Khas-khas, Bena, Gandhar; Sugandhimula (S) – *Vetiveria zizanioides* (L.) Nash.; Vetiver (E); Khus-khus (E); Gramineae; tall perennial grass. Cultivated for its aromatic roots, which are the source of vetiver oil that is used in perfumery, cosmetics and syrups. Oil is also used in medicines for treating vomiting, flatulence, colic, lumbago, sprains and rheumatic pain. Dried roots are used as padding to make thick door-screens and window-curtains which on wetting make the rooms cool during summer and also add fragrance. Leaves are used for thatching and for the manufacture of paper.

Khatmitthi – *Oxalis pes-caprae* L.; Bermuda butter cup (E); Oxalidaceae; herb. leaves are used as vegetable and in chutneys.

Khatta – *Citrus aurantium* L.; Seville orange (E), Sour orange (E); Rutaceae; small tree. Fruits are acidic, edible, and are used for confectionery, marmalades, and squashes. Fruit peel, leaves and flowers yield an essential oil used in perfumery. The variety called *bergamia* Watt., yields bergamot oil from fresh fruit-rinds, and petit grain oil from leaves which are used in the manufacture of cosmetics and soaps. Plant also serves as a hardy root-stock for grafting mandarin-orange, lemon, sweet-orange and grape-fruit.

Khatta-palak – *Rumex acetosa* L.; Garden sorrel (E); Polygonacee; herb. Leaves are used as pot-herb and as salad. Dried root powder is diuretic and is used for combating diarrhoea and bleeding. Herb is also used for bronchial disorders and skin ailments.

Khatte chawal; Laghulonika (S) – *Portulaca quadrifida* L.; Portulacaceae; succulent herb. Plant is used in medicines for the treatment of asthma, cough, ulcers, inflammation and urinary discharges. Poultice of the plant is used on haemorrhoids.

Khatti buti – *see* Amrul.

Khejri – *see* Chaunkra.

Khel – *see* Kartah.

Khesari, Kesari; Sandika (S) – *Lathyrus sativus* L.; Jarosse (E); Chickling pea (E); Papilionaceae; hardy annual herb. Cultivated in some parts of India for fodder. Seeds are consumed as a pulse by poor classes. If used as a principal diet over long periods, it can cause lathyrism or paralysis of the lower limbs due to the presence of β-N-oxalyl amino alanine, a neurotoxin and β-amino propio nitrile, an oesteo-toxin, which cause the crippling that may persist. The former i.e. BOAA has been implicated as the cause of lathyrism in humans. Fatty oil from the seeds is cathartic, but poisonous. Protein from the seeds is used in the preparation of adhesives used for sticking plywood.

Kheta chirayeta – *see* Barik chirayeta.

Kheu, Suthara – *Melanorrhoea usitata* Wall.; Burmese lacquer tree (E); Anacardiaceae; tree. Trees are tapped for lacquer called thitsi, a natural varnish which is used as a preservative for wood and leather and for water-proofing cloth, paper and boats. Oleo-resin from the tree is used in leprosy and also considered to be an anthelmintic. Wood is used for construction work, bridges, rafters, railway carriages, implements and furniture.

Khewnau, Jahrphali – *Ficus samicordata* Buch-Ham ex J.E. Smith.; Moraceae; tree. Fruits are edible, and are also preserved as jam. Root-juice is used in bladder complaints. Bark is the source of fibre used for ropes. Tree serves as a host to lac-insect. Leaves are lopped for fodder.

Khilut, Tilluk, Retwa – *Sclerostachya fusca* (Roxb.) A. Camus.; Gramineae; robust grass. Culms are used for making screens and light fencing. Cellulose content is suitable for the manufacture of wrapping paper, cardboards and other cellulose products.

Khinna – *see* Khirun.

Khip – *see* Jhamo; *see also* Mahur.

Khira; Sukasa (S) – *Cucumis sativus* L.; Cucumber (E); Cucurbitaceae; trailing annual herb. Cultivated for its tender green fruits which are used fresh for salads. Seeds are considered to be cooling, tonic and diuretic, and are rich in an edible fatty oil.

Khirni – *Manilkara kauki* (L.) Dubard (syn. *Mimusops kauki* L.); Kauki tree (E); Sapotaceae; tree. Cultivated for its edible fruits. Ripe fruits are ovoid, orange red in colour and sweet. Seeds are considered as tonic and the wood is used for furniture and implements. Root and bark are used for diarrhoea in infants. Another species *M. hexandra* (Roxb.) Dub. also known by the same Hindi name also bears edible fruits, but is chiefly used as a root-stock for grafting 'chiku' or sapodilla.

Khirun, Khinna, Kendwa – *Sapium insigne* Trimen.; Euphorbiaceae; robust deciduous tree. Wood is used for making packing boxes, floats, toys, and match boxes. Leaves are lopped for fodder.

Khokali, Kuppi; Harita-manjari (S) – *Acalypha indica* L.; Indian Acalypha (E); Euphorbiaceae; annual herb. Plant constitutes the drug used for treating bronchitis, croupy laryngitis, asthma, haemoptysis and rheumatism. Active principles include the alkaloid acalyphine and a cyanogenetic glucoside. Fresh leaf-juice acts as an emetic and is also used for cutaneous disorders.

Khopra – *see* Nariyal.

Khorial, Supota – *Parkia roxburghii* G. Don.; Mimosaceae; small tree. Tender pods are edible. Seeds are consumed after roasting. Whole fruit is used for treating gastric disorders. Bark and leaf infusion is used for skin ailments.

Khubani, Zardalu – *Prunus armeniaca* L.; Apricot (E); Rosaceae; tree. Fruits are very nutritious and consumed both fresh and dried. Kernel of some varieties is sweet and edible. Kernels yield a fatty oil, used in cosmetics and pharmaceuticals. The left over seed-cake is unfit as a stock-feed because of the presence of amygdalin and is used only as manure. Seed-cake also yields an essential oil identical with bitter-almond oil.

Khubasi, Sonchala – *Malva rotundifolia* L.; Dwarf mallow (E), Cheese-cake flowers (E); Malvaceae; herb. Tender shoots are used as salad; plant is used as pot-herb and fodder. Dried leaves and seeds are demulcent and used in piles. Seeds are also used in the treatment of cough, bronchitis, haemorrhoids and skin diseases.

Khubkalan, Jangli sarson – *Sisymbrium irio* L.; London rocket (E); Cruciferae; annual herb. Leaves are used as pot-herb, and are rich in minerals and vitamins specially vitamin C and β-carotene. Seeds are used for combating asthma and also considered as a rubefacient. Fatty oil from the seeds is used as a lubricant and in the manufacture of soaps.

Khulkhuri – *Hydrocotyle sibthorpioides* Lam.; Hydrocotylaceae; herb. Plant is considered to be a diuretic and vermifuge and is used for treating digestive, cutaneous and pulmonary disorders and also rheumatism. Roots are used for liver complaints and leaves for treating boils.

Khumbi – *Agaricus campestris* L. [syn. *Psalliota campestris* (L.) Fr.]; Field mushroom (E); Agaricaceae; fleshy saprophytic fungus. Fruiting bodies called mushrooms, are consumed at the mature button stage and are considered to be a rich source of protein and vitamins B complex, C, D and K.

Khurasani ajvayan; Dipya (S), Parasikaya (S) – *Hyoscyamus niger* L.; Henbane (E); Solanaceae; herb. Dried leaves and flowering tops comprise the source of the drug henbane, which is used as a sedative for asthma, whooping cough and nervous disorders. It is poisonous when taken in large doses leading to giddiness and delirium; chief alkaloids *viz.* hyoscyamine and hyoscine are narcotic, mydriatic and anodyne in action.

Khurbanti – *see* Nilkanthi.

Khursa – *see* Kulfa.

Khurti-ki-phali – *see* Guar.

Kikar, Babul – *Acacia nilotica* (L.) Willd. ex Del. ssp. *indica* (Benth.) Brenan. (syn. *Acacia arabica* Willd.); Babul Acacia (E); Mimosaceae; tree found in dry and arid zones, and considered to be a very useful afforestation plant. Three varieties *viz.*, *vediana* Cooke., *cupressiformis* Steward and 'telia babul', are known. Bark is a rich source of tannin which is used in tannng industry. Gum (gum acacia) from the tree is widely used in calico printing, dyeing, sizing, and in white-washing and distempering solutions. Being demulcent it finds use in pharmacy and medicine and in lozenges and sweetmeats. Gum is also used as a substitute of gum arabic. Wood is used for agricultural implements, axles, spokes, shafts and as fuel. Tender shoots and pods are used as fodder.

Kilbli – *Colvillea racemosa* Boj ex Hook.; Colville's glory (E); Caesalpiniaceae; tree. Cultivated as an ornamental usually for hedges and for its bright orange flowers.

Kimsuka – *see* Palas lata.

Kimu – *see* Himu.

Kingani – *see* Baikal.

Kinkar, Bouli – *Acacia jacquemontii* Benth.; Mimosaceae; thorny small tree with yellow, fragrant flowers. It is considered to be good as a sand-binder and useful for planting in arid zones. Wood yields gunpowder charcoal. Bark yields tannin. Gum is edible and tender branches are used as fodder.

Kinoo – *Citrus reticulata* Blanco. (product of intraspecific cross between the *willow-leaf* and *king* varieties of the common mandarin); Kinoo mandarin (E); Rutaceae; small tree. Fruit is delicious, very juicy and eaten fresh as dessert. Fruit pulp is rich in sugars, minerals and vitamin C. Fruit peel is rich in citrus oil, pectin and carotene.

Kiramar; Dhumra-patra (S) – *Aristolochia bracteolata* Lamk.; Bracteated-birthwort (E); Aristolochiaceae; bitter prostrate herb. Root decoction is used medicinally to expel roundworms. Leaf juice with castor oil is used for eczema. Seeds contain a non-drying fatty oil. Plant contains aristolochic acid.

Kirata (S) – *see* Kirayat.

Kirata-tikta (S) – *see* Chirayeta.

Kirath – *see* Vilayati lassan.

Kirayat, Kalmegh; Kirata (S) – *Andrographis paniculata* Wall ex Nees.; Creat (E). King of bitters (E); Acanthaceae; annual herb. Drug known as 'kalmegh' comprises stems, leaves and inflorescence and is considered a bitter tonic; it is used for debility, dyspepsia, dysentery, sluggish liver, fever, bronchitis, itch and piles. Leaves and roots are anthelmintic. Herb is often used as a substitute for chirayeta.

Kirmala; Gadadhari (S) – *Artemisia maritima* L.; Worm-seed (E); Santonica (E); Compositae; aromatic undershrub with the leaves being white underneath. The Indian var. *thomsoniana* C.B. Clarke contains the alkaloid santonin. The parts used include the dry unopened flower-heads and immature leaves. The drug santonin is used for expulsion of roundworms and threadworms. Herb decoction is used as a febrifuge. The varieties *'neercha'* and *'seski'* are rich in an essential oil.

Kirua – *see* Kari.

Kiryat-charayatah – *see* Chirayeta.

Kishmish – *see* Angoor.

Kiwach, Goncha; Atamagupta (S) – *Mucuna prurita* Hook.; Cowitch (E), Cowhage (E); Papilionaceae; twining annual. Cultivated for its tender young leaves and pods which are used as vegetable. Roots act as a tonic, diuretic, and purgative and are used in dropsy, kidney and nervous disorders, and externally in ointments for treating elephantiasis. Seeds are considered to be aphrodisiac, and are also used as nervine tonic.

Kiwi-phal – *Actinidia chinensis* Planch.; Kiwi fruit (E), Chinese gooseberry (E); Actinidiaceae; straggling woody shrub. Although native to China, the plant has been successfully introduced in Himachal Pradesh (India) from New Zealand. Fruit is edible, tasty, nutritious with juicy pulp and good keeping quality; it is used raw as a dessert fruit or preserved into jam, jelly and marmalade and has excellent economic potential as a promising fruit crop.

Kochi – *see* Shikakai.

Koda – *see* Chamror.

Kodhab – *Cadaba fruticosa* (L.) Druce (syn. *C. farinosa* Forsk.); Capparidaceae; small tree. Wood is used for turnery. Root and leaf decoction is used for uterine obstruction, and their poultice is used for sores. Plant is considered to be anthelmintic and antisyphilitic.

Kodo, Kodra; Kodrava (S) – *Paspalum scrobiculatum* L.; Kodo millet (E); Gramineae; herb. Cultivated for fodder and also grains which can be used after storage for six months. Stem juice is reported to be used to treat corneal opacity.

Kodra – *see* Kodo.

Kodrava (S) – *see* Kodo.

Koi – *see* Bhenght.

Koka – *see* Bhenght.

Kokam, Vishambil – *Garcinia indica* (Dupetit-Thouars) Choisy; Kokam butter tree (E), Brindonia tallow tree (E); Mangosteen oil tree (E); Guttiferae; tall tree. Ripe sweet fruits are edible, also made into syrups and jellies, and considered as cardiotonic and anthelmintic. Seeds are the source of kokam butter and an edible fat considered as an emollient and astringent; it is used in ointments for skin ailments, pharmaceuticals, and for the manufacture of soaps and candles.

Kokan – *see* Lal-murghka.

Kokaraye; Shveta-dhataki (S) – *Calycopteris floribunda* (Roxb.) Lamk.; Combretaceae; diffuse shrub. Leaves act as an anthelmintic, laxative and astringent. Leaf-juice is used for controlling excessive thirst.

Kokilaksha (S) – *see* Talimakhana.

Kolkanda (S) – *see* Ban piyazi.

Komal – *Koelzella pabularia* (Lindl.) Hiroe. (syn. *Prangos pabularia* Lindl.); Umbelliferae; perennial herb. Roots are diuretic and also used for treating itch, indigestion and irregular menstruation. They are the source of an essential oil and are rich in coumarin compounds. Fruits are considered to be laxative, carminative, aphrodisiac, stimulant, diuretic and liver tonic. Dried plant is used as a stock-feed.

Kondai – *see* Kondari.

Kondari, Kondai – *Flacourtia sepiaria* Roxb.; Flacourtiaceae; small tree. Fruits are edible; wood is used for making charcoal and for construction work. Bark decoction in sesame oil is used topically for rheumatism. Leaves are lopped for fodder.

Konpal sehund; Trikantaka (S), Vajradruma (S) – *Euphorbia tirucalli* L.; Indian tree spurge (E), Milk bush (E); Euphorbiaceae; small tree with succulent stems without spines found in arid wasteland. Latex or milk is used for treating neuralgia, asthma, cough, toothache and rheumatism; it is also used locally for warts. Roots are used for stupefying fish. Being rich in hydrocarbons, and easily grown on marginal, wasteland and arid lands, it offers immense potential as a promising petro-crop.

Kooshmanda (S) – *see* Petha.

Kootu – *see* Kutu.

Korake–*see* Chakwat.

Koshaphala (S)–*see* Bindak.

Koshapushpi (S) – *see* Kanshurra.

Koshataki (S) – *see* Kali tori.

Koshta, Mithapat, Tossa – *Corchorus olitorius* L.; Jews mallow (E); Tossa jute (E); Tiliaceae; erect sparsely branched shrub. Cultivated for its fibre obtained by retting of stems and used for making sacs, coarse packing-cloth, rugs, ropes and twines. Infusion of leaves acts as a tonic and febrifuge.

Kotagandhal, jilpai; Iswara (S) – *Ixora arborea* Roxb.; Torchwood Ixora (E); Rubiaceae; small tree. Branches are made into torches, and wood is used for building work, turnery and engraving. Fruits are edible. Decoction of bark has tonic properties and is used for anaemia.

Koushikaha (S) – *see* Guggul.

Kramighna phal – *Maesa indica* Wall.; Myrsinaceae; small tree. Fruits are anthelmintic and edible and are also used as fish poison. Leaves are used in curries. Roots are used to treat syphilis. Wood is used for fencing, house-posts and fuel.

Krisna-aguru (S) – *Vepris bilocularis* (Wight & Arn.) Engl.; Rutaceae; large evergreen tree. Wood is used for making cart wheels, spokes and helves. Wood boiled in oil is used for rheumatism, leprosy and asthma. Root decoction is used for biliousness.

Krishnabija (S) – *see* Nilkalmi.

Krishna-kamboji (S) – *see* Buinowla.

Krishna keli (S) – *see* Gulabash.

Krishnasara (S) – *see* Gab.

Krishna-toot – *see* Shah-toot.

Krishna-tulsi – *see* Tulsi.

Kshetraparpata (S) – *see* Daman papra.

Kshira champa (S) – *see* Khair champa.

Kshiradruma (S) – *see* Peepal.

Kshudra-pashanabheda (S) – *see* Pashana-bhedak.

Kuchila lata – *Strychnos colubrina* L.; Strychnaceae; woody climber found in S. India. Leaves and roots decoction in oil is used for rheumatic inflammation. Wood paste is used in dyspepsia. Roots are anthelmintic and purgative and are also used for skin ailments. Alkaloids strychnine and brucine are present.

Kuchla, Bailewa; Chipita (S) – *Strychnos nux-vomica* L.; Nux-vomica (E); Strychnaceae; deciduous tree. Dry ripe, bitter seeds are the source of the drug 'kupilu' or nux vomica which is used as a tonic, and for nervous disorders and paralysis. Seeds form part of the prescriptions for treating colic and scalp infections. Leaf poultice is used for sloughing wounds. Bark decoction is used in epilepsy. Wood is termite-free, and is used for agricultural implements. Juice of fresh wood is used in dyspepsia, fever and dysentery. Alkaloids strychnine and brucine are present in all parts of the plant but are very concentrated in the seeds which can be deadly poisonous.

Kuchle-ka-malang – *Viscum monoicum* Roxb. ex. DC.; Viscaceae; partial parasitic shrub. Plant becomes a powerful narcotic, when parasitic on 'Kuchla' i.e. nux-vomica trees and acquires properties similar to it, and also used as its substitute.

Kudaliya – *Desmodium triflorum* (L.) DC.; Papilionaceae; trailing and much branched herb. The plant is considered to be good as a soil-binder and as fodder. It is also suitable as green turf for lawns and pastures. Leaves are used for curing convulsions, diarrhoea and dysentery.

Kudumi – *Polyalthia cerasoides* (Roxb.) Bedd.; Annonaceae; small tree. Fruits are edible. Wood is used for construction work, rafters, packing boxes and boats.

Kuji, Kunja, Kwiala; Sewati (S) – *Rosa brunonii* Lindl.; Himalayan musk rose (E); Rosaceae; climbing shrub. Flower petals are very fragrant and are used for extraction of 'attar' or otto of roses. Wood is good for walking-sticks.

Kukar-makri, Durpa-tandar – *Polygonum amplexicaule* D. Don.; Polygonaceae; herb. Rootstocks are rich in tannin and serve as the source of the drug 'anjubar' which is used in Ayurvedic and Unani systems of medicine. Plants are used as fodder.

Kukua-lata, Mulluta – *Thunbergia grandiflora* (Roxb. ex Rottl.) Roxb.; Thunbergiaceae; woody climber. Cultivated as an ornamental for its beautiful flowers and foliage. Leaf decoction is used in gastric disorders and leaves are considered to be a rich source of potassium.

Kukuradru (S) – *see* Kakranda.

Kukurbicha, Kakarundah – *Grewia hirsuta* Vahl. (syn. *G. polygama* Mast.); Tiliaceae; shrub. Fruits are edible and are used medicinally in diarrhoea and dysentery.

Kukurkat – *see* Bhaulan.

Kulai – *Chlorophytum tuberosum* Baker; Liliaceae; undershrub. Roots are edible.

Kulanjan – *Alpinia officinarum* Hance; Lesser galangal (E); Zingiberaceae; perennial herb. Rhizomes are aromatic, pungent and with spicy odour and they are used in curry powders and for flavouring tobacco and liquor. They are also considered to be stimulant and carminative.

Kulanjan (S) – *see* Bara-kulanjan.

Kulantha (S) – *see* Kulthi.

Kulfa, Bara-laniya, Khursa; Brihalloni (S) – *Portulaca oleracea* L.; Common purslane (E); Portulacaceae; herb. Tender shoots are used as pot-herb and in soups. Herb considered as a diuretic, is used in liver, spleen, bladder and kidney disorders. It is also used in remedies for treating dysuria, dysentery, ulceration of mouth, sore nipples and cardio-vascular diseases. Herb is rich in minerals specially potassium salts.

Kulthi; Kulaththa (S) – *Dolichos biflorus* L.; Horse-gram (E); Papilionaceae; trailing herb. Cultivated for fodder. Seeds are edible after cooking or frying, and are considered to be tonic, astringent and diuretic.

Kulu – *see* Gulu.

Kumach, Tohar sem – *Mucuna cochinchinensis* (Lour.) A Cheval; Lyon bean (E); Papilionaceae; trailing herb. Cultivated as a cover crop, for fodder and green manure. Pods are used as vegetable after removing skin.

Kumal – *see* Ulatkambal.

Kumali – *Leea edgeworthii* Santapau; Leeaceae; shrub. Roots, leaves and fruits are edible.

Kumbhi (S) – *see* Kalikatbhi.

Kumbhika (S) – *see* Jalkhumbi.

Kumbi – *see* Peeli kapas and Kalikatbhi.

Kumeria, Parwa, Shurval, Sura – *Heteropogon contortus* (L.) Beauv. ex Roem et Schult.; Bellary grass (E), Spear grass (E); Gramineae; perennial grass. Plants are considered to be good soil-binder and are used both for fodder and silage. Roots act as a stimulant and diuretic. Culms are used for mats.

Kumpaiman – *see* Bairola.

Kumra – *see* Safed kaddu.

Kumta; Sneta khadira (S) – *Acacia senegal* (L.) Willd.; Gum-arabic Acacia (E); Mimosaceae; small tree; Stem bark exudes the true gum arabic which has miscellaneous uses *viz.* in confectionery, chewing gum, pharmaceuticals, adhesives, sizing of textiles and paper, and lithographic printing. Being a demulcent, its use extends to ointments and lotions for burns, sores, and inflammation, and as a suspending agent of hair-setting creams. Roots are used for nodular leprosy and dysentery. Bark is the source of fibre for ropes. Wood is used for implements and leaves are used as fodder.

Kumud, Pandharen kamal; Kumuda (S) – *Nymphaea alba* L.; European white water-lily (E); Nymphaeaceae; perennial aquatic herb. Decoction of fresh rhizomes is used for diarrhoea. Fresh flowers and fruits decoction is also used for diarrhoea. Parched seeds and boiled rhizomes are edible. Rhizomes contain the alkaloid nymphaeine, which has a sedative effect in small doses while large doses can be paralytic. They are also used for tanning.

Kumuda (S) – *see* Kumud.

Kun-chandana (S) – *see* Bari-ghumchi.

Kundali (S) – *see* Kantagur-kamai.

Kundphul; Vasanta (S) – *Jasminum multiflorum* (Burm. f.) Andr.; Downy jasmine (E); Oleaceae; ornamental scandent shrub. Cultivated for its beautiful densely profuse umbellated flowers. Dried leaf poultice is used for ulcers.

Kundri, Tarali – *Melothria heterophylla* (Lour.) Cogn.; Cucurbitaceae; climbing herb. Roots are stimulant and purgative and are considered invigorating in spermatorrhoea and dysuria. Leaf juice is used locally for getting rid of inflammation caused by 'bhilawa' or marking-nut juice. Fruits and leaves are edible.

Kundru, Kanduri – *Coccinia grandis* (L.) Voigt.; Ivy gourd (E), Kovai fruit (E); Cucurbitaceae; climbing robust herb. Cultivated for its green fruits which are used as vegetable. Leaves and tender shoots are used as pot-herb. Juice of roots and leaves is considered to be useful in diabetes.

Kungku, Barphali – *Euonymus tingens* Wall.; Spindle wood (E); Celastraceae; small tree. Inner bark is the source of a dye. Bark is used for treating chronic constipation, indigestion and eye trouble. Wood is used for carving.

Kungyi, Kharenti, Bala – *Sida cordifolia* L.; Country-mallow (E); Malvaceae; shrub. Roots are astringent, diuretic and tonic, and are used as a component of the Ayurvedic prescription termed 'Bala-chatustya' (mixture of roots of four different plants) *viz.*, 'Mahabala' (*S. rhombifolia*), 'Bhumibala' (*S. veronicaefolia*), 'Bala' (*S. cordifolia*) and 'Atibala' (*Abutilon indicum*). Root infusion is used for hematuria, cystitis, urinary disorder, facial paralysis, sciatica and leucorrhoea. Seeds are demulcent and are used in bowel complaints. Stem yields a rough fibre. Presence of the alkaloid ephedrine has been reported from the plant.

Kuni (S) – *see* Kamrup.

Kunis – *Alnus nitida* Endl.; Himalayan black cedar (E); Betulaceae; large tree. Wood is used for building purposes, tea-chests and match-sticks. Bark is the source of tannin and a dye.

Kunja – *see* Kuji.

Kunjuya, Lotloti – *Urena lobata* L. var. *sinuata* King; Malvaceae; shrub. Stem is the source of a fibre used for making fishing lines, and ropes. Leaf decoction is used for bladder and intestinal inflammation, and flower infusion for curing bronchitis; root extract is used externally for lumbago and as a skin emollient.

Kunlai – *see* Virtuli.

Kunzi – *see* Gulkhair.

Kuppi – *see* Khokali.

Kura – *see* Gwaladarim.

Kurchi – *see* Kutaja.

Kureli, Jhangi – *Hydrilla verticillata* (L.f.) Royle; Hydrocharitaceae; submerged or floating aquatic herb. The plant is extremely useful as an oxygenator for fish-ponds and also serves as food for some types of fish. Plants are also considered to be a good green manure.

Kuri, Kuriya – *Urochloa panicoides* Beauv.; Gramineae; herb. Cultivated as a fodder crop. Grains are also edible.

Kuriya – *see* Kuri.

Kurkur-jiwah – *Leea indica* (Burm. f.) Merr.; Leeaceae; shrub. Leaves are used as pot-herb, and also as green manure. Mucilaginous fresh roots are used to cure diarrhoea, dysentery and colitis.

Kurry-patta – *see* Mitha-neem.

Kuru – *see* Katki.

Kusar – *Jasminum malabaricum* Wight; Oleaceae; large scandent shrub. Cultivated for its fragrant flowers. Leaf juice is reported to be used for the treatment of cataract.

Kusha – *see* Dab.

Kushta (S) – *see* Kuth.

Kushth-nashini (S) – *see* Babchi.

Kussunt – *Maughania strobilifera* (L.) J. St. Hill. ex Jacks. (syn. *Flemingia strobilifera* R. Br.); Papilionaceae; undershrub, with distinct persistent large bracts. Roots are used as a sedative to relieve pain, and for the treatment of hysteria and epilepsy.

Kustumburi (S) – *see* Dhania.

Kusum – *Schleichera oleosa* (Lour.) Oken. (syn. *Pistacia oleosa* Lour.); Macassar oil tree (E), Lac tree (E), Ceylon oak (E); Sapindaceae; tree. Wood is used for agricultural implements, cart wheels, shafts, axles and construction work; it is also considered to be good for fuel and charcoal. Fruits are edible, raw ones are pickled. Seeds yield an oil called macassar oil used in soap manufacture, and as a lubricant. It is also used for hair dressing, culinary purposes, skin ailments and locally on rheumatic joints. Oil-cake is used as manure. Bark yields tannin and its paste is used for ulcers and inflammations. Flowers are the source of a dye. Leaves and tender shoots are lopped for fodder. Tree serves as a host to 'kusumi' lac insect.

Kusumbh, Kardi, Karrah, Kusumbha (S) – *Carthamus tinctorius* L.; Safflower (E); Compositae; herb. Cultivated extensively as an oil-seed crop. Fruits (achenes) yield an oil which after refining serves as a very good cooking medium. Oil is also used for the manufacture of paints, varnishes, linoleum, soaps and applied locally to sores and rheumatic joints. Oil-cake is used as a stock-feed. Flower-heads or capitula yield a yellow dye which is used for colouring food, butter and cloth.

Kusumbha (S) – *see* Kusumbh.

Kutaja, Kurchi, Karwa-indrajau; Kalinga (S) – *Holarrhena antidysenterica* (L.) Wall. ex DC.; Easter tree (E), Ivory tree (E); Apocynaceae; small tree. Seeds, leaves and bark are used for curing diarrhoea and dysentery. Bark called conessi bark is used for treating amoebic dysentery, and contains the alkaloid conassine, tannin and a gum-resin. Seeds known as 'karwa-indrajau' are used for similar purpose. Fatty oil from the seeds is used as an anthelmintic. Wood is used for small carpentry.

Kuth; Kushta (S) – *Saussurea lappa* C.B. Clarke; Costus (E); Compositae; herb. Roots considered as carminative and stimulant are used for combating bronchial asthma, cough, rheumatism and skin ailments. Alcoholic extract of roots is very rich in an alkaloid and an essential oil; it is considered to be very useful in vagotonic asthma. Essential oil from the roots is used in perfumery and cosmetics. Roots show anti-fungal activity and are also used as a moth-proof for woollen clothes.

Kutki – *see* Karu, *see also* Katki and Shavan.

Kuttra – *Limnophila aromatica* (Lam.) Merr.; Scrophulariaceae; aromatic herb found on damp ground. Leaves are used raw as salad or as a pot-herb. Plant yields an essential oil, and possesses turpentine-like odour. Plant juice is considered to be antiseptic and a febrifuge. *Limnophila indica* (L.) Druce is also known by the same Hindi name and possesses camphor like odour.

Kutu, Kootu – *Fagopyrum esculentum* Moench; Buckwheat (E); Brank (E); Polygonaceae; herb. Cultivated as a minor grain-crop. Grains are made into porridge or flour for making bread. Grains are also used as a poultry feed. Hulls are the source of a dye. Leaves are a rich source of rutin which is used for decreasing capillary fragility.

Kuwar-buti – *Agave vera-cruz* Mill.; Blue elephant aloe (E); Agavaceae; xerophytic perennial with long narrow leaves on a condensed stem. Cultivated for fencing and as a soil binder. Leaves are the source of a fibre which is used for making mats and cordage.

Kwiala – *see* Kuji.

L

Lablab – *Hedera nepalensis* Koch.; Nepal ivy (E); Araliaceae; perennial evergreen, woody climber. Leaves are used for fomentation of enlarged glands. Fruits act as a cathartic and stimulant. Infusion of fruits is used in treating rheumatism. The intensely haemolytic active principle α-hederin, a glycoside is present. Seeds yield a semi-drying oil.

Laghududhika (S) – *see* Chhoti dudhi.

Laghulonika (S) – *see* Khatte chawal.

Laghuparnika (S) – *see* Murhari.

Laghupushpa madhukar (S) – *see* Bililotan.

Laghushlesh mataka (S) – *see* Gondi.

Lahichan – *see* Gual.

Lahouri-hurmul – *see* Harmal.

Lahra – *see* Bajra.

Lahsun – *see* Lassan.

Lai – *see* Pahari rai.

Lajalu – *Neptunia prostrata* (Lamk.) Baill.; Mimosaceae; annual aquatic herb. Pods and young stems are used as vegetable. Herb is astringent. Stem juice is used for curing earache, and that of the root for treating syphilis.

Lajja (S) – *see* Chui mui.

Lajwanti – *see* Chui mui.

Lakhmana; Lakshmana (S) – *Mandragora officinarum* L.; Mandrake (E); Solanaceae; herb. Roots are hypnotic with similar properties as belladona; they are used as anaesthetic and sedative, and contain the alkaloid mandragorine.

Lakshmana (S) – *see* Lakhmana.

Lakshmanphal – *see* Hanuman phala.

Lal ambari – *see* Patwa.

Lal barela – *see* Bhiunli.

Lal bichhua – *Fleurya interrupta* Gaud.; Urticaceae; herb with stinging hair. Root decoction is diuretic. Leaves are applied topically to carbuncles.

Lal botal-brush, Botal-brush – *Callistemon lanceolatus* DC.; Bottle-brush (E); Myrtaceae; small tree. Cultivated as an ornamental for its characteristic flowers, evergreen beautiful foliage and drooping branches; it is often planted in groves or as an avenue tree.

Lal champa – *Plumeria rubra* L.; Frangipani (E); Apocynaceae; small tree. Cultivated as an ornamental. Latex is used for tooth cavities and toothache.

Lal chandan; Rakta chandana (S) – *Pterocarpus santalinus* L.f.; Red sandalwood (E); Papilionaceae; tree. Wood is highly valued and is used for construction work and for dyeing cotton, wool and leather. Wood paste is used on inflammations and on the forehead to treat headache. Fruit decoction is used to cure chronic dysentery. Leaves are lopped for fodder.

Lal chini – *Amoora spectabilis* Miq.; Meliaceae; tree. Wood is suitable for plyboards, furniture and decorative work; it is also used for making railway carriages.

Lal-chitra; Rakta-chitraka – *Plumbago indica* L.; Plumbaginaceae; undershrub. Cultivated as an ornamental for its beautiful red flowers. Roots are used in the treatment of leucoderma, leprosy and syphilis. Plumbagin, the active principle acts in small doses as a stimulant on the central nervous system and the secretion of bile, sweat and urine.

Lalchuni – *Calophyllum soulattri* Burm f.; Nicobar canoe tree (E); Guttiferae; tall tree. Wood is used for planking, rafters, masts, boxes and plywood.

Laldana – *see* Sal.

Lal dudhi – *Euphorbia hirta* L.; Euphorbiaceae; erect to prostrate annual herb. The entire plant is used as an ingredient of medicines used for asthma, cough, urino-genital disorders, colic and dysentery. Latex is used on warts.

Lal indrayan, Mahakal; Shvetpushpi (S) – *Trichosanthes bracteata* (Lam.) Voigt.; Cucurbitaceae; trailing or climbing annual herb. Roots are used as paste on carbuncles and also in veterinary medicine. Fruit paste mixed with coconut oil is used for treating sores.

Lal jhari – *Geranium wallichianum* D. Don.; Wallich crane's bill (E); Geraniaceae; prostrate herb. Roots are used for tanning; they are considered to be astringent and are used for getting rid of toothache.

Lal-jhau, Farash – *Tamarix aphylla* (L.) Karst.; Athel tamarisk (E); Tamaricaceae; tree. Often cultivated as an ornamental, and for providing shelter belts and wind breaks. Wood is used for construction work, carts and agricultural implements. Twigs are used for making baskets. Bark is astringent and is used for cutaneous infections and eczema. Galls termed 'chhoti main' are used for tanning and as a mordant in dyeing; they are also used in gargles. The name 'Lal-jhau' is also used for *Tamarix dioica* Roxb. which has similar uses.

Lal jumrool – *Syzygium aqueum* (Burm. f.) Alston.; Watery rose apple (E); Myrtaceae; small tree found in East India. Ripe fruits are consumed fresh or made into syrup.

Lal kachnar – *see* Kaliar.

Lal kadsumbal – *see* Makhan sem.

Lal kumra – *see* Kaddu.

Lal lasora – *Cordia sebestena* L.; Geiger tree (E), Scarlet Cordia (E); Ehretiaceae; tree. Cultivated as an ornamental for its orange red flowers.

Lal mirch – *Capsicum annuum* L. var. *acuminatum* Fingh.; Red pepper (E), Chilli (E); Solanaceae; annual or perennial herb. Cultivated for its fruit which yields the dry chilli powder of commerce used extensively as a spice. Fresh green chillies are also used in chutneys and curries and made into pickle. Capsicum fruit contains the pungent principle capsaicin. It is used medicinally in counter-irritant preparations for rheumatism, neuralgia and lumbago.

Lal-murghka, Kokan, Morsikha; Mayura shikha (S) – *Celosia argentea* L. var. *cristata* Voss.; Cock's comb (E); Amaranthaceae; annual herb. Cultivated as an ornamental.

Lal post, Poste-ke-bija – *Papaver rhoeas* L.; Corn poppy (E), Papaveraceae; annual herb. Cultivated as an ornamental for its beautiful red flowers. Petals act as an expectorant, sedative and anodyne and their tincture is used for colouring medicines. All parts contain rhoeadine; latex from the capsules is narcotic. Seeds yield a fatty oil.

Lal-sabuni, Santhi, Shveta-punarnava (S) – *Trianthema portulacastrum* L.; Horse purslane (E); Aizoaceae; prostrate herb with succulent leaves. The leaves are diuretic and used in oedema, dropsy and disorders of liver and kidney. Decoction of the herb is used as a vermifuge and in rheumatism. Roots are cathartic and abortifacient and are used in amenorrhoea and asthma.

Lal-sag, Bari-chaulai, Chaulai sag – *Amaranthus tricolour* L.; Tampala (E), Chinese spinach (E), Amaranth (tender) (E); Amaranthaceae; herb. Cultivated for its leaves and tender shoots which are used as pot-herb and have high vitamin A and C content. Plant is astringent and is used in diarrhoea and dysentery. Decoction of the plant is used as a gargle for throat and mouth ulcers.

Lamajjaka (S) – *see* Lamjak.

Lamjak; Lamajjaka (S) – *Cymbopogon jwarancusa* Schult.; Gramineae; perennial grass. Leaves are rich in an essential oil with peppermint flavour. They are used in rheumatism, gout, dyspepsia and cough. Roots are used to cure fevers.

Lampa, Surwala – *Chrysopogon aciculatus* (Retz.). Trin.; Gramineae; perennial grass. Culms are used for thatching. Grains when consumed by grazing animals can cause mouth ulceration.

Langali (S) – *see* Langalia.

Langalia, Langali (S) – *Hydrolea zeylanica* Vahl.; Hydrophyllaceae; procumbent herb. Leaves are antiseptic. Leaf poultice is used on callusing ulcers.

Lani, Loonak – *Salsola baryosma* (R & S) Dandy; Saltwort (E); Chenopodiaceae; herb. Plant is used as camel fodder. Leaves yield 'manna'. Plant ash is used for curing itch.

Lanjai, Sangkupi; Vanajai (S) – *Clerodendrum inerme* (L.) Gaertn.; Verbenaceae; straggling shrub. Cultivated as an ornamental. Leaves are used as a febrifuge.

Lansa – *Aglaia domestica* (Correa emend Jack) Pallegrin; Langsat (E), Duku (E); Meliaceae; tree. Cultivated for its edible fruit. Wood is used for rafters and tool handles. Decoction of the bark, and resin from the peel of fruits are used for diarrhoea and dysentery. Peels contain an essential oil and are used as incense and mosquito repellent.

Lapetua – *see* Bachita

Laptuna – *Setaria verticillata* (L.) Beauv.; Bristly foxtail (E), Bur (E); Gramineae; herb. Cultivated for its grain which is used as food in arid regions; mature plants are too bristly for cattle feed but young plants can be used for fodder.

Lashtia, Masethi – *Tephrosia candida* (Roxb.) DC.; White Tephrosia (E); Papilionaceae; shrub. Often cultivated as an ornamental, wind-break and for green manuring and mulching in coffee, tea, coconut and rubber plantations. Plant shows insecticidal and piscicidal properties due to the presence of rotenoids. Bark and leaves are used as fish poison.

Lashuna (S) – *see* Lassan.

Lasora, Chokargond; Uddalaka (S), Bahuvaraka (S) – *Cordia dichotoma* var. *wallichii* (Cl.) Maheshwari; Clammy cherry (E), Sebesten (E); Ehretiaceae; small tree. Cultivated for fruits which are used as vegetable and also pickled. Fruits are also used medicinally for urinary and chest disorders. Wood is used for boats and agricultural implements and bark yields tannin.

Lassan, Lahsun; Lashuna (S) – *Allium sativum* L.; Garlic (E); Alliaceae; perennial herb, cultivated for its bulbs consisting of 'cloves', which are used as a spice, condiment and gastric stimulant. Bulbs are used medicinally for flatulence, dyspepsia and colic and in many remedies used for treating cough, fever and rheumatism. The active principle allicin is antibacterial and has inhibitory action on gram-negative bacteria specially of paratyphoid, typhoid and enteritis group. The juice of bulbs is used externally for curing earache and skin ailments.

Lata–achhuk; Pitadaru – *Morinda umbellata* L.; Rubiaceae; climbing shrub. Ripe fruits are edible and green fruits are used in curries. Roots are the source of a red dye called 'mang-kudu' which is used for batik paintings on fabrics; the colouring principles are morindin and morindone. Root and leaves decoction is used for diarrhoea and dysentery.

Latahai, Vasuka (S) – *Indigofera enneaphylla* L.; Papilionaceae; herb. Juice of the herb is antiscorbutic and diuretic and is used in the treatment of chronic venereal disorders. Herb decoction is used in epilepsy.

Latakasturicum (S) – *see* Kasturi dana.

Latapalasha (S) – *see* Palas lata.

Latjira, Puthkunda; Apamarga (S) – *Achyranthes aspera* L.; Prickly chaff flower (E); Amaranthaceae; herb or undershrub. Decoction of the plant is used for treating cough, bronchial infection, and renal dropsy.

Latkan – *see* Sinduria.

Latkua – *see* Kataphal.

Latmahuria, Gangetiya – *Digera muricata* (L.) Mart.; Amaranthaceae; herb. Tender shoots are used as pot-herb, and the plant is also grazed by cattle. Flowers and seeds infusion is used for checking urinary discharges.

Latman – *Deeringia amaranthoides* (Lamk.) Merr.; Amaranthaceae; herb or undershrub. Sometimes cultivated as an ornamental for its bright red panicles of flowers. Tender shoots are used as pot-herb; leaves are rich in alkaloids and applied to sores.

Laugauni – *see* Didhen.

Lauki – *see* Ghia.

Laung; Lavanga (S) – *Eugenia caryophyllus* (Spreng.) Bullock & Harrison [syn. *Syzygium aromaticum* (L.) Merr. & Perry]; Clove (E); Myrtaceae; evergreen tree. Dried flower buds are used as a spice and condiment, and are highly prized for their essential oil called clove oil which is used extensively for flavouring food products, fermented beverages, and as an ingredient of tooth-pastes, mouth washes, gargles and chewing gums. It is also used as a local analgesic in carious cavities and toothaches. Clove oil is also used as a clearing agent in histological work and for scenting soaps and toiletries. Large amount of synthetic vanillin used in ice-cream flavouring is manufactured from eugenol which is obtained from clove oil.

Launku – *Sechium edule* (Jack) Sw.; Chocho (E), Chayote (E); Christophine (E); Cucurbitaceae; trailing herb. Cultivated in different regions of India for its edible fruits. Tender shoots and flowers are used as pot-herb. Roots are the source of starch.

Lavana-valli (S) – *Asystasia gangetica* (L.) T. Anders; Acanthaceae; herb or undershrub. Cultivated as an ornamental for its beautiful blooms. Plant juice is used for treating swellings and rheumatism. Tender leaves are rich in thiamine.

Lavanga (S) – *see* Laung.

Lavni-anona – *see* Ramphal.

Leauri – *Cupressus torulosa* D. Don.; Himalayan cypress (E); Cupressaceae; large tree. Wood is the source of coniferous timber, which is used for furniture, construction work, flooring and ceiling. Wood shavings are used as packing material. Leaves are fragrant and rich in an essential oil.

Lichi – *Litchi chinensis* (Gaertn.) Sonn.; Leechee (E); Sapindaceae; small tree. Cultivated mainly for its delicious fruit with fleshy sweet edible aril, eaten fresh or canned. Seeds are used as an anodyne in neuralgic disorders. Bark is the source of tannin.

Lichora – *see* Gorakh amli.

Loban – *see* Luban.

Lobhia, Chowli; Nishapava (S) – *Vigna unguiculata* (L.) Walp.; Cowpea (E); Papilionaceae; Tender trailing herb. Cultivated for its young tender pods used as vegetable and its mature seeds used as a pulse. Plant is good as a green-manure crop and after harvesting of pods, serves as stock-feed. Starch from seeds is used for sizing of textiles. Seeds are antibilious and considered to be good in treating hepatic disorders.

Lodh; Lodhra (S), Marjana (S) – *Symplocos paniculata* Miq.; Sapphire berry (E); Symplocaceae; small tree. Leaves and bark are the source of a yellow dye, and are also used as a mordant with 'madar'. Wood is used for carving, and seeds yield an oil. Other species *viz.*, *S. racemosa* Roxb. and *S. sumuntia* Buch.-Ham. are also known as Lodh in Hindi and their bark and leaves are also sources of a yellow dye.

Lodhra (S) – *see* Lodh, *see also* Bholia.

Lohari – *see* Bistendu.

Lokat – *Eriobotrya japonica* (Thunb.) Lindl.; Loquat (E), Japan medlar (E); Rosaceae; evergreen tree. Cultivated for its yellow-orange juicy and fleshy fruits which are consumed fresh or made into jam and jelly. Flower decoction is used as an expectorant.

Lomasaa (S) – *see* Jatamansi.

Lonia – *see* Chhoti lani.

Loonak – *see* Lani.

Lotloti – *see* Kunjuya.

Luban, Loban – *Styrax benzoin* Dryand; Benzoin tree (E); Styracaceae; evergreen small tree. Incised bark yields a resin called gum-benzoin which is used medicinally as a diuretic, carminative and expectorant, and also used in inhalants for respiratory catarrh; it is also used for healing sores and ulcers in veterinary medicine. Benzoin is the source of benzoic acid and is used to fix odour of perfumes, cosmetics, toiletries and pharmaceuticals. Its usage extends to the manufacture of varnishes and laminated plastic sheets.

Luchra, Kansa – *Chionachne koenigii* (Spreng.) Thw.; Gramineae; tall grass. Fruits are used for rosary beads, and for making ornamental trays and baskets.

Lunak – *see* Chhoti lani.

M

Maalati, Gandhamalati (S) – *Aganosma caryophyllata* (Roxb. ex Sims.) G. Don.; Apocynaceae; climbing shrub. Cultivated as an ornamental. The plant is used as an anodyne and sedative in Ayurvedic medicine for treating neuralgia and sciatica.

Maamsi (S) – *see* Jatamansi.

Machni – *Lolium temulentum* L.; Darnel grass (E); Gramineae; annual or perennial herb. Plant is used as fodder only up to seed-setting stage. Mature grains are toxic due to fungal infection caused by *Endoconidium temulentum* Pritt & Deloer.

Machola; Subhar (S) – *Arthrocnemum indicum* (Willd.) Moq.; Chenopodiaceae; herb. Plant is found in coastal swamps, and is also cultivated on saline soils to reduce salinity. Leaves are used as salad or pickled; their juice is used to reduce pain caused by scorpion sting. Plant ashes are used as mordant in dyeing.

Mada (S) – *see* Mari.

Madala (S) – *see* Maharukh.

Madama – *see* Kakandan.

Madana (S) – *see* Mainphal.

Madana-ghanti, Guthari – *Borreria articularis* (L.f.) F.N. Williams; Rubiaceae; herb. Plant makes good fodder. Leaf-juice is used for gall-stones and haemorrhoids. Seeds are used in combating diarrhoea and dysentery.

Madanmohan, Attardana – *Clerodendrum japonicum* (Thunb.) Sweet; Glory tree (E); Verbenaceae; shrub. Cultivated as an ornamental for its extremely sweet-scented flowers. Extract of leaves mixed with black pepper is used for colic pain.

Madar – *see* Akada,

Madayantika (S) – *see* Mehndi.

Madhavi (S) – *see* Madhvi lata.

Madhavi lata, Aneta, Kampti; Madhavi (S) – *Hiptage benghalensis* (L.) Kurz.; Malpighiaceae; evergreen climbing shrub. Plant is cultivated as an ornamental for its fragrant white and yellow flowers. Leaf juice is insecticidal, and is also used for cutaneous infections. Wood is used for tool handles; bark yields tannin. Plant is used for treating asthma and rheumatism. Leaves are lopped for fodder.

Madhuka (S) – *see* Mulhatti.

Madhupaka (S) – *see* Kharbuja.

Madhuraphala (S) – *see* Baer.

Madhurica (S) – *see* Saunf.

Maghi – *see* Kali sarson.

Magrabu – *see* Ananta mul.

Mah – *see* Urad.

Mahabala – *see* Bhiunli.

Mahabaribach – *see* Narkachur.

Mahabi – *see* Hirruseeah.

Mahadev-ka-phul – *see* Satpura.

Mahagani – *Swietenia mahagoni* (L.) Jacq.; West Indian mahogany (E); Meliaceae; tree. Cultivated as a timber plant, and is also good for hedges. Timber is highly prized for panelling, carved furniture, wood-work, veneers, plywood, and cabinet work. Bark acts as an antipyretic and astringent and is rich in tannin.

Mahakal – *see* Lal indrayan.

Mahanim – *see* Toon.

Mahanimba – *see* Bakain.

Maharukh, Arua; Madala (S) – *Ailanthus excelsa* Roxb.; Tree of heaven (E); Simaroubaceae; tall tree. Cultivated as an avenue tree and also for protection as shelter belts and wind breaks. Wood is used for making plywood, veneers, toys, packing boxes and printing paper. Bark acts as an antispasmodic and expectorant and is used in asthma and bronchitis. Root bark contains alkaloids. Leaves are lopped for fodder and they are also used for rearing 'eri' silkworms.

Mahendravaruni (S) – *see* Indrayan.

Mahoor – *see* Bish.

Mahua, Mohwa – *Madhuca indica* J.F. Gmel.; Mahua tree (E), Illipe butter (E); Sapotaceae; tall tree. Plant is cultivated for its flowers and seeds. Seeds yield mahua oil which is used as a cooking medium and for the manufacture of laundry-soap. Oil is also used medicinally for rheumatism and skin ailments. Oil-cake is used as manure, and is also reported to possess insecticidal and piscicidal properties. Flowers are very rich in sugars and are eaten raw or cooked; they are also fermented and distilled to produce alcohol and vinegar. Spent flowers are used as stock-feed. Wood is considered suitable for agricultural implements, furniture, house building and sports goods.

Mahur, Khip – *Orthanthera viminea* Wight & Arn.; Asclepiadaceae; bushy leafless shrub. Stems are the source of a fibre which is used for making ropes. Flower-buds are used as vegetable.

Mainakanta – *see* Muyna.

Mainphal; Madana (S) – *Randia spinosa* Poir.; Common emetic nut (E); Rubiaceae; shrub or small tree. Cooked or roasted fruit is edible; pulp is used in dysentery. Extract of the fruit is insecticidal and insect repellent, and is also used as a synergist. Fruit is the source of a yellow dye and is used in calico printing as colour-intensifier. Unripe fruits and roots are used as fish-poison. Seeds are the source of a fat; they are also used as an appetizer and tonic. Bark infusion is used internally to relieve body pain and externally for rheumatism. Wood is used for making bobbins, blocks for calico-printing and walking-sticks. Leaves are lopped for fodder.

Mainphal – *see also* Moyena.

Majith – *see* Manjit.

Majnun – *Salix babylonica* L.; Weeping willow (E); Salicaceae; tree. Cultivated along banks of rivers and lakes, and is also grown as an ornamental. Tender branches are used for basketry. Wood is used for fences, building work and sports goods. Saw-dust is used for making activated charcoal. Leaves contain a crude protein and the enzyme salicase; their infusion is prescribed in rheumatism. Leaves are also used as a stock-feed.

Majuphal, Mazu, Muphal; Keetavasa (S) – *Quercus infectoria* Olivier; Dyers' Oak (E); Gall oak (E); Fagaceae; small tree. Galls from the plant called 'mayaphal' or gall nut are used for tanning, preparation of ink, dyeing and mordanting. Galls are also used in various preparations for treating cough, diarrhoea, dysentery, bleeding piles, intestinal haemorrhages, eczema, sore throat and in hair dyes. They are rich in ellagic acid, gallo-tannic acid and pentadigalloyl. Bark is astringent and is used in eczema.

Makai – *see* Makka.

Makal – *see* Indrayan.

Makhana – *Euryale ferox* Salisb.; Fox nut (E), Gorgon nut (E); Euryalaceae; prickly aquatic herb. Seeds are edible both as raw and roasted, and are considered to be tonic, highly nutritive and easily digestible. Seed flour is used as a substitute for arrowroot.

Makhan katori – *Ficus krishnae* C. DC.; Krishna's fig (E); Moraceae; tree. Each leaf base is characteristically joined to form a shallow cup-like structure. Cultivated for shade and as an ornamental tree.

Makhan-sem, Lal kadsumbal – *Canavalia gladiata* (Jacq.) DC.; Sword bean (E); Papilionaceae; large climber. Fruits or pods are extensively used as vegetable. Plant is also grown for green manure and as a cover crop, and is a rich source of the enzyme urease.

Makka, Makai, Bhutta – *Zea mays* L.; Maize (E), Corn (E); Gramineae; tall annual grass. Cultivated as a food crop. Mature grain is high in nutritional value and is used as popcorn, corn flakes, corn soup, or ground into flour and used for unleavened bread, pies, puddings, confectionery and salad dressing. Maize starch is used for the production of corn syrup, dextrose and as a sizing material in paper and textiles industry. The germs or embryos of dried mature grains serve as the source of an edible oil called corn oil which is used extensively as a cooking medium. Maize gluten yields zein which is used as the source of a synthetic fibre called vicara with the combined properties of cotton and wool. Cobs left after harvesting the grains are used for the preparation of furfural. Baby-corncobs are used as salad.

Makoh; Bahukantaka (S), Srigalakoli (S) – *Ziziphus oenoplia* Mill.; Jackal jujube (E); Rhamnaceae; small tree. Ripe fruits are edible. Bark contains tannin, cyclopeptide alkaloids zizyphine A and B, and betulinic acid. Roots are used in indigenous medicine for hyperacidity and expulsion of roundworms. Fruits are used medicinally for stomach ache.

Makoi; Kakamachi – *Solanum nigrum* L.; Black nightshade (E); Solanaceae; small herb. Fresh plant extract is used for cirrhosis of liver and the infusion of tender shoots with leaves is given for dropsy and also applied to anthrax pustules. Berries act as a tonic, cathartic and diuretic and are used to treat fevers, diarrhoea, heart diseases and eye trouble. Immature fruits contain glycoalkaloids. Decoction of the herb is narcotic, diuretic, antispasmodic and antiseptic. Fresh leaf juice produces dilation of the pupils of the eye.

Makola, Masuri – *Coriaria nepalensis* Wall.; Coriariaceae; shrub. Leaves are the source of tannin; they also serve as food for silkworms. Fruit is edible but can cause colic pain.

Makra – *Dactyloctenium aegyptium* (L.) Beauv; Crow-foot (E); Gramineae; annual herb. Plant is used as fodder. Grains are consumed as food in times of scarcity.

Makshikavisha (S) – *see* Jarayupriya.

Makusal – *see* Chilauni.

Makushtaka (S) – *see* Moth.

Malaya jaam – *Syzygium malaccense* (L.) Merr. & Perry.; Malaya apple (E); Myrtaceae; tree. Fruits are edible and are also made into jam and pickle. Bark is astringent and is used for treating thrush and in the preparation of mouth washes. Root acts as a diuretic and is also used for curing itch. Pulverized dry leaves are used for treating cracked tongue.

Malijhan, Jallur – *Bauhinia vahlii* Wight & Arn.; Camel's foot climber (E); Caesalpiniaceae; woody climber. Bark is the source of tannin and fibre which is used for making ropes. Leaves are used for thatching and for making disposable 'pattals' or platters. Seeds are eaten raw or fried.

Malka masur – *see* Masur.

Malkangni; Jyotishmati (S) – *Celastrus paniculata* Willd.; Celastraceae; large climber. Seeds are the source of an oil considered as a nerve stimulant and also used on rheumatic joints. The active principle present is the alkaloid celastrine. Seeds are also considered to be an aphrodisiac and tonic.

Mallika (S) – *see* Bela.

Malta – *see* Musambi.

Malti – *Jasminum flexile* Vahl.; Oleaceae; climbing shrub. Cultivated as an ornamental for its white sweet-scented flowers.

Malya (S) – *see* Kasuri methi.

Mamira, Pitmula – *Coptis teeta* Wall.; Gold thread (E); Ranunculaceae; small perennial herb with rhizomes. The underground yellow, knotted, bitter and aromatic rhizomes are used for treating debility, atonic dyspepsia, asthma, nervous diseases, jaundice, flatulence, and eye troubles. Active principles are berberine and coptine.

Mamiran, Mamiri, Pinjari – *Thalictrum foliolosum* DC.; Ranunculaceae; erect perennial herb. Root extract, decoction and powder are highly valued for ophthalmia; they are also used as bitter tonic, diuretic and purgative and for atonic dyspepsia. Roots are rich in berberine.

Mamiri – *see* Mamiran.

Mamphal – *Annona muricata* L.; Sour sop (E), Guanabana (E); Annonaceae; small evergreen tree. Fruit which is more sour than custurd apple, is also fibrous, juicy and aromatic, and is usually used for making cordials and drinks. Green bark is used as a purgative. Infusion of leaves and flowers is used in kidney trouble.

Mamri – *see* Kali tulsi.

Manaka (S) – *see* Mankand.

Manda – *Cudrania cochinchinensis* (Lour.) Kudo & Masam ex Sauer; Moraceae; spiny shrub. Wood is the source of a yellow dye. Tender leaves and ripe fruits are edible.

Mandal, Mandua; Rajika (S) – *Eleusine coracana* (L.) Gaertn.; Finger millet (E), Ragi (E); Gramineae; annual or perennial grass. Cultivated as a cereal crop. Grain is also used in cakes, sweatmeats, puddings and in the preparation of alcohol and beer. Extract of the germinated grains is used for dehairing hides. Straw is used as fodder.

Mandania – *see* Mundani.

Mandara – *see* Dadap.

Mandara (S) – *see* Ak.

Mandla, Balraja – *Eleusine indica* Gaertn.; Goose grass (E), Fowl-foot grass (E); Gramineae; annual herb. Plant is used as fodder and soil-binder. Culms are used for making hats.

Mandua – *see* Mandal.

Mandukaparni (S) – *see* Brahmi.

Manduparni (S)–*see* Thuno.

Mangustan – *Garcinia mangostana* L.; Mangosteen (E); Guttiferae; evergreen cultivated tree. Seed aril is consumed as dessert or made into preserves. Rind of the fruit is astringent with 7-14 per cent tannin, and is used in diarrhoea, dysentery and cutaneous diseases. Seeds are the source of a fatty oil. Wood is used for building purposes and cabinet work.

Manjari (S) – *see* Tulsi.

Manjariki (S) – *see* Ban-tulsi.

Manjit, Majith; Kala-meshika (S) – *Rubia cordifolia* L. sensu Hook. f.; Indian madder (E); Rubiaceae; herb. Roots are the source of a red dye which is used for dyeing carpets, cotton fabrics and Ayurvedic medicines. Roots are carminative, tonic, expectorant, astringent and are used in several Ayurvedic medicines for curing cough, indigestion, inflammation, ulcers, hepatic and urinal tract obstructions and fractures; they are also used for freckles of skin and rheumatism. The decoction of leaves and stem is used as a vermifuge. The colouring matter present in the roots is a mixture of munjistin and purpurin.

Mankanda, Manaka (S) – *Alocasia indica* (Roxb.) Schott.; Giant taro (E); Araceae; perennial large herb with underground modified stem. Corms and tubers at the end of suckers are used as vegetable after boiling. Corms are also pulped for the extraction of starch. Tubers are diuretic and act as a mild laxative. Leaf juice is considered to be astringent.

Mansala (S) – *see* Amrud.

Manya (S) – *see* Amarkand.

Marainda – *see* Dhanua.

Maravuli – *see* Sakarkanda.

Mari, Ramgoah; Mada (S), Dirgha (S) – *Caryota urens* L.; Fish-tail palm (E), Wine palm (E); Palmae; tall feather-leaved palm. Pith of the palm yields sago or kittul starch. Sap from tapping the inflorescence gives toddy and palm-sugar. Leaf-sheaths yield kittul fibre which is used for making ropes, brooms, brushes, baskets and as a stuffing material.

Maricha (S) – *see* Kali mirch.

Marisha (S) – *see* Chaulai.

Marjana (S) – *see* Lodh.

Marmandai – *Pluchea lanceolata* Oliver & Hiern; Compositae; undershrub. The plant is used as fodder. It is also used medicinally in rheumatoid arthritis.

Marorphali, Bhendu; Avartani (S), Mriga-shinga (S) – *Helicteres isora* L.; East Indian screw tree (E); Sterculiaceae; shrub or small tree. Bark is the source of a fibre which is used for cordage and ropes. Stalks yield good quality paper-pulp. Root juice is used for gastric disorders. Leaves are lopped for fodder.

Maru – *see* Moru.

Marua – *see* Ban-tulsi.

Marul, Murahri, Murva; Maurvi (S) – *Sansevieria roxburghiana* Schult f.; Indian bowstring hemp (E); Agavaceae; perennial herb. Succulent leaves yield a strong fibre used for making bowstrings, mats, cloth and cordage. Rhizomes are used in indigenous medicine for treating gonorrhaea, heart diseases, itch, rheumatism, leprosy, glandular enlargement, bile disorder and fever. Active principle present is sansiverine.

Masa, Musadadhi – *Bulbostylis barbata* (Rottb.) Clarke; Cyperaceae; annual herb. Herb infusion is used for curing dysentery.

Masethi – see Lashtia.

Masha (S) – *see* Urad.

Mashaparni (S) – *see* Mashoni.

Mashoni; Mashaparni (S) – *Teramnus labialis* Spreng.; Papilionaceae; slender climbing hairy herb. Plants are used for cover crop, green manure and fodder. Herb is used for nervous disorders, catarrh and rheumatism. Fruits are considered to be stomachic and astringent.

Masser – *see* Masur.

Masur, Malka masur, Masser – *Lens culinaris* Medik.; Lentil (E); Papilionaceae; annual herb. Cultivated as a pulse crop for its edible seeds. Plant after harvesting the pods is used for fodder both in fresh and dried condition.

Masuri – *see* Makola.

Matamar, Chapri, Sanka – *Paspalidium flavidum* (Retz.) A. Camus.; Gramineae; Perennial semi-aquatic herb. Plants have lower parts of the culms often spongy and serve as good quality fodder.

Matar; Satila (S) – *Pisum sativum* L. var. *arvense* (L.) Poir.; Garden pea (E); Papilionaceae; spreading or climbing cultivated herb. Seeds are used as vegetable and also as a pulse. Plant after harvesting the pods is used as fodder. Fresh pod-shells are also used as stock-feed. Peas contain 28 per cent or more protein along with minerals and vitamins and are highly nutritive. Experimental trials on pea-oil show possibility of its potential as a contraceptive for preventing pregnancy. The active principle present is m-xylohydroquinone. The drug proved to be non-toxic with no side effects in preliminary trials.

Matazor, Sarangum – *Phytolacca acinosa* Roxb.; Indian poke (E); Phytolaccaceae; perennial herb. Cultivated in the hilly regions for its leaves and tender shoots which are used as vegetable. Fruits are used as a condiment.

Mathaniya – *see* Bamna.

Maula – *see* Bando.

Mauli – *see* Banpalati.

Maulsari, Bakul (S) – *Mimusops elengi* L.; Spanish cherry (E); Sapotaceae; large spreading tree. Cultivated as an ornamental. Small beautiful flowers are very fragrant, made into garlands and yield a delicate perfume called 'maulsari attar'. Ripe fruits are edible. Kernels yield a fatty oil. Wood is very strong and used for boats, bridges, crushers, carts, agricultural implements and building purposes. Leaves are lopped for fodder. Dried flowers are used as snuff. Pounded seeds are used to get rid of constipation. Fruit pulp and the crushed bark are used for treating diarrhoea and dysentery.

Maurvi (S) – *see* Marul.

Mayura-shikha (S) – *see* Lal murghka.

Mayur-pankh – *see* Mor-pankhi.

Mayur-pankhi – *Actiniopteris dichotoma* Bedd.; Peacock's tail (E); Actiniopteridaceae; fern with fan-like fronds. Plant is used as an antiseptic and anthelmintic and is also accredited with anti-fertility properties.

Mazari – *Nannorrhops ritchieana* H. Wendl.; Mazari palm (E); Palmae; a gregarious low palm growing in clusters. Fruits and the inflorescence are consumed as vegetable. Leaves are the source of a fibre which is used for making baskets, hats, hand-fans, ropes and cordage.

Mazenga – *see* Timar.

Mazu – *see* Majuphal.

Meda, Katmarra, Patoia – *Litsea monopetala* (Roxb.) Pers.; Lauraceae; tree. Seeds are the source of a fat used for candles and in ointments for treating rheumatism. Wood is used for making furniture, plywood, implements and packing boxes. Leaves are used to rear 'muga' silkworms. Bark is rich in tannin, and is used for curing diarrhoea.

Meda (S) – *see* Dori.

Meda-tumri, Garsilug, Garshuma – *Pittosporum eriocarpum* Royle; Pittosporaceae; tree restricted to N.W. Himalayas. Wood is used for making toys, and it also yields an essential oil. Bark is expectorant and is used in chronic bronchitis and skin ailments.

Medh – *see* Garbijaur.

Mehal, Mol – *Pyrus pashia* Buch-Ham. ex D. Don; Rosaceae; small tree. Wood is used for making tobacco pipes and walking-sticks. Plants are hardy and are used as root-stocks for grafting 'nakh' or pear.

Mehndi, Henna; Mendika (S), Madayantika (S), Raktgarbha (S) – *Lawsonia inermis* L.; Henna (E), Egyptian privet (E); Lythraceae; small tree or much-branched shrub. Leaves are the source of an orange-red semi-permanent dye and their paste is used in the orient, to stain palms and feet in artistic designs on special festive occasions. Leaf powder is also used in herbal preparations for hair-dyes, and in ointments for skin inflammation, boils and burns. Leaves are reported to possess antibiotic activity against some microorganisms. Flowers are fragrant and small, and serve as the source of otto of henna which is used in perfumery. Leaf-paste is also used as a hair conditioner.

Meki, Takmak – *Cucumis melo* L. var. *agrestis* Naud.; Small gourd (E); Cucurbitaceae; annual herb. Fruit is edible.

Mendika (S) – *see* Mehndi.

Meradu, Miragu – *Polygala chinensis* L.; Polygalaceae; herb. Leaf infusion is used in the treatment of chronic bronchitis, asthma and catarrhal infections. Roots are used for dizziness and fever.

Merasinghi, Gur-mar; Meshashringi (S) – *Gymnema sylvestre* (Retz.) Schult.; Asclepiadaceae; woody climber. Leaves if chewed, destroy the sense of taste for both sweet and bitter substances, due to the presence of gymnemic acid. Reported to be useful as an anti-diabetic. Leaf powder acts as a diuretic and cardiac stimulant.

Meshashringi (S) – *see* Merasinghi.

Methi; Asumodhagam (S), Chandrika (S), Methika (S) – *Trigonella foenum-graecum* L.; Fenugreek (E); Papilionaceae; small annual herb. Cultivated for its leaves and tender shoots which are used as pot-herb. Seeds are used as a condiment in curry powders. Seeds are considered to be carminative and tonic and are used as an emollient in intestinal inflammation; they are also used in poultices for ulcers and boils. Seed mucilage is used in commercial coating-bases as a surface-sizing material. They are also the source of diosgenin, a precursor of steroids.

Methika (S) – *see* Methi.

Meyna – *see* Moyena.

Miana – *see* Chandausi.

Michai – *Ipomoea turbinata* Lag. [syn. *I. Muricata* (L.) Jacq.] Convolvulaceae; twining shrub. Swollen pedicels of flowers are consumed as vegetable. Seed oil is rich in behenic acid. Seeds act as a cathartic.

Mini-chambelli – *see* Akasneem.

Minjurgorwa – *Vitex peduncularis* Wall ex Schauer; Verbenaceae; tree. Wood is used for posts, beams, crushers, oars and carving. Leaves are considered to be antibacterial and the infusion of leaves and bark is used for malaria and other fevers.

Miragu – *see* Meradu.

Mirchai – *see* Nilkalmi.

Mirtenga – *Protium serratum* (Wall ex Colebr.) Engl.; Indian red pear (E); Burseraceae; tree. Fruit is edible. Tree serves as a host to 'kusumi' strain of lac insect. Wood pulp is used for the manufacture of wrapping paper.

Mishran – *Pedicularis pectinata* Wall.; Scrophulariaceae; semi-parasitic herb. Plant acts as a diuretic. Leaves are haemostatic, and are used to check spitting of blood.

Mitha alu – *see* Shakarkandi.

Mitha dudia – *Polygonatum verticillatum* All.; Liliaceae; herb. Rhizomes are edible, and are considered to be a strength giving food. A glucoside of the digitalis group is present in the plant; it is also used as a diuretic.

Mitha-indrajau – *see* Indrajau.

Mitha kaddu, Kansiphal, Sitaphal – *Cucurbita moschata* (Duch.) Poir.; Pumpkin (E); Cucurbitaceae; annual, spreading and climbing herb. Cultivated for its fruit which is used as vegetable, and is also made into jam.

Mitha karela – *Cyclanthera pedata* (L.) Schrad.; Cucurbitaceae; annual climbing herb. Cultivated in the hilly regions and is an introduced plant. Fruits are used as vegetable.

Mitha kirayat, Pahari kiretta – *Swertia angustifolia* Buch-Ham; ex D. Don.; Gentianaceae; herb. Plant is used as a substitute for 'chirayeta' but is inferior in its effectiveness.

Mitha neem, Kurry patta, Gandhela; Surabhininiba (S) – *Murraya koenigii* (L.) Spreng.; Curry leaf plant (E); Rutaceae; large shrub or small tree. Cultivated for its leaves which are used for flavouring curries, chutneys and many other dishes. They also yield an essential oil used for fixing heavy perfumes in soaps. Root juice is used for treating kidney pain and leaf juice for combating vomiting, diarrhoea and dysentery. Fruits are edible.

Mitha nimbu – *Citrus aurantifolia* (Christm) var. *limetta;* Sweet lime (E); Rutaceae; shrub. Cultivated for its edible fruit. Rooted stem cuttings serve as stock for grafting mandarin oranges.

Mithapat – *see* Koshta.

Mochkand – *see* Bhangra.

Mogra – *see* Bela.

Mohin – *see* Jhingan.

Mohwa – *see* Mahua.

Moka, Ban palas, Ghant – *Schrebera swietenioides* Roxb.; Weaver's-beam tree (E); Oleaceae; tree. Cultivated for timber which is used for making the beams of weaver's looms, shuttles, posts, poles, agricultural implements, carts, wheels and wooden utensils. It is also used for making charcoal. Fruits are used for treating hydrocele, leaves for spleen enlargement, root for leprosy and bark for boils and burns. Crushed roots are used to kill larvae in cattle wounds.

Mokha – *Momordica balsamina* L.; Balsam apple (E); Cucurbitaceae; climbing herb. Tender fruits are either cooked as vegetable, or stewed and pickled. Plant is considered to be a tonic and stomachic, and the fruits are cathartic. Fruits contain momordicin. Plant is also used as camel fodder.

Mol – *see* Mehal.

Mombatti – *Parmentiera cereifera* Seem; Candle tree (E); Bignoniaceae; small tree. Cultivated as an ornamental for its beautiful candle-like flowers. The plant is also grown for hedges.

Moonj – *see* Dolsar.

Morang elaichi, Bari elaichi–*Amomum aromaticum* Roxb.; Bengal cardamom (E); Zingiberaceae; perennial herb. Fruits and seeds are used as a condiment like 'Bari elaichi' or Greater cardamoms. Seeds yield an essential oil which is used as a stimulant and stomachic, and also for inflammation of eyelids. Seed-decoction is used for gum infections.

Mored – *see* Chambar-maya,

Morha – *see* Cheen.

Morhal, Morkhal – *Vatica lanceaefolia* Blume; Mascal wood (E); Vatica (E); Dipterocarpaceae; small tree. Bark is the source of an aromatic oleoresin which is used as an incense and for flavouring tobacco. Wood is used for constructional work and railway sleepers.

Morkhal – *see* Morhal.

Morpankhi, Mayur pankh – *Thuja orientalis* L. (syn. *Biota orientalis* Endl.); Oriental arbor-vitae (E); Cupressaceae; shrub with a dense crown. Cultivated as an ornamental in parks and gardens, often kept trimmed in beautiful oval or spherical shapes and planted in symmetrical rows. Twigs and leaves are the source of tannin and an essential oil which is used as a tonic and diuretic. Fruiting bodies and roots also yield an essential oil while seeds yield a fatty oil.

Morsikha – *see* Lal murghka.

Moru, Maru – *Quercus dilatata* Lindl.; Fagaceae; tree found in W. Himalayas. Wood is used for construction work, implements, turnery, spokes of wheels, and sleepers. Bark and leaves are rich in tannin. Leaves are lopped for fodder.

Moth; Makushtaka (S) – *Vigna aconitifolia* (Jacq.) Marechal (syn. *Phaseolus aconitifolius* Jacq.); Moth bean (E), Mat bean (E); Papilionaceae; herb. Cultivated for its seeds used as a pulse and tender pods used as vegetable. Plant after harvesting the pods is used for green-manuring and also serves for soil conservation.

Motha; Mustaka (S) – *Cyperus rotundus* L.; Nut grass (E); Cyperaceae; perennial herb. Dried rhizomes are known as souchet.

Rhizomes are the source of an essential oil which is used as an insect repellent, for scenting soaps and in perfumery. They are astringent, carminative, diuretic, expectorant, stomachic and nerve tonic, and are used in many Ayurvedic preparations.

Mothitrina – *see* Bora.

Motia – *Jasminum officinale* L.; Jasmine (E); Oleaceae; bushy shrub when kept pruned. Cultivated as an ornamental for its small white, extremely sweet-scented flowers, very popular for making garlands usually worn by women to adorn their hair and for worshipping and festival decorations in India. Flowers also serve as the source of an essential oil used in perfumery.

Moyena, Mainphal, Meyna – *Vangueria pubescens* Kurz.; Rubiaceae; large shrub. Young leaves are consumed as vegetable. Fruits are also edible.

Mradupatra (S) – *see* Guchha-pushp.

Mriga-shinga (S) – *see* Marorphali.

Mubaraka – *see* Hansraj.

Muchkand – *Pterospermum canescens* Roxb.; Sterculiaceae; tree. Flower paste mixed with rice and vinegar is used for hemicrania or headache affecting only one side of the head. Charred flowers and bark mixed with 'kamela' powder are used for smallpox eruptions. Bark is used to clarify jaggery. Fruits are preserved as jam. Another species *P. acerifolium* Willd. is also known by the same Hindi name; *see* Kanak champa.

Mudga (S) – *see* Mung.

Mudgaparni (S) – *see* Mugam.

Muduna – *see* Muyna.

Mudunirbisha – *see* Kanjanbura.

Mugam, Mugani; Mudgaparni (S) – *Vigna trilobata* (L.) Verdcourt (syn. *Dolichos trilobatus* L.); Papilionaceae; herb. The plant is cultivated for fodder.

Mugani – *see* Mugam.

Mugdhee – *see* Juhi.

Mugrela – *see* Kalonji.

Mukhajali – *Drosera peltata* Sm. (syn. *D. lunata* Buch.-Ham.); Droseraceae; insectivorous herb with glandular peltate leaves. Herb is the source of a crystalline pigment which is used for dyeing silk. Crushed leaves are used as a blistering agent; they are also used as a tonic and anti-syphilitic.

Mukhatari, Mustaru – *Grangea maderaspatana* (L.) Poir.; Compositae; prostrate or suberect herb. Leaf infusion is used as an antispasmodic and stomachic.

Mukulaka (S) – *see* Chilgoza.

Mulaka (S) – *see* Muli.

Mulhatti; Madhuka (S), Yasti-madhu (S) – *Glycyrrhiza glabra* L.; Licorice (E), Liquorice (E); Papilionaceae; perennial herb. Cultivated for its valuable roots. Root powder is used in 'pan' or betel leaf chewed as a popular masticatory. Roots are used in medicine as an expectorant, tonic and for cough, sore-throat and gastric ulcers. The sweet principle present is glycyrrhizin – a glycoside. Root extract is used to stabilize fat dispersion in the manufacture of chocolates, ensure flexibility in chewing-gums and add foam and sparkle to beer. Licorice forms an important sweetening, flavouring and moisture conditioning agent in tobacco industry. After extraction of the water-soluble matter, the second extract of the spent pulp with caustic soda, is utilized as a foam-stabilizer in fire-foam liquids for fire extinguishers. It also finds use as a spreading agent in the preparation of insecticides.

Muli; Mulaka (S) – *Raphanus sativus* L.; Radish (E); Cruciferae; annual herb. Cultivated for its tuberous fleshy roots which are eaten fresh in salads or cooked as vegetable. Fruits are also used both raw and cooked. Leaves are consumed as pot-herb. Fresh leaf-juice is used as a diuretic and laxative. Roots are used in liver, gall bladder, piles, chronic diarrhoea, urinary complaints and neuralgic headaches. Seeds act as an expectorant, carminative and diuretic. Fatty oil from the seeds is used for soap manufacture and for making crayons. Seed-cake is used as a manure and can be used as a stock-feed only after removal of isothiocyanates.

Mulluta – *see* Kukua-lata.

Muna, Munna – *Crotalaria laburnifolia* L.; Papilionaceae; undershrub. Cultivated as an ornamental for its large yellow flowers. Infusion of the plant is used as a gargle for sore-throat.

Munakka – *see* Angoor.

Mundi, Gorakhmundi; Hapusa (S) – *Sphaeranthus indicus* L.; Compositae; aromatic herb. Plant juice is used in gastric and hepatic disorders. Roots as well as pulverized seeds are anthelmintic. Root decoction is used for chest infections and considered to be antitubercular. Aqueous extract is lethal to certain varieties of cockroaches. Herb is also used as a fish-poison. Flowers are considered as tonic. Herb is also the source of an essential oil.

Mung, Pessara; Mudga (S) – *Vigna radiata* (L.) Wilczek (syn. *Phaseolus aureus* Roxb.); Green-gram (E); Papilionaceae; twining herb. Cultivated as a major pulse-crop. Tender pods are used as vegetable. Seeds, used as pulse are often fried and used as a snack. Sprouted seeds are used in salads either raw or steamed. They are also used for vertigo. Soaked seed-paste is used for preparing many delicacies in the Indian cuisine. Plants are used as a cover-crop, green manure and stock-feed after harvesting the pods.

Mungaskajur – *Solanum spirale* Roxb.; Solanaceae; undershrub. Roots are considered to be diuretic and narcotic. Ripe fruits are eaten raw or after cooking; unripe berries are poisonous. Leaves are consumed as pot-herb.

Mugna – *see* Sainjna.

Mung-phali – *Arachis hypogaea* L.; Groundnut (E), Peanut (E); Papilionaceae; trailing or suberect herb. Cultivated for its fruits called pods which develop underground. Kernels or seeds are rich in protein, vitamins and oil. Seeds are consumed as such or after roasting; they are also used for making peanut butter and confectionery. Groundnut or peanut oil is used as a popular cooking medium, in the form of refined oil or hydrogenated fat. The oil is predominantly rich in monounsaturated fatty acids. High grade oil is used in pharmacy and low grades in the manufacture of soaps and varnishes. Oil-cake is highly nutritive and used as a stock-feed and manure. Other commercial products are peanut ice-creams, and groundnut milk. Peanut protein is used for the manufacture of a synthetic textile fibre called ardil. The pod shells or hulls are used in the manufacture of insulation blocks, cork-substitutes, and coarse particle-boards; they are also used as fuel and fertilizer. Green aerial parts after harvesting the pods make excellent fodder and green manure.

Mungra – *see* Singri.

Munj, Ban, Sentha, Sarkanda – *Erianthus munja* Jesw. (syn. *Saccharum munja* Roxb.); Gramineae; tall grass. Stem is the source of a fibre used for making mats, baskets, cordage and ropes. Leaves are used for thatching and paper-pulp. Stems are used for making low priced stools, chairs, screens and winnowing trays. Plant is considered to be a good soil-binder and as the source of furfural.

Munmuna, Jhunjhuni-ankari – *Vicia hirsuta* (L.) S.F. Gray; Tiny vetch (E); Papilionaceae; herb. The plant is cultivated for fodder. Leaves are used as pot-herb.

Munna – *see* Muna.

Muphal – *see* Majuphal.

Murad, Vilayati mehndi – *Myrtus communis* L.; Myrtle (E); Myrtaceae; small tree. Cultivated for its leaves and flowers which yield an essential oil which is used in perfumery. Green ripe fruits and dried fruits are used as a condiment, and are also considered as a carminative and used in combating diarrhoea, dysentery, gastric ulceration and rheumatism. Myrtle oil considered as an antiseptic, disinfectant and rubefacient is used externally for respiratory disorders and rheumatism. Seeds are the source of a fatty oil and wood is used for turnery.

Murahri – *see* Marul.

Murchi – *see* Dhanua.

Murhari; Laghuparnika (S) – *Clematis triloba* Heyne ex Roth.; Ranunculaceae; climbing shrub. Plant stems are the source of a fibre. Plant contains anemonin and is used in leprosy.

Murkia puleri – *Arundinella setosa* Trin.; Gramineae; annual herb. Plant is used for making brooms.

Murkula, Pathor – *Marsdenia roylei* Wight; Asclepiadaceae; climbing shrub. Stems are the source of a strong silky fibre which is used for making ropes, fishing lines and fishing nets.

Murva – *see* Marul.

Murwa – *Majorana hortensis* Moench. (syn. *Origanum majorana* L.); Sweet marjorum (E); Labiatae; herb. Cultivated for its leaves and flowering tops, which are considered as a stimulant and carminative; they are the source of an essential oil which is used in perfumery and manufacture of liqueurs and soaps. Oil is also used externally for treating toothache, sprains and stiff and paralysed limbs.

Musadadhi – *see* Masa.

Musakani; Mushakarni (S) – *Merremia gangetica* (L.) Cuzodont. (syn. *Ipomoea reniformis* Choisy.); Convolvulaceae; herb. Plant acts as a diuretic and is used in treating cough, neuralgia and rheumatism. Leaves are used as pot-herb.

Musali-kant – *see* Kali musli.

Musambi, Malta – *Citrus sinensis* (L.) Osbeck.; Sweet orange (E); Rutaceae; small tree. Cultivated for its sweet, juicy and nutritious fruits rich in vitamin C, and highly valued as a dessert fruit. Several varieties are grown. All parts are aromatic. Peels yield an essential oil called orange oil which is used for flavouring food products and in cosmetics for skin-acne, toiletries, perfumery, and pharmaceutical preparations to conceal their unpleasant odours. Flowers yield neroli oil and tender shoots and leaves yield petitgrain oil.

Mushakarni (S) – *see* Musakani.

Mushali (S) – *see* Kali musli.

Mushan – *Iseilema laxum* Hack.; Gramineae; perennial grass. Plants are considered as good soil binder and are also used as fodder.

Mushel – *Iseilema anthephoroides* Hack.; Gramineae; perennial grass. Plants provide excellent fodder relished by cattle till it is in flowering condition.

Mushkapur – *see* Kapur.

Mushkbala – *Valeriana jatamansi* Jones.; Indian valerian (E); Valerianaceae; herb. Dried rhizomes are used in incense, perfumes and medicines for treating nervous disorders, hysteria and emotional disturbances. Their decoction is used as a sedative. Aromatic rhizomes yield an essential oil used as an adjunct to certain flavours for tobacco and also as a tonic. They are the source of valepotriates (monoterpenic derivatives) which are used as tranquillizers and also used in several Ayurvedic preparations.

Mushkiara – *Sambucus ebulus* L.; Dwarf elder (E); Sambucaceae; small shrub found in Kashmir. Fruits are the source of a blue dye which is used for dyeing leather and yarn. Berries, leaves and roots are purgative and the inner bark is diuretic. Leaves are also used as an expectorant.

Mushkwalee, Tagar – *Valeriana officinalis* L.; Valerian (E), Garden heliotrope (E); Valerianaceae; herb. Rhizomes and roots constitute the drug valerian which is used as a depressant for the central nervous system, and relieve hysteria and coughing. Rhizomes are also the source of an essential oil used as a stimulant and tonic; it is also used in perfumery and for adding flavour to beer and tobacco.

Mushkdana – *see* Kasturi dana.

Musna – *see* Sabuni.

Mustaka (S) – *see* Motha.

Mustaru – *see* Mukhatari.

Muta bela, Saptalla (S), Navamallika (S) – *Jasminum arborescens* Roxb. (syn. *J. roxburghianum* Wall.); Tree jasmine (E); Oleaceae; climbing shrub. Cultivated as an ornamental for its white scented flowers. Fruits are edible.

Muyna, Muduna, Mainakanta; Pundrika (S) – *Meyna laxiflora* Robyns (syn. *Vangueria spinosa* Hook f.); Rubiaceae; large shrub or small tree. Leaves and fruits are edible. Dry fruit is narcotic, and is used for treating dysentery and boils. Seeds are the source of a fatty oil.

Mwari – *see* Nwari.

N

Nadarang – *see* Kanchari.

Nagadamini (S) – *see* Nagdona.

Naga-kesara (S) – *see* Nag-kesar.

Naga-patra (S) – *see* Pindar.

Nagarmotha, Nargmusta (S) – *Cyperus scariosus* R. Br.; Nut grass (E); Cyperaceae; perennial herb. Rhizomes yield an essential oil which is used as a fixative for perfumes. Oil is also used as a hair tonic and as a substitute for patchouli oil.

Nag-champa, Nagesar, Nag-kesar; Nageshwara (S) – *Mesua ferrea* L.; Iron-wood tree (E); Guttiferae; tree with white fragrant flowers. Wood is used for posts, construction work, bridges, railway sleepers, crushers, boats, agricultural implements and cabinet work. Seeds are the source of an oil used for rheumatism and skin ailments. Flowers and flower buds are used in cosmetics and contain an essential oil and the bitter principle mesual. Flowers are also used for getting rid of cough and the flower buds for dysentery. Dried stamens are fragrant and are used for stuffing pillows.

Nagdona; Nagadamini (S) – *Artemisia nilagirica* (Clarke.) Pamp.; Indian wormwood fleabane (E); Compositae; aromatic shrub. Tender leaves and flower-heads are considered to be anthelmintic and antispasmodic, and are used in asthma and nervous diseases; they are also the source of an essential oil used for flavouring. Roots are antiseptic, tonic and antispasmodic.

Nagesar – *see* Nag-champa.

Nageshwara (S) – *see* Nag-champa.

Nag-kesar; Naga-kesara (S) – *Mammea longifolia* Planch. & Triana [syn. *Ochrocarpus longifolius* (Wight.) Benth & Hook. f.]; Alexandrian laurel (E); Guttiferae; tree. Dry flower buds are the source of a red dye used for dyeing silk fabrics. Buds are astringent, carminative and tonic, and are used in treating dyspepsia and haemorrhoids. Fruits are edible. Wood is used for construction work. *See also* Nag-champa.

Nagphani, Hathhathoria – *Opuntia elatior* Mill.; Prickly pear (E); Slipper thorn (E); Cactaceae; large succulent prickly xerophytic cactus. Cultivated for fencing, and also as an ornamental on rockeries. Fruits are edible and rich in fermentable sugars. Stem yields a coarse fibre and has the potential for making paper pulp. Crushed pulp is used as poultice on inflammation and guinea-worm abscesses. Baked fruit and fruit syrup act as an expectorant, and are used in curing whooping cough. Plant can be used for making farm-yard manure.

Nag-phul – *see* Badhara.

Nahani-khapat – *Abutilon theophrastii* Medic.; Indian mallow (E); Malvaceae; small shrub. Stem is the source of a strong, lustrous but coarse fibre with jute-like properties called China jute. Fibre is used for making rugs, ropes, sacks and paper. Seed decoction is used as a remedy for sore-eyes, fistula and dysentery; seeds also yield a semi-drying oil.

Nak-chhikni; Chhikika (S) – *Centipeda minima* (L.) A. Br. & Aschers.; Compositae; prostrate herb. Seeds and leaves are the source of a snuff used in colds. Seeds are vermifuge, and also contain an essential oil. Herb infusion is used in ophthalmia.

Nakh – *Pyrus communis* L.; Pear (E); Rosaceae; small tree. Fruits are edible. Fruit juice is used fresh, canned or made into beverages.

Nakhari (S) – *see* Ghiabato.

Nakra (S) – *see* Pitpapara.

Nakuli, Gandhata (S) – *Saccolabium papillosum* Lindl.; Orchidaceae; epiphytic herb. Roots are considered to be specific for treating rheumatism and are often substituted for 'anantamul' or Indian sarsaparilla.

Nal – *see* Narkul.

Nala, Narasala; Devanala (S) – *Lobelia nicotianaefolia* Roth ex Roem. & Schult.; Campanulaceae; herb, found in S. India. Plants are antiseptic and rich in the alkaloid lobeline, and are often used as a substitute for *Lobelia inflata* L. which forms the chief source of the drug lobelia used in asthma and chronic bronchitis, and cultivated to some extent in the hills of India.

Nalita (S) – *see* Patsan.

Nandi-vriksha (S) – *see* Toon.

Nanka – *Monochoria vaginalis* (Burm. f.) Presl.; Pontederiaceae; rhizomatous aquatic herb. Tender twigs with leaves are used as pot-herb. Roots are used for curing gastric disorders, toothache and asthma. Leaf juice is used for getting rid of cough.

Narakiya – *Gironniera cuspidata* (Bl.) Kurz.; Ulmaceae; large evergreen tree. Fruit is edible. Wood is used for rafters, construction work and planks. Leaves are lopped for fodder.

Narangi – *see* Santara.

Narasala – *see* Nala.

Narbans – *see* Bans kaban.

Narcha – *see* Pat.

Nargis – *Narcissus tazetta* L.; Narcissus (E); Amaryllidaceae; herb with underground bulb. Plant is cultivated as an ornamental for its beautiful sweet scented flowers. Fragrant flowers are the source of an essential oil which is used in perfumery directly or blended with jasmine and other perfumes.

Nargmusta (S) – *see* Nagarmotha.

Narhal – *see* Baranal.

Narikela (S) – *see* Nariyal.

Nariyal, Gola, Khopra; Narikela (S) – *Cocos nucifera* L.; Coconut (E); Palmae; tall palm. Cultivated in the hot damp coastal areas of India specially Kerala, Tamil Nadu and Karnataka, and has immense commercial value. Fruit-milk or nuclear endosperm from the large green young fruit called 'dab' provides a very nutritious and refreshing drink while the mature kernel consisting of fleshy endosperm gives 'copra' which on fine grating is used in confectionery, bakery, chutneys and special culinary preparations. 'Copra' is also the source of coconut oil which is used as a cooking medium, and in several other industries such as cosmetics, toiletries, detergents and lubricants. Copra residue or oil-cake is used as a stock-feed, poultry feed, and manure. Fibre from the husk or mesocarp of the fruit called coir is used commercially in the manufacture of carpets, door mats, rugs, wall hangings and thermal insulation boards. Inferior fibre grades are used for making ropes, and the coir dust is used as a mulch, rooting medium and compost. Hard endocarp of shells is used for vessels, scoops, musical instruments, 'hookah' base, buttons, combs, bangles, gas absorbent charcoal, and filler in plastics. Inflorescence is tapped for toddy which provides a fresh drink or is converted into palm jaggery or palm sugar. 'Arrack' is produced after fermenting and distilling toddy. Leaves are used for thatching, screens, baskets and hats. Midribs of leaves are used for making brooms, and baskets. Palm-cabbage or terminal buds are eaten raw or cooked, and are a delicacy. Straight unbranched tree trunks are used for posts or as fuel.

Narkachur, Maha-baribach – *Zingiber zerumbet* (L.) Rosc. ex Sm.; Zerumbet ginger (E); Zingiberaceae; perennial herb. Cultivated for its rhizomes which are used as a spice and condiment and medicinally for curing cough, stomach ache, asthma and skin ailments. Rhizomes are fragrant and are the source of an essential oil which is used to perfume soaps and toiletries.

Nar-kachura – *see* Kali-haldi.

Narkul, Nal – *Phragmites karka* (Retz.) Trin. ex Stend.; Common reed-grass (E); Gramineae; perennial herb. Culms are used for thatching, fencing, and in the preparation of chairs, baskets, mats, paper, and pipes for flutes and 'hookah' or tobacco pipe. Young plants are used for fodder.

Narsal – *see* Baranal.

Nashpati – *Pyrus pyrifolia* (Burm. f.) Nakai var. *culta* (Mak.) Nakai; Chinese pear (E); Rosaceae; small tree. Cultivated for its edible fruits which are sweet, gritty and rich in sugars. Fruit is eaten raw or canned.

Nasut – *see* Pangra.

Naval susarini – *Merremia vitifolia* (Burm. f.) Hallier. f. (syn. *Ipomoea vitifolia* Bl.); Bombay nawal (E); Convolvulaceae; trailing herb. Root is used for treating stomach ache and plant juice for inflamed eyes. Plant is also used to treat urethral discharges.

Navamallica (S) – *see* Muta bela.

Neel; Nilika (S), Nilla (S) – *Indigofera tinctoria* L.; Indigo (E); Papilionaceae; small shrub. Cultivated as a green manure or cover crop; it is also one of the sources of indigo. Plant extract is used as a remedy for nervous diseases and epilepsy. Roots are used in hepatitis and urinary disorders. Leaf juice is used as a prophylactic for hydrophobia. Plant extract is also used in ointments for treating haemorrhoids and sores.

Neela-vriksa (S) – *see* Nila vriksha (S).

Neela vriksh – *Cryptocarya wightiana* Thw.; Lauraceae; evergreen tree. Wood is used for building purposes, rafters and match-sticks. The leaves are boiled in oil and used topically in elephantiasis.

Neeli gulmohar – *Jacaranda mimosifolia* D. Don.; Jacaranda (E); Bignoniaceae; small tree. Cultivated as an avenue and ornamental tree for its dense crown, beautiful foliage and blue-mauve flowers in terminal panicles. Bark and leaves are used as a remedy for syphilis. Wood is fine textured and is used for making tool handles.

Neeli nargandi, Udi-sambhalu; Nila-nirgundi (S) – *Justicia gendarussa* L.f.; Acanthaceae; evergreen shrub. Cultivated as an ornamental, and is also grown for hedges. Leaf decoction is used for combating rheumatism, facial paralysis and cephalagia. Leaf juice is used to check internal haemorrhage and fresh leaves are used topically on rheumatic swelling.

Neel kamal – *see* Nilkamal.

Neem; Arishta (S), Nimba (S) – *Azadirachta indica* A. Juss.; Margosa tree (E); Meliaceae; large tree with dense crown. The tree is regarded as one of the sacred plants of the Hindus and is cultivated in parks, homes and on road-sides in India to provide cool shade and purify the air. It has immense medicinal value. Leaves are used for healing of wounds and in tooth pastes; dried leaves are used as an insect-repellent and insecticide. Bark is rich in tannin and is used for curing nausea, vomiting and skin ailments. Gum exudate from the bark is used in dyeing of silk and as a stimulant. Plant contains azadiractin which has insecticidal property and appears to be non-toxic to humans. Other alkaloids include margosine, nimbidin, nimbin and nimbinin. Nimbidin the bitter principle present in neem-seed oil called margosa oil is used in medicinal cosmetics, gargles, soaps and creams for skin diseases. Seed-oil after removal of the bitter principles is suitable for hydrogenation and is used as an antiseptic, illuminant and in soap manufacture. Green twigs chewed at one end to make 'datun', a sort of tooth brush are used in rural India for cleaning teeth and making the mouth germ free. Ripe fruits are edible and sweet. Timber is used for making agricultural implements. Recent researches point to the possible use of neem oil as a potential contraceptive in Third World countries, as it has been found to be a strong spermicide. Other components show promise as oral birth control pills for men. It is rightly termed as one of the wonder plants bestowed to us by mother nature, for 'neem' possesses many compounds that can be used to treat bacterial infections, control lice, and kill parasites in human digestive tract, blood and lymph system. The tree is important for reforestation in tropical regions, as a source of neem-seed oil and oil-cake which is used for manuring and disinfecting the soil, and as an asset to dental hygiene.

Neelopalam (S) – *Monochoria hastata* (L.) Solms; Pontederiaceae; rhizomatous aquatic herb. Tender shoots and leaves are used as pot-herb. Leaf juice is used as a remedy for boils. Pounded rhizomes are used for treating scaly or flaky dry-skin crust and the plant is considered to be a tonic.

Neem-chameli – *see* Akasneem.

Neemda, Newarpati – *Buddleja asiatica* Lour.; Butterfly bush (E); Buddlejaceae; tall evergreen shrub. Cultivated as an ornamental in parks for its fragrant, tiny, white flowers in spikes. Flowers are eaten. Smoke emanating from burning leaves is used as an anaesthetic for pain in boils. Crushed roots are used for the preparation of a fermented drink.

Neer-brahmi, Brahmi, Jalnimba; Nira-brahmi (S) – *Bacopa monnieri* (L.) Pennell; Thyme leaved gratiola (E); Scrophulariaceae, prostrate herb found in damp, marshy areas. Entire plant is considered to be a potent nerve tonic and diuretic cardio-tonic, used in combating epilepsy and nervous disorders including insanity. Active principles include the alkaloids herpestin and brahmine.

Neimal, Nelmal; Kataka (S) – *Strychnos potatorum* L.f.; Clearing-nut tree (E); Strychnaceae; tree. Seeds act as an emetic, stomachic and tonic and are used in diarrhoea, gonorrhoea and diabetes. Seeds are used to make water germ-free for drinking and are considered to be useful in conjunctivitis and other eye troubles. They also yield a gum used for sizing in textile and paper industry. Fruits are edible.

Nelmal – *see* Neimal.

Neoza – *see* Chilgoza.

Nepali dhaniya – *see* Timur; *see also* Tumru.

Nepal nimb – *see* Sanipat.

Newarpati – *see* Neemda.

Nikumba (S) – *see* Undarbibi.

Nila-nirgundi (S) – *see* Neeli nargandi.

Nilapushpa (S) – *see* Banafshah.

Nila-vriksha (S), Neela-vriksa (S) – *Diospyros candolleana* Wight; Ebenaceae; tree found in W. Ghats. Root-bark decoction is used medicinally for painful rheumatic joints and swellings.

Nilika (S) – *see* Neel.

Nilkalmi, Kaladana, Mirchai; Krishnabija (S) – *Ipomoea nil* (L.) Roth.; Convolvulaceae, twining, hairy shrub. Dried seeds are used as a purgative and as a substitute for jalap seeds (*Exogonium purga* Benth.). Seeds also yield a fixed oil.

Nilkamal, Neel kamal, Nilopala (S) – *Nymphaea stellata* Willd.; Indian blue water-lily (E); Nymphaeaceae; perennial aquatic herb. Tender leaves and rhizomes are used as vegetable. Flower decoction is considered to be a narcotic. Infusion of rhizomes acts as a diuretic and is used for urinary infections. Powdered rhizomes are used for treating piles, dyspepsia and diarrhoea.

Nilakanthi, Khurbanti – *Ajuga bracteosa* Wall. ex Benth.; Labiatae; herb with blue-lilac flowers in spikes. Leaves are aromatic and stimulant. Herb is considered to be a tonic, astringent and diuretic, and is used in combating rheumatism, gout and palsy.

Nilkattai – *see* Kadhera.

Nilla (S) – *see* Neel.

Nilli – *Indigofera sumatrana* Gaertn.; Papilionaceae; small shrub. Cultivated as a green manure and cover crop.

Nilopala (S) – *see* Nilkamal.

Nim – *see* Neem.

Nimba (S) – *see* Neem.

Nimbu – *see* Kagzi nimbu.

Nimuka; Vanatiktika (S) – *Stephania japonica* (Thunb.) Miers. var. *discolor*; Menispermaceae; climbing shrub. Tubers are used in the treatment of fever, dyspepsia, stomach ache, diarrhoea and urinary diseases. Important alkaloid present is aknadine.

Nini, Banspati – *Oplismenus burmannii* (Retz.) Beauv.; Gramineae; small grass found in dense pure mats. It is used as fodder when fresh and young, and is also good for hay.

Nira-brahmi (S) – *see* Neer-brahmi.

Nirbisi – *see* Jadwar.

Nirgandi, Sambhalu; Nirgundi (S) – *Vitex negundo* L.; Chaste tree (E); Verbenaceae; shrub. Cultivated for reclaiming forest land and also for hedges. Leaves are aromatic, vermifuge and tonic and the leaf decoction is used in rheumatism and medicinal baths for skin diseases, sores, and sprains. Roots are considered to be diuretic, febrifuge, anthelmintic and tonic; they are used in treating dyspepsia, dysentery, piles, bladder irritation and rheumatism. Leaves and roots act as a tranquillizer and are used as important constituents of the Ayurvedic preparations such as 'Nirgandi-kalpa', 'Vishagarbha taila' and 'Nirgundi-taila'. Flowers are astringent and are used as a remedy in gastric and liver disorders. Plant possesses insecticidal properties and twigs are used in basketry.

Nirgandi-kanda – *Alectra parasitica* A. Rich. var. *chitrakutensis* M.A. Rau; Scrophulariaceae; herb found parasitic on the roots of 'Nirgandi' (*Vitex negundo* L.). Rhizomes are used for treating constipation, paralysis, leprosy, tuberculosis and for expelling intestinal worms. Important chemicals present are azafrin, mannitol and several alkaloids.

Nirgundi (S) – *see* Nirgandi.

Nirvisha (S) – *see* Bhada-motha.

Nishapava (S) –*see* Lobhia.

Nisomali (S) – *see* Bannalia.

Nisoth, Pitohri; Trivrit (S) – *Operculina turpethum* (L.) Silva Manso [syn. *Ipomoea turpethum* (L.) R. Br.]; Indian jalap (E); Convolvulaceae; twining herb. Root bark the source of turpeth, is a substitute for true jalap and is used as a strong purgative. The active principle turpethine is a glucosidic resin found in the root bark.

Nivaara (S) – *see* Janglidal.

Nwari, Mwari; Asphota (S), Vanamalli (S) – *Jasminum angustifolium* Vahl.; Wild jasmine (E); Oleaceae; evergreen shrub. Cultivated as an ornamental for its extremely sweet-scented delicate white flowers which bloom in profusion during summer. Root extract is used locally for getting rid of ringworm. Leaf juice is used as an emetic in cases of poisoning.

O

Odabrini – *Smithia sensitiva* Ait.; Papilionaceae; herb. Tender shoots and leaves are used as pot-herb. Plant is used as fodder either in fresh condition or as hay. Herb infusion is used for relieving difficulty in passing urine.

Okharadi (S) – *see* Gandhi-buti.

Olak – *see* Ulatkambal.

Oulota – *Tetracera scandens* Merr. (syn. *Delima sarmentosa* L.); Dilleniaceae; shrub. Leaves are used for treating boils, and are also used for polishing metal-ware. Roots are used for healing burns and stems are used for making fences.

P

Pabuna – *see* Chambar-maya

Pacholi, Peholi – *Pogostemon perilloides* (L.) Mansf.; Patchouly (E); Labiatae; herb. Cultivated for its fragrant leaves, which yield an essential oil called Bombay-patchouli oil used in the manufacture of soaps. Dried leaves are used for keeping the woollens moth-free. Herb acts as a diuretic and the infusion of leaves is used for getting rid of cough. Root decoction is used for treating dropsy.

Padaria, Paral, Patla – *Stereospermum suaveolens* DC.; Bignoniaceae; tree. Wood is used for general construction work, cabinet work, furniture, and good quality charcoal. Stem bark is considered as a tonic and diuretic. Root bark is one of the ingredients of 'Dasamula' an Ayurvedic prescription. Leaves are lopped for fodder.

Padauk – *Pterocarpus dalbergioides* Roxb.; Andaman redwood (E), Burmese rosewood (E); Papilionaceae; tree. Wood is highly valued for panelling, balustrades, cabinet work, furniture, decorative work and veneers.

Paddam, Phaya; Padmaka (S) – *Prunus cerasoides* D. Don.; Himalayan wild cherry (E); Rosaceae; tree. Fruits are used for making brandy, and are also edible. Stony endocarp is used for making rosaries and necklaces. Kernels yield an oil. Bark is the source of tannin.

Pader, Padri, Parral – *Stereospermum personatum* (Hassk.) Chatt.; Yellow snake tree (E), Trumpet-flower (E); Bignoniaceae; tree. Wood is used for building work, canoes, oars, ploughs, shafts, furniture, fancy-goods, excellent charcoal, match-boxes and plywood. Root decoction is used in combating cough and asthma. Leaves are lopped for fodder.

Padiri – *Bignonia crispa* Buch-Ham.; Bignoniaceae; tree. Cultivated as an ornamental for its beautiful flowers.

Padma (S) – *see* Kamal.

Padmaka (S) – *see* Paddam.

Padma-pushkara (S) – *see* Keore-ka-mul.

Padri – *see* Pader.

Pahari-gandana – *Marrubium vulgare* L.; Hoarhound (E); Labiatae; herb found in Kashmir. Flowering tops and dried leaves constitute the drug sold as 'farasiym' in the Indian market which is used as a home remedy for cough, colds and rheumatism.

Pahari kikar – *Acacia eburnea* Willd.; Mimosaceae; tree. Wood is used for tool handles and for burning in kilns.

Pahari kiretta – *see* Mitha kirayat.

Pahari nimbu – *see* Bara nibu.

Pahari pan – *see* Pahari pipar.

Pahari pipar, Pahari pan – *Piper mullesus* Buch-Ham.; Pahari pipar (E); Piperaceae; climbing shrub. Leaves are the source of a volatile oil with lime-like fragrance.

Pahari pudina – *Mentha spicata* (L.) Huds.; Spearmint (E); Labiatae; perennial herb. Cultivated in several places for its leaves which yield spear-mint oil, used for flavouring chewing gums, toothpastes, confectionery and pharmaceuticals. Leaf infusion with sugar is used for treating hysteria and gastric troubles in infants. Herb is considered to be a carminative, antispasmodic and stimulant.

Pahari rai, Lai – *Brassica juncea* (L.) Czern. & Coss. var. *rugosa* (Roxb.) Tsen & Lee.; Cabbage-leaved mustard (E); Cruciferae; annual herb. Cultivated in the terai regions for its leaves and tender shoots which are used as vegetable and are also pickled. Leaves are considered as anthelmintic and antidysenteric. Seeds are the source of a fatty oil and also a volatile oil. The decoction of seeds is used for indigestion, cough and lumbago.

Pakar, Gagjaira – *Ficus rumphii* Blume; Moraceae; medium-sized tree. Cultivated as an evergreen ornamental. Ripe fruits are edible. Fruit juice is used for treating asthma and for killing worms. Bark is the source of a fibre used for cordage. Leaves are lopped for fodder.

Pala – *Carmona microphylla* (Lam.) G. Don. (syn. *Ehretia microphylla* Lam.); Ehretiaceae; shrub or small tree. Roots are used as a remedy for syphilis and general debility. Leaf decoction is used in cough and gastric disorders.

Palak, Isfanaj, Palangsag, Palanki; Palakyam (S), Palangkya (S) – *Beta vulgaris* L. var. *orientalis* (Roth) Moq., also var. *palonga*; Indian spinach (E); Chenopodiaceae; annual herb native to India. Cultivated for its leaves which are used in salads, soups and curries; they are also used as vegetable and in various Indian dishes and snacks. Leaves are a good source of chlorophyll and are considered rich in vitamins and minerals. Leaves are diuretic and leaf lipids are antibacterial in action. Fruits are used to treat bowel inflammation and fevers. Another species *Spinacia oleracea* L. is also known by the same Hindi name.

Palak, Isfanaj, Palangsag, Palanki – *Spinacia oleracea* L.; Spinach (E); Chenopodiaceae; cultivated herb. Uses similar to Indian spinach or Palak.

Palak juhi, Yuthuka-parni (S) – *Rhinacanthus nasuta* (L.) Kurz.; Acanthaceae; shrub. Bruised leaves and fresh roots crushed and mixed with lime are used locally for getting rid of ringworm, dhobi's itch and eczema. Roots are accredited with antiseptic and aphrodisiac properties and possess rhinacanthin. Seeds are fragrant, and are used for scenting clothes.

Palakyam (S) – *see* Palak.

Palandu (S) – *see* Piaz.

Palanggini – *see* Trinpali.

Palangkya (S) – *see* Palak.

Palangsag – *see* Palak.

Palanki – *see* Palak.

Palas – *see* Dhak.

Palasha (S) – *see* Dhak.

Palas lata, Kimsuka; Latapalasa (S) – *Butea superba* Roxb.; Papilionaceae; woody climber. Flower is the source of a yellow dye. Gum exuded by the stem is used in poultices and tonics. Leaf juice is used for treating heat-rash in children. Shoot decoction is used in piles. Seeds are the source of a fatty oil, and are also used as an anthelmintic and sedative. Leaves are lopped for fodder.

Palawat – *Phoenix pusilla* Gaertn.; Wild date (E); Palmae; bushy palm, occurring along Coromandel coastal region. Terminal bud and fruits are edible. Stem yields starch for sago. Tree is the source of a gum used in urinary trouble and diarrhoea. Leaf rachis is used for basketry and leaves are used for thatching and making mats.

Paludar, Badar, Rewar – *Abies pindrow* Royle; Himalayan silver fir; Pinaceae; tall evergreen tree, found in W. Himalayas. Wood is light and strong, and is used for furniture, planking, construction work, flooring, cabinet work, packing boxes and for good quality news-print paper and rayon-grade pulp.

Pan, Tambuli; Tambula (S) – *Piper betle* L.; Betel pepper (E); Piperaceae; climbing shrub. Cultivated for its leaves, which are very popular as a masticatory in the Indian sub-continent, and are chewed with many additives *viz.*, lime, 'kaththa' or catechu, chips of areca nut, fennel, lesser cardamoms, powdered liquorice, desiccated coconut powder, 'gulkand' (a special preparation of rose-petals and sugar) and cloves. Some people add finely chopped and scented chewing tobacco as a mild intoxicant. The leaf is a stimulant, cleanses the mouth, imparts a pleasing aroma to the breath and is considered as a blood purifier, gastric stimulant and an effective prophylactic in the Ayurvedic texts. The leaf has religious sanction and is incorporated as one of the articles of worship along with whole areca nut in many religious rituals of the Hindus. Of the trinity Hindu Gods, Lord Vishnu is said to be enamoured by 'pan' or betel leaf, Brahma by 'supari' or areca nut and Shiva by lime, all three of which are important ingredients in the preparation of the leaf as a popular masticatory. Decoction of the leaves is used for healing of wounds and the essential oil from the leaf is considered to be a carminative and is used for respiratory catarrh.

Panar – *see* Katul.

Panas – *see* Kathal.

Panasa (S) – *see* Kathal.

Pandaren kamal – *see* Kumud.

Panevar – *see* Chakunda.

Pangar – *see* Bankhor.

Pangra, Dauldhak, Nasut – *Erythrina suberosa* Roxb.; Papilionaceae; small tree. Often cultivated in gardens as a hedge plant. Wood is used for making ladles, small jars, water troughs, drums and lacquered boxes. It is also suitable for match-sticks. Bark is the source of fibre used for cordage, and cork which is used for making cork-sheets suitable for insulation boards and screw-cap cork-liners. Bark-ash is used for dyeing.

Paniala, Bhillar – *Bischofia javanica* Blume; Bishop wood (E); Java cedar (E); Bischofiaceae; tree. Bark is the source of tannin, and a red dye which is used for dyeing rattan cane baskets. Fruits are edible; seeds yield a drying oil. Wood is used for boats, rafters, bridges, house posts, sleepers and good quality writing paper.

Paniamla, Talispatri; Talisha (S) – *Flacourtia jangomas* (Lour.) Raeusch.; Puneala plum (E); Flacourtiaceae; small spreading tree. Cultivated for its fruits used either fresh or made into jams and marmalades. Fruits are also considered useful in liver complaints and biliousness. Wood is used for agricultural implements. Seeds yield a fixed oil. Tender shoots and leaves are astringent and are used for controlling diarrhoea. Infusion of bark is used as a gargle for sore throat and also used as a mouth-wash.

Pani-bel – *Ampelocissus latifolia* (Roxb.) Planch. (syn. *Vitis latifolia* Roxb.); Vitidaceae; woody climber. Root decoction is used for dysentery. Fresh juice of tender leaves is used for indolent ulcers and dental troubles. Fruits are edible.

Pani-ka-sambhalu, Safed sambhalu – *Vitex trifolia* L.; Verbenaceae; tree. Flower and leaves are aromatic. Flowers are administered with honey for certain fevers which are accompanied by vomiting. Leaves are antiseptic, insecticidal and anti-bacterial in action, and are also used locally for sprains and rheumatic swellings. Fruits are rich in vitricine and are used for checking amenorrhoea.

Pani-maricha – *Polygonum hydropiper* L.; Water pepper (E), Pepper-wort (E); Polygonaceae; perennial herb. Plant is used as a flavouring for foods, and also acts as a stimulant, diuretic, and haemostatic. Herb infusion is used in uterine disorders and the liquid extract as an oral contraceptive. Roots are considered as a tonic, carminative, anthelmintic and diuretic; and root juice is used for skin ailments. Dry powdered herb is used as a fish-poison. Fresh leaf juice is used as a remedy for toothache. Herb is the source of a yellow dye which is used for colouring wood.

Panirak, Kasbeeze-mradupatra – *Malva parviflora* L.; Mallows (E); Malvaceae; herb. Plant is a rich source of vitamin A and minerals specially iron and calcium and is used as a pot-herb. Infusion of the leaves is used as a nerve tonic and a taenicide. Seeds are demulcent and are used for treating cough and ulcers in bladder. Roots are used for washing woollens and for shampooing hair.

Panjan – *see* Sandan.

Panjiri-ka-patta – *Anisochilus carnosus* (L.) Wall.; Labiatae; herb. Plant is aromatic, and considered to be a stimulant and expectorant, and is used for treating colds and cough. Plant yields an essential oil, and the leaf juice is given in urticaria following liver disorders. Leaves are also used as vegetable.

Panjuli – *see* Buinowla.

Pankaja (S) – *see* Kamal.

Panlata – *Derris trifoliata* Lour.; Papilionaceae; large climber. Plant is considered to be an antispasmodic, anti-irritant and stimulant. Roots are the source of an insecticide. Stems are flexible and are used for rough cordage, and leaves are lopped for fodder.

Pansra – *see* Binda.

Panwar – *Cleome brachycarpa* Vahl ex DC.; Capparidaceae; herb. Plant is used in the preparation of ointments used for external applications for treating scabies, inflammations and rheumatism. Leaves are used for the treatment of leucoderma.

Papari – *see* Kathachampa.

Papata (S) – *see* Kathachampa.

Papaya – *see* Papeeta.

Papeeta, Papaya – *Carica papaya* L.; Papaya (E), Papaw (E); Caricaceae; small tree with fruits borne directly on the unbranched stem near the crown. Cultivated for its fruit. Raw green immature fruits on scratching the rind exude a milky latex, very rich in papain a proteolytic enzyme which is used commercially in bating of hides, clearing of beer, tenderizing of meat, and for the preparation of chewing gum and shrink-resistant wool. It is further used in some cosmetics to get rid of blemishes and freckles on the skin, as an anthelmintic and as an aid to digestion in some pharmaceutical preparations. Leaves and seeds yield carpaine, an alkaloid which is used as a diuretic, heart stimulant, and amoebicide. Ripe fruits have sweet and juicy flesh rich in sugar, vitamins, carotene and papain and are considered very nutritious and digestive.

Paphar, Papura, Ban-pindalu – *Gardenia latifolia* Ait.; Box-wood gardenia (E); Rubiaceae; small tree. Cultivated in gardens for hedges. Wood is used as a substitute for box-wood, and for light furniture, toys, shuttles, engraving and turnery articles.

Papotan – *see* Tulati patti.

Papra, Bankakri, Bhavanbakra, Rikhpat – *Podophyllum hexandrum* Royle; Indian Podophyllum (E); Podophyllaceae; perennial herb found in high altitudes in the Himalayas. Irregular, twisted and knotted rhizomes are the source of a drug called 'giriparpat' or Indian Podophyllum which yields a medicinal resin called podophyllin with podophyllotoxin as the active principle, and is used as a purgative and effective vermifuge. It is also considered to be one of the possible cancer-fighting drugs. Fruit is cucumber-like and edible.

Papri – *see* Chikri.

Papura – *see* Paphar.

Paral – *see* Padaria.

Paras-pipal, Parsipu, Gardha-bhanda (S) – *Thespesia populnea* (L.) Soland ex Corr.; Portia tree (E), Umbrella tree (E); Malvaceae; small tree. Often cultivated as a road-side tree. Wood is used for furniture, cabinet work, boats, musical instruments, agricultural implements and turnery articles. Bark provides a fibre for making ropes. Bark, flowers, fruits and leaves are used in remedies for skin ailments. Seeds are the source of a fatty oil, used for cutaneous diseases. Bark, fruits and roots are used for dysentery and haemorrhoids. Seeds act as a purgative. Fruits and flowers are the source of a yellow dye. Leaves are lopped for fodder.

Paraspipal; Plaksha (S) – *Ficus arnottiana* Miq.; Moraceae; tree. Bark and leaves are used for treating skin ailments. Leaves are lopped for fodder.

Paravalli (S) – *see* Kali dudhi.

Parbati jeera – *see* Par bel.

Parha – *Stephania glabra* (Roxb.) Miers.; Menispermaceae; climbing shrub with peltate leaves. Large underground tubers are used in combating asthma, pulmonary tuberculosis and intestinal disorders and contain several alkaloids with diverse activities *viz.*, palmitine, stepharine, cycleanine and hyndarine.

Parijata (S) – *see* Dadap, *see also* Raktamadar.

Parpat – *Mollugo cerviana* (L.) Ser.; Tel (E); Molluginaceae; herb. Plant is considered to be an antiseptic, stomachic and febrifuge and is used as a cure for gonorrhoea. Roots are boiled in oil and used for external application on painful joints to get relief in rheumatism and gout.

Parpata – *see* Daman-papra.

Parral – *see* Pader.

Parsipu – *see* Paras-pipal.

Parusha (S) – *see* Phalsa.

Parvataranda (S) – *see* Bagbherenda.

Parwa – *see* Kumeria.

Parwal, Potol, Putulika (S) – *Trichosanthes dioica* Roxb.; Pointed gourd (E); Cucurbitacee; scandent herb. Cultivated for its small green fruit popular as a vegetable. Fruit is nutritive and easily digestible, and is also made into sweetmeats. Leaves are used as pot-herb. Seeds yield a fatty oil, and seed extract is haemagglutinating in activity.

Parwatti, Illarbillar – *Cocculus pendulus* (Forsk.) Diels.; Menispermaceae; shrub found in dry regions. Roots possess tonic properties and are used for the treatment of intermittent fevers; they are also used as a fish-poison.

Pasati – *Talinum triangulare* Willd.; Surinam purslane (E); Fame flower (E); Portulacaceae; herb. Cultivated in South India as an introduced plant from Sri Lanka for its tender shoots and leaves which are used as vegetable. Fresh green parts are very rich in vitamins, but due to the presence of appreciable quantities of hydrocyanic acid and oxalates, the herb should not be used unless cooked properly.

Pashana-bhedak, Surra; Kshudra-pashanabheda (S) – *Homonoia riparia* Lour.; Euphorbiaceae; shrub found among rocks in river beds or streams. Roots are diuretic and laxative and are used for urinary disorders, stones in bladder, and piles. Tender leafy tops are used as vegetable. Leaves are also used medicinally for skin ailments. Leaf juice is used as an astringent to strengthen gums and teeth among some tribals and for blackening of teeth which is considered to be an added asset to their beauty.

Pashanabhedi – *see* Pathurchur.

Pat, Titapat, Narcha; Kalasaka – *Corchorus capsularis* L.; White jute (E); Tiliaceae; tall thin-stemmed shrub. Cultivated for the fibre called white jute obtained after retting of its stems. The fibre is used extensively for gunny bags, packing cloth, coarse cloth, curtains, upholstery, carpets, ropes, twines, base of linoleum carpets, cloth for padding, wall plastering, jute-wool cheap blankets, and paper manufacture. Jute-stick is used in the manufacture of grease-proof paper and active carbon for medicinal charcoal.

Patakona – *see* Chirpoti.

Patala – *see* Bakarcha.

Patalagaruda (S) – *see* Akasgaddah.

Patalagarudi (S) – *see* Jamti-ki-bel.

Patang – *Haematoxylon campechianum* L.; Logwood (E), Campeachy wood tree (E); Caesalpiniaceae; thorny shrub or small tree. Cultivated as an ornamental in gardens and also makes a nice hedge. The colouring constituent haematoxylin is present along with tannins in the heartwood. It is a precursor which on mild oxidation produces the actual dye called haematine, a violet coloured crystalline substance tinged with metallic green lustre. Depending on the mordant being used it is capable of producing colours ranging from blue to black. The logwood extract with iron salts as mordant, is used extensively to impart a permanent black colour to cottons, silks, woollens, furs and leather. Haematoxylin is also employed in histological work for permanent staining of cell nuclei and thin sections of biological tissues in preparing microscopic slides. It is also used in the manufacture of some inks. The wood is considered to be an astringent and tonic and its decoction is used for controlling diarrhoea, dysentery, leucorrhoea and atonic dyspepsia. It is also used for making small fancy articles. Another plant called Bakam (*Caesalpinia sappan* L.) is also known by the same Hindi name.

Patang – *see* Bakam.

Patat-ki-bel – *see* Akanadi.

Patchouli – *Pogostemon cablin* (Blanco) Benth.; Patchouli (E); Labiatae; herb. Cultivated for its fragrant leaves which yield the essential oil called patchouli oil, which is very much in demand for scenting soaps, cosmetics, incense, tobacco and for masking the foul odour of depilatory creams. The oil also has antibacterial properties. Fresh leaf-infusion is used for normalizing menstrual disorders.

Patee-badam, Deshi-badam; Grahadruma (S) – *Terminalia catappa* L.; Indian almond tree (E); Combretaceae; tree. Cultivated for its edible kernel. Kernels are also the source of an oil used as a substitute for almond oil. Oil cake is used as pig-feed. Fruits yield a black dye. Fruit and bark are used for tanning. Wood is used for rafters, posts and beams and is considered to be a good quality timber. Leaf juice is used in cutaneous infections and in creams and lotions for rheumatic joints. Bark is a cardiotonic and diuretic and is used in dysentery. Leaves are used to rear 'tassar' silkworms. Tree is the source of Indian-almond gum.

Patera – *Typha australis* Schum & Thonn.; Lesser Indian reed mace (E); Typhaceae; tall marshy perennial. Soft sweet core of spike, flowers, young shoots and rhizomes are edible. Leaves are woven into various articles, and the silky florets are used as a stuffing material. Rhizomes are considered to be astringent and diuretic.

Pathar phori; Shilapushpa (S) – *Didymocarpus pedicellata* R. Br.; Gesneriaceae; herb. Leaves serve as a cure for stones in kidney and bladder. Pedicin, a fish-toxin, is present as a crystalline substance in the leaves.

Pathor – *see* Murkula.

Pathur-chatta – *see* Zakhm-haiyat.

Pathurchur, Amroda; Pashanabhedi (S) – *Coleus amboinicus* Lour.; Indian borage (E); Labiatae; hairy herb. Cultivated for its fragrant leaves which are used for flavouring dishes. Leaf decoction is used for treating chronic cough, asthma and urinary disorders.

Leaves are the source of an essential oil which contains carvacrol.

Pathurua bhelagni – *Polygonum glabrum* Willd.; Polygonaceae; herb found along margins of lakes, ponds and ditches. Tender shoots and leaves are used as pot-herb. Infusion of leaves is used in colic pain. Root stocks are used as a remedy for general debility, jaundice and piles.

Pati – *Cyperus serotinus* Rottb. var. *inundatus* (Roxb.) Kukenthal; Cyperaceae; perennial herb. Rhizomes possess stimulant and tonic properties.

Patkarru – *Roylea cinerea* (D. Don) Baill.; Labiatae; tall hoary undershrub. Leaf decoction is used as a febrifuge and tonic.

Patla – *see* Padaria.

Patoia – *see* Meda.

Patol – *see* Jangli seb.

Patrasnuhi (S) – *see* Katathohar.

Patsan, Ambari, Pitwa; Nalita (S) – *Hibiscus cannabinus* L.; Ambari hemp (E); Bimlipatam jute (E); Mesta (E); Malvaceae; bushy undershrub. Stems yield coarse mesta fibre which is used for making rough sack cloth, cordage, paper-pulp, canvas and fishing nets. Seeds yield a fatty oil used in soap and paint industry. Oil is also used for manufacturing linoleum and varnishes, and after refining it is used for edible purposes. Tender shoot and leaves are used as pot-herb and also as cattle-feed.

Patta-gobi, Band-gobi, Karamkalla – *Brassica oleracea* L. var. *capitata* L.; Cabbage (E); Cruciferae; herb with extremely condensed stem and closely packed leaves to form a head. Cultivated for its aerial head which is used raw as salad or cooked as vegetable or soup. Leaves are rich in vitamins and minerals; sinigrin a glycoside is also present.

Pattaranjaka (S) – *see* Bakam.

Patthiri – *see* Rampatri.

Patuasag – *see* Kalmi sag.

Patwa, Lal ambari – *Hibiscus sabdariffa* L.; Roselle (E); Red sorrel (E); Malvaceae; shrub. Cultivated for the fibre called roselle obtained from the stems and used as a jute substitute. Tender shoots and leaves are used as vegetable and condiment. Fleshy fruiting calyces which are rich in pectin, are used in the preparation of jellies and sauces. Calyx infusion is used as a refreshing and digestive beverage, with a mild laxative and cooling action. Seeds yield a fatty oil and the oil-cake is used as cattle-feed.

Paunda – *see* Ganna.

Pavna – *see* Sedwa.

Peela bhangra, Bhanra; Kesaraja (S), Bhringaraja (S) – *Wedelia chinensis* (Osbeck.) Merr.; Compositae; herb. Leaves are used to promote hair growth and also for dyeing hair. Roots are the source of a black dye. Leaf decoction is used as a remedy for alopecia and cough. Herb infusion is used in uterine haemorrhages and menorrhagia. Leaves are used in many herbal hair-dyes and hair-oils.

Peela hisalu – *Rubus pedunculosus* D. Don.; Rosaceae; shrub. Fruits are succulent and edible with pleasant taste.

Peeli badkhadi – *see* Latlatia.

Peeli chameli, Peeli juhi; Svarnajuthica (S) – *Jasminum humile* L.; Yellow jasmine (E); Oleaceae; evergreen shrub. Cultivated as an ornamental for its bright yellow fragrant flowers which are the source of an essential oil used in perfumery. Root juice is used for curing ringworm. Root is also the source of a yellow dye. Milky juice of the stem bark is used for treating sinus trouble.

Peeli champa – *see* Peeli champak.

Peeli champak, Peeli champa – *Michelia nilagirica* Zenker; Yellow champak (E); Magnoliaceae; small tree found in the Nilgiri and adjacent hill ranges. Wood is used for construction work, panels, beams, rafters and furniture. Flowers and bark are the source of an essential oil which is used in perfumery. Bark is also rich in tannin.

Peeli juhi – *see* Peeli chameli.

Peeli kachnar; Phalgu (S); Pita kanchana (S) – *Bauhinia tomentosa* L.; Yellow Bauhinia (E); Caesalpiniaceae; shrub or small tree with conspicuous yellow flowers with a purple centre. Often cultivated as an ornamental. Wood is used for making tool handles. Bark is the source of a fibre. Root bark is medicinal, and is used for curing inflammation of liver. Fruits are considered as diuretic and seeds as tonic. Seeds are the source of a fatty oil called ebony oil.

Peeli kapas, Kumbi – *Cochlospermum religiosum* (L.) Alston; White silk-cotton tree (E); Cochlospermaceae; tree. Seed surface fibre is used for stuffing. Seeds contain a fatty oil. Tree yields an edible gum called 'gond-katira' or katira gum which is used in calico printing, ice-creams, cigar paste and finishing of leather.

Peeli kaner; Ashvaghna (S), Haripriya (S) – *Thevetia peruviana* (Pers.) K. Schum.; Yellow oleander (E), Lucky nut tree (E); Apocynaceae; shrub or small tree. Cultivated as an ornamental. All parts of the plant especially milky latex and kernels are poisonous and possess glycosides as active principles. Kernels are used in treating rheumatism and dropsy and also as a purgative and abortifacient. Root paste is applied to tumours. Bark and leaves act as an emetic and cathartic. Kernels are a rich source of cardiac glycosides which are considered to be useful in heart diseases, of which peruvoside is considered as the most important.

Peeli sarson – *see* Sarson.

Peepal; Ashvattha (S), Kshiradruma (S), Bodhivriksha (S) – *Ficus religiosa* L.; Peepul tree (E), Bo-tree (E); Moraceae; large tree with dense spreading crown. Cultivated as a road-side tree for shade and is considered sacred by the Hindus and Buddhists. The plant is mentioned in sacred scriptures and depicted in temple sculptures. It is one of the few plants which shows high degree of tolerance to atmospheric pollutants, purifies air and is regarded in high reverence. Bark is rich in fibre and tannin, and the bark-infusion is antibacterial; it is used for treating ulcers and skin ailments. Fruits are laxative, and leaves are lopped for fodder. The tree has many legends associated with it, the most important being the attainment of 'nirvana' or salvation by Lord Buddha while meditating under the 'Bodhi tree'.

Peholi – *see* Pacholi.

Peka, Chau – *Bambusa tulda* Roxb.; Bamboo (E); Gramineae, tall erect woody grass. Mature culms are used for building purpose, basketry, and paper manufacture. Young tender culms are used as vegetable.

Pessara – *see* Mung.

Petha, Kooshamanda (S) – *Benincasa hispida* (Thunb.) Cogn.; Ash gourd (E), White pumpkin (E); Cucurbitaceae; large trailing herb. Cultivated for its large oval fruit. Young fruits are used as vegetable. Mature fruit flesh (pulp) is cut into pieces and made into a confectionery called 'petha'. Seeds yield a fatty oil which is considered to be anthelmintic. Fruit pulp decoction is laxative, diuretic, nutritive and tonic; it is used for treating cough, respiratory disorders, internal haemorrhages, dyspepsia, piles and diabetes in the indigenous systems of medicine.

Phalgu (S) – *see* Peeli kachnar.

Phalsa, Shakri-phalsa, Parusha (S) – *Grewia subinaequalis* DC.; Phalsa (E); Tiliaceae; small tree with spreading crown; Cultivated for its small sweet delicious fruits, eaten fresh or made into squashes and a refreshing cool drink. Fruit is rich in sugars, minerals and vitamins and is considered to be nutritive, cooling, astringent and stomachic. Wood is used for implements. Bark is the source of a fibre and is also used for combating rheumatism in tribal medicine.

Phang – *Rivea hypocrateriformis* (Lamk.) Choisy; Midnapore creeper (E); Convolvulaceae; climbing shrub. Root-decoction is administered after child-birth. Tender shoots and leaves are used as vegetable.

Phang nijat; Phanji (S) – *Rivea ornata* (Roxb.) Choisy; Convolvulaceae; straggling shrub, with large white fragrant flowers. Flowers and tender shoots are used as vegetable. Plant juice is used in ointments for curing piles and phthiriasis.

Phanija (S) – *see* Jima.

Phanji (S) – *see* Phang nijat.

Phaphra – *see* Kaspat.

Pharash, Telingachina – *Lagerstroemia indica* L.; Crape-myrtle (E); Lythraceae; shrub. Cultivated as an ornamental. Bark decoction is used as a stimulant and fever reducing agent. Roots act as an astringent. Fruits-infusion is used for local application in aphthae of mouth. Seeds are narcotic. Bark, leaves and flowers are considered to be purgative. Plant is mildly salt-spray tolerant and is considered to be good for beach planting.

Pharsa – *see* Dhamni.

Pharsia – *Grewia sclerophylla* Roxb. Tiliaceae; tree. Wood is used for posts and field implements. Stem yields a fibre. Root is used for treating cough and irritable bladder and root decoction for soothing the skin.

Phaya – *see* Paddam.

Phenila (S) – *see* Reetha.

Phog – *Calligonum polygonoides* L.; Polygonaceae; evergreen shrub found in arid and semi-arid regions. Flower buds are used for treating sun-stroke. Decoction of the root with catechu is used as a gargle for sore-gums. Tender green leaf-like phyllodes are used as camel fodder and thick branches are used as fuel.

Phool gobi – *Brassica oleracea* L. var. *botrytis* L.; Cauliflower (E), Broccoli (E); Cruciferae; annual herb. Cultivated for its immature, dense and highly condensed inflorescence called curds which is used as a vegetable or made into soups and pickles. Leaves and condensed stems are used as stock feed.

Phoont – *see* Kachri.

Phulan – *see* Didhen.

Phulla – *see* Ban tambaku.

Phulvara, Phulwa – *Diploknema butyracea* (Roxb.) H.J. Lam. (syn. *Bassia butyracea* Roxb.); Indian butter tree (E), Bassia fat (E); Sapotaceae; large tree found in the Himalayan ranges. Fruits are edible. Seeds are the source of a fat called 'phulwa' butter which is used either in the manufacture of margarine, candles and soaps or used directly as a cooking medium and illuminant. 'Phulwa' butter is also used as a substitute of cocoa butter in the manufacture of chocolates. Oil-cake is used as manure and after removal of toxins serves as poultry- or stock-feed. Bark and oil-cake are both used as a fish poison.

Phulwa – *see* Phulvara.

Phusera, Gogsa – *Maesa argentea* Wall.; Myrsinaceae; shrub. Berries are eaten by people living in the hills.

Phutki – *Melastoma malabathricum* L.; Indian Rhododendron (E); Melastomataceae; shrub. Leaves and flowers are eaten. Fruits are the source of a black dye while the roots and leaves yield a pink dye. Decoction or paste of root and bark is used for curing wounds and skin ailments. Plant is used for controlling diarrhoea and dysentery. Leaves are used to rear 'atlas' silkworms.

Piaman – *see* Dugdugia.

Piaz – *see* Piyaz.

Pilkhan – *Ficus virens* Ait. var. *sublanceolata* (Miq.) Corner and *Ficus virens* Ait. var. *virens*; Moraceae; tree with dense crown. Both the varieties are cultivated as avenue trees, and for shade in public places. Leaves are lopped for fodder and are relished by animals. Tree is very popular for making bonsai.

Pilu – *see* Bara pilu.

Pindalu – *see* Katul.

Pindalu (S) – *see* Chupri alu.

Pindar; Nagapatra – *Crinum asiaticum* L.; Amaryllidaceae; perennial robust herb with underground bulb. Cultivated as an ornamental for its evergreen foliage and fragrant flowers. Seeds are purgative. Bulb acts as a laxative, and is used in biliousness and urinary disorders. Fresh roots are emetic.

Pindara – *see* Bhillaura.

Pindava – *see* Dikamli.

Pind khajur – *see* Khajur.

Pinjari – *see* Mamiran.

Pipal – *see* Pipli.

Piplamul – *see* Pipli.

Pipli, Pipal, Piplamul; Pippali (S) – *Piper longum* L.; Long pepper (E); Piperaceae; climbing shrub. Cultivated for its fruit which is used as a spice and condiment and also used in indigenous medicine for treating colds and bronchitis. Roots called 'piplamul' and fruits called 'pipli' are used for reducing inflammation and as an analgesic for muscular pains. Fruits are used internally as a carminative, sedative, abortifacient and for removing obstruction in the gall bladder and bile duct.

Pippali (S) – *see* Pipli.

Pippalyang, Tarcharbi, Vilayati shisham – *Sapium sebiferum* (L.) Roxb.; Chinese tallow tree (E); Euphorbiaceae; tree. Cultivated as an ornamental. Fruits are the source of a fat called Chinese vegetable tallow which is obtained from the waxy cover on the seeds and is used in the manufacture of soaps, candles, and cosmetics. It is edible after refining and is used as a substitute for animal tallow. The kernels yield a drying oil known as stillingia oil used for the manufacture of varnishes, paints and plastics. The oil is considered to be emetic and purgative, and is used for cutaneous infections. Oil-cake is used as a stock-feed and fertilizer. Wood is used for making toys and cricket bats. Root bark acts as a purgative. Root decoction is tonic and used in dyspepsia. Leaves are the source of a black dye and are also used to rear 'eri' silkworms.

Pismarum, Satari – *Ruta chalepensis* L.; Rutaceae; herb. Cultivated for its aromatic leaves which are used in stews and salads. Leaves yield an essential oil which is used as a substitute for garden rue oil obtained from *Ruta graveolens* L. Plant is considered to be an antispasmodic and nerve stimulant and is used for the treatment of inflammation of the mucous membranes in infants.

Pissu-mar buti – *Boenninghausenia albiflora* (Hook.) Reichb. ex Meissn.; Rutaceae; perennial herb found in the Himalayas and

Khasi hills. Leaves when crushed emit a strong disagreeable smell and is used to ward off fleas. Essential oil obtained from the leaves is also used as a flea-repellent.

Pista – *Pistacia vera* L.; Pistachio (E), Green almond (E); Pistaciaceae; small tree. Cultivated in the hilly regions of North India for its edible seeds which are used as a dry fruit after roasting. Due to its high price very thin slices are usually sprinkled on top of certain confectionery to add to its appearance and taste.

Pitaalu – *see* Ratalu.

Pitadaru (S) – *see* Lata-achhuk.

Pita kanchana (S) – *see* Peeli kachnar.

Pita-kara – *Donella roxburghii* (G. Don.) Pierre ex Lecomte; Star apple (E); Sapotaceae; evergreen tree. Fruits are edible. Wood is used for match-box and match-stick industry.

Pitasara – *see* Bijasal.

Pithari (S) – *see* Seri.

Pithia – *see* Bachita.

Pithvan; Atiguha (S), Prisniparni (S) – *Uraria lagopodioides* (L.) Desv.; Papilionaceae; erect undershrub. Plant is used in Ayurvedic medicine as one of the constituents of 'Dasamula'. Herb decoction with milk acts as an abortifacient. Herb is considered to be a carminative, diuretic, expectorant and nervine tonic, and is used for combating cough, asthma, dysentery, bleeding piles, and rheumatism.

Pitmari; Kandalu (S) – *Naregamia alata* Wight & Arn.; Goanese ipecacuanha (E); Meliaceae; shrub. Creeping roots are expectorant and emetic and are used in chronic bronchitis, rheumatism and dysentery. Leaf decoction is useful in counteracting biliousness. Plant is also used in prescriptions for treating enlarged spleen, anaemia and intermittent fevers.

Pitmula – *see* Mamira.

Pitni baer – *see* Unnab.

Pitohri – *see* Nisoth.

Pitpapara, Shahterah; Araka (S), Nakra (S) – *Fumaria vaillantii* Loisel. (syn. *Fumaria indica* Pugsley; *Fumaria parviflora* ssp. *Vaillantii* Hook f.); Fumitory (E); Fumariaceae; annual herb. Dried plant is used in many Ayurvedic preparations. Plant is anthelmintic, diuretic, laxative and expectorant and is used in treating dyspepsia, liver troubles, cough, colds, skin infections and alcoholism. The drug called 'shahterah' is also used in Unani medicine and is obtained from both *Fumaria officinalis* L. and *Fumaria parviflora* Lam.

Pitti – *see* Bika-kalibel and Rai-dhani.

Pitwa – *see* Patsan.

Piyala – *Buchanania axillaris* (Desr.) Ramam; Buchanan's mango (E); Anacardiaceae; tree. Fruits are edible. Wood is used for making packing boxes.

Piyaz, Piaz; Palandu (S) – *Allium cepa* L.; Onion (E); Alliaceae; herb. Cultivated as an annual for its mature and immature bulbs, used raw or cooked as vegetable or put in curries for seasoning food. Bulbs are expectorant, diuretic and stimulant, and are used in cough, colds, flatulence and dysentery. Chief principle present is glycollic acid. Roasted onions are also applied as poultice.

Piyazi – *Allium schoenoprasum* L.; Chive (E); Alliaceae; perennial herb. Often cultivated for its bulbs and leaves which are used as a condiment.

Plaksha (S) – *see* Kahimal; *see also* Paraspipal.

Podina – *see* Pudina.

Pohna – *see* Ponai.

Poi – *Basella alba* L. (syn. *B. rubra* L.); Ceylon spinach (E); Basellaceae; twining perennial herb. Cultivated for its tender stem and succulent leaves which are used as pot-herb. Pulped leaves are used as poultice. Leaf juice is used as a mild laxative. Fleshy fruits yield a sap which is used for colouring sweets and jellies.

Pola – *see* Choupultea.

Ponai – *see* Bhanjuri.

Pooah, Puya – *Maoutia puya* (Hook.) Wedd.; Urticaceae; shrub. Stem bark is the source of a strong fibre called 'puya' hemp which is used for making twines and fishing nets.

Poogiphalam (S) – *see* Supari.

Post – *see* Afim.

Poste-ke-bija – *see* Lal post.

Potol – *see* Parwal.

Prasarani (S) – *see* Gandhali.

Prasarna – *see* Haranpadi.

Prasniparni (S) – *see* Dabra.

Prisniparni (S) – *see* Pithvan.

Priyangu – *Aglaia elaeagnoidea* (Juss.) Benth.; Meliaceae; large tree. Wood is heavy and with a natural lustre and is used for ornamental furniture and implements. Flowers are fragrant and are used in perfumery. Fruits are edible, and considered to be astringent and are used for treating inflammation, leprosy and mild fever.

Pudina, Podina – *Mentha arvensis* L.; Field mint (E); Labiatae; perennial herb. Cultivated for its fragrant leaves. Plant is stimulant, digestive, carminative and cooling and is used in many Ayurvedic preparations. Infusion of leaves is used in rheumatism. Leaves are the source of an essential oil. Fresh leaves crushed along with certain spices are consumed in the form of chutney or made into a dry powder which is used to flavour yoghurt and certain cool refreshing drinks.

Pudu – *see* Budu.

Puga (S) – *see* Supari.

Pula – *see* Choupultea.

Pullung, Warras – *Heterophragma quadriloculare* (Roxb.) K. Schum.; Bignoniaceae; tree. Wood is used for rafters, posts, planks and cabinet-work. It also yields a thick tar which is used in cutaneous diseases. Root decoction is prescribed as an antidote in viper bite.

Punarnava (S) – *see* Sant.

Pundarika (S) – *see* Muyna.

Punia – *see* Gual.

Punir – *see* Akri.

Punjki – *see* Samudulan.

Punk – *Combretum roxburghii* Spreng; Combretaceae; Large climber. Stems are used for basketry. Leaves are considered to be a febrifuge.

Punnagchampa – *Alpinia zerumbet* Burtt & R.M. Smith; Light galangal (E), Shell flower (E); Zingiberaceae; ornamental herb. Cultivated for its fragrant flowers which are borne on long drooping racemes. Rhizomes and leaves yield an essential oil. Rhizomes are also used as a condiment and as a substitute for 'Bara kulanjan' or Greater galangal.

Purtuk – *Astragalus hamosus* L.; Papilionaceae; large shrub. Plant is considered to be a laxative and demulcent and is useful in counteracting the irritation of mucous membranes, and nervine disorders.

Pussur – *Xylocarpus molluccensis* (Lamk.) Roem. (syn. *Carapa moluccensis* Lamk.); Carapa (E); Meliaceae; tree found in the Andamans. Wood is used for making house posts, boats and furniture. Seed is the source of carapa oil which is used for the manufacture of soaps and also serves as an illuminant. Bark is rich in tannin and is used for tanning and toughening fishing nets. Another species *Xylocarpus granatum* Koen., a tree found in the swampy forests of India is also known by the same Hindi name and yields valuable, hard, dark-red coloured wood which is suitable for making boats and furniture, and bark which is used for treating diarrhoea, dysentery and abdominal disorders.

Puth kunda – *see* Latjira.

Putikaranja – *see* Karanju.

Putranjiva, Jiaputa – *Putranjiva roxburghii* Wall.; Indian amulet plant (E); Child life-tree (E); Euphorbiacee; tall tree. Cultivated as an evergreen avenue tree or as a hedge plant. Wood is used for agricultural implements. Nuts are made into rosaries and necklaces and are often put on children as an amulet for their long life. The decoction of leaves and nuts is used for treating colds, fever and rheumatism. Leaves are lopped for fodder.

Putulika (S) – *see* Parwal.

Puya – *see* Pooah.

R

Rai – *see* Asal rai.

Raiba – *Cenchrus ciliaris* L.; Bunch grass (E); African foxtail (E); Gramineae; much tillered perennial grass. Plant is used as fodder both fresh and as hay and is considered to be very nutritious.

Raichkand trivritta – *Merremia tuberosa* (L.) Rendle (syn. *Ipomoea tuberosa* L.); Spanish arbour-vine (E); Convolvulaceae; twining or prostrate herb. Cultivated for its tuberous roots termed Brazilian jalap which are used as a strong purgative.

Rai-dhani, Pitti – *Ventilago denticulata* Willd.; Rhamnaceae; scandent shrub. Stem bark is the source of a fibre used for cordage. Bark-juice is reported to cure deafness. Pulverized bark is used on sprains. Seeds yield a fatty oil which is used as a cooking medium.

Raitung – *see* Tung.

Rajakoshataki (S) – *see* Tori.

Rajana – *see* Rangan.

Rajataru (S) – *see* Amaltas.

Rajika – *see* Mandal.

Rajmah – *see* Frash bean.

Rajnigandha, Gulcheri, Gulshabbo – *Polianthes tuberosa* L.; Tuberose (E); Amaryllidaceae; herb with underground bulbs. Cultivated for its beautiful white, extremely sweet scented flowers which are highly esteemed for garlands, cut flower arrangements, and bouquets. Flowers are the source of an essential oil with very delicate odour called tuberose-oil which is used in perfumery. Bulbs are considered as an emetic and diuretic.

Rakasgaddah – *see* Akasgaddah.

Rakat-rohan – *see* Rohan.

Raktachandana (S) – *see* Lal chandan.

Raktachitraka – *see* Lal chitra.

Raktaka (S) – *see* Rangan.

Raktamadar, Dadap, Parijata (S) – *Erythrina variegata* var. *orientalis* (L.) Merr. (syn. *E. indica* Lamk.); Coral tree (E); Papilionaceae; tree. Cultivated as an ornamental for its beautiful scarlet-red flowers and also grown as a live-support for black-pepper vines. Tender shoots and pods are edible. Flowers yield a red dye. Stem bark is the source of cordage fibre. Leaves are lopped for fodder.

Rakta-skandana (S) – *see* Vrana patta.

Raktavalli (S) – *see* Bika-kalibel.

Raktgarbha (S) – *see* Mehndi.

Ral – *see* Safed damar; *see also* Sal.

Ramalo – *Macaranga indica* Wight; Euphorbiaceae; tree. Bark serves as the source of a crimson-red gum which is used for taking impressions of coins, medallions etc., for making casts. Wood is suitable for match-stick industry and paper pulp.

Ram baigan; Garbhada (S) – *Solanum stramonifolium* Jacq.; Solanaceae; prickly herb. Plant is used in indigenous medicine as a remedy for cough, sore throat, bronchitis, asthma, rheumatism and dropsy. Root decoction is given to improve digestion, and relieve labour-pains. Seed fumes are used to treat toothache. Berries are used in curries to improve appetite and help digestion.

Rambha (S) – *see* Kela.

Ramchana – *see* Amal bel.

Ram dana – *Amaranthus caudatus* L.; Amaranth seed (E), African spinach (E); Amaranthaceae; tall herb. Cultivated for its tender shoot, leaves and seeds. Tender shoots along with leaves are used as pot-herb and are very rich in vitamins and minerals. Seeds known as 'chaulai' or 'Ram dana' are consumed as food in various ways after puffing and are considered very nutritious.

Ram-dataun – *Smilax perfoliata* Lour.; Smilacaceae; prickly climber. Cultivated as an ornamental. Roots are used medicinally as a substitute for sarsaparilla. Jangli aushbah, is also known by the same Hindi name.

Ram-dataun – *see also* Jangli aushbah.

Rametha – *Lasiosiphon eriocephalus* Decne.; Thymelaeaceae; large shrub. Bark yields a fibre, and is also suitable for paper pulp. Leaves in paste-form are applied to swellings. Bark and leaves are used to stupefy fish.

Ramgoah – *see* Mari.

Ramkurthi – *see* Bhat.

Rampatri, Patthiri–*Myristica malabarica* Lamk.; False nutmeg (E), Bombay mace (E); Myristicaceae; small tree. Seeds and aril of seeds are odourless and are used as an adulterant for the genuine 'jaiphal' or nutmeg and 'javitri' or mace. Seeds are the source of a crude fatty oil called pundi oil which is used in rheumatism and also as an illuminant. Bark yields a gum-resin. Wood is suitable for making furniture, match-sticks and packing boxes.

Ramphal, Lavni-anona – *Annona reticulata* L.; Bullock's heart (E), Common custard apple (E); Annonaceae; small tree. Cultivated for its fruit which is edible but considered inferior to 'sharifa' or custard apple. Raw fruits act as an anthelmintic and seeds are the source of an oil used for making soap. Seed oil is considered insecticidal. Bark is a powerful astringent.

Ramsar; Chamri-ke-bel, Bhadramunja (S) – *Vallaris solanacea* (Roth) O. Kuntze (syn. *Peltanthera solanacea* Roth.); Apocynaceae; shrub with white, fragrant flowers. Cultivated as an ornamental. Bark is a bitter astringent, strengthens loose teeth, and is used in Ayurvedic medicinal oil known as 'Vishagarbha taila'. Seeds are the source of a fatty oil. Latex from the plant, a mild irritant is used on sores and wounds. Flowers and fruits are edible.

Ram til – *see* Kala til.

Ram tulsi; Vriddhutulsi (S) – *Ocimum gratissimum* L.; Shrubby basil (E); Labiatae; shrub. Often cultivated for its strongly scented leaves used as a mosquito repellent and for biological control of mosquitoes. Leaves yield an antibacterial essential oil which is used for curing toothache, earache and stomach ache in children. Plant has antiseptic, tonic, digestive, stimulant, diuretic, soothing, expectorant and anthelmintic properties and is often used in the form of tea and cough mixtures. Leaves are also used in fumigations given for treating paralysis and rheumatism. Seeds are used for curing dysentery, neuralgia and urinary disorders.

Ranavali – *see* Kanocha.

Ranbaigan – *see* Titbaigan.

Ranbhendi, Vilayati bhendi – *Malachra capitata* L.; Cork wood (E); Malvaceae; herb. Stem is the source of a coarse fibre used for making gunny bags, coarse cloth, ropes and twines. Roots are used as a febrifuge and in medicinal lotions and oils used for rubbing on painful rheumatic joints. Leaves are considered as an anthelmintic.

Ranbhindi – *Abelmoschus ficulneus* (L.) Wight. & Arn. (syn. *Hibiscus ficulneus* L.); White wild musk-mallow (E); Malvaceae; herb. Green stems are the source of a mucilaginous extract used for clarifying sugarcane juice. Seeds are fragrant, and serve as the source of an essential oil used for flavouring. Stems yield a rough fibre used for making ropes and twines.

Randhuni – *see* Ajmud.

Rangan, Rajana, Rookmini; Bandhuka (S); Raktaka (S) – *Ixora coccinea* L.; Jungle flame Ixora (E); Rubiaceae; shrub. Cultivated for hedges and as an ornamental plant for its beautiful red flowers produced in clusters. Flowers are used medicinally for curing dysentery, severe cough associated with bleeding and leucorrhoea. Roots are antiseptic, astringent, sedative and stomachic, and are used in diarrhoea, dysentery, hiccups and loss of appetite.

Rangoon-ki-bel – *Quisqualis indica* L.; Rangoon creeper (E); Combretaceae; climbing shrub. Cultivated as an ornamental for its beautiful clusters of pinkish-red fragrant flowers. Seeds are anthelmintic and soporific. Roasted seeds are used in treating rickets, diarrhoea and fever. Seeds decoction in oil is applied topically in skin diseases. Seeds are the source of a fatty oil which is purgative in action. Flexible stem is used for making baskets and fish-traps.

Rasagaduhi (S) – *see* Guggul.

Rasaut, Darhald; Daruharidra (S) – *Berberis aristata* DC.; Indian barberry (E); Berberidaceae; spiny shrub found in the hills. Root bark is the principal source of 'rasaut' which is considered as a carminative, blood purifier, ophthalmic and tonic, and is used in the treatment of hepatitis, diarrhoea, bilious disorders, remittent fevers, uterine troubles, skin diseases and infections of the eyes. Active principles present are berberine, oxycanthine and umbellatine. Other species used as sources of 'rasaut' are – *Berberis asiatica* Roxb. and *B. lycium* Royle. Fruits are used as a mild laxative for children.

Rasbhari, Tankari, Tipari – *Physalis peruviana* L.; Cape gooseberry (E); Solanaceae; annual herb. Cultivated for its juicy, fleshy and orange coloured edible berries enclosed within a papery persistent calyx, and used fresh or made into jam. Seeds are the source of a semi-drying oil. Leaves are used in abdominal disorders.

Rasna, Vanda; Atirasa (S), Bhujangakshi (S) – *Vanda tessellata* (Roxb.) Hook ex G. Don; Orchidaceae; epiphytic herb. Thick white fleshy roots are a bitter astringent and are used for treating bronchitis, dyspepsia, fevers and rheumatism; they are also used in medicated oils applied to painful inflamed rheumatic joints. Roots are reported to show antibacterial and antitubercular action. Leaf juice is used for ear trouble.

Ratakohomba, Sivanimba (S) – *Indigofera aspalathoides* Vahl ex DC; Wiry indigo (E); Papilionaceae; perennial herb, found in South

India. Tender shoots, leaves and flower decoction is used in indigenous medicine for combating leprosy and cancerous infections; the plant is also used in the preparation of medicated oils for treating dandruff, skin ailments and syphilis.

Ratalu, Gaithi, Pitaalu – *Dioscorea bulbifera* L.; Air potato (E); Potato yam (E); Dioscoreaceae; perennial herbaceous climber with tuberous roots. Leaf axils produce fleshy succulent bulbils or tubers which can be consumed only after elimination of calcium oxalate and poisonous alkaloids. Dried and powdered tubers are applied to ulcers and also used in remedies for curing piles and dysentery.

Ratanjot – *Onosma hispidum* Wall ex D. Don; Boraginaceae; hispid undershrub. Roots serve as one of the sources of 'ratanjot' used as a red colouring for foodstuffs, oils and medicinal products. However, the genuine 'ratanjot' used commercially and available in the Indian market, is the dye-yielding root of *Arnebia nobilis* Reichb. f. The root of the Indian species *Arnebia hispidissima* (Laehm.) DC. also yields a red dye but is used for colouring hair oils only.

Ratanjyot – *see* Bagbherenda.

Ratanpurus; Amburuha (S), Charati (S) – *Hybanthus enneaspermus* (L.) F.v. Muell; Violaceae; herb. Roots are considered as tonic and diuretic and are used in urinary and bowel disorders.

Rat-ki-rani – *Cestrum nocturnum* L.; Night jessamine (E); Solanaceae; diffuse shrub trained as a climber. Cultivated as an ornamental for its extremely sweet scented clusters of flowers which open in the night, and fill the air with their aroma.

Ratmandi – *see* Chhota kulpha.

Ratnagandi (S) – *see* Gulutora.

Ratti, Gunchi, Chirmiti; Gunja (S) – *Abrus precatorius* L.; Indian liquorice (E), Jecquirity seeds (E); Papilionaceae; climbing shrub. Roots and leaves are rich in glycyrrhizin and their decoction is used for getting rid of cough and colds. Roots act as an emetic, diuretic and tonic. Seeds are used in the prescriptions for nervous system disorders and contain the poisonous principle abrine: bruised seeds are highly poisonous. The attractive, red coloured seeds with black hilum are used for making necklaces, bracelets and fancy articles and were used as standard small weights by the jewellers in India in olden times.

Reetha; Ritha; Arishtha (S), Phenila (S) – *Sapindus emarginatus* Vahl; Soapnut (E); Sapindaceae; tree. Fruits are valued as a detergent and are used for washing hair, silks and woollens. Saponins are present in the fruit pericarp, which are used in soaps, tooth pastes, and as foam stabilizers in shampoos, deodorants, germicides and fire extinguishing preparations. Fruits are tonic, astringent, and emetic, and are used in remedies for asthma, stomach ache following indigestion, diarrhoea, lumbago and paralysis of limbs. Fruits and root-bark are also used as fish-poison. Seed-shell is the source of a black dye. Kernels yield a fixed oil which is used as a source of oleic acid and for the manufacture of soap.

Retwa – *see* Khilut.

Revand-chini – *see* Dolu.

Revatchini (S) – *see* Dolu.

Rewar – *see* Paludar.

Rikhpat – *see* Papra.

Rion – *Marsdenia tinctoria* R. Br.; Asclepiadaceae; undershrub. Cultivated for a coarse fibre obtained from its stem and used for making ropes. Leaves are the source of an indigo like dye and are also used for curing stomach ache.

Rissa – *see* Badavard.

Ritha – *Erioglossum rubiginosum* (Roxb.) Blume; Sapindaceae; tree. Tender shoots and leaves are used as pot-herb. Fruits are edible. Wood is used for making rice-pounders and for other purposes. Seed decoction is used as a remedy for whooping cough.

Ritha – *see* Reetha.

Riu – *Cotoneaster acuminata* Lindl; Rosaceae; shrub found in the hills. Stem is used for making turnery articles like umbrella handles, golf-clubs, walking-sticks and some agricultural implements. Twigs are used for basketry.

Rogan-banafshah – *see* Banafshah.

Rohan, Rakat-rohan – *Soymida febrifuga* A. Juss.; Indian red-wood (E); Meliaceae; tree. Bark yields a fibre of red colour which is used for making ropes. Gum exuded from the tree trunk is a good adhesive. Bark is also rich in tannins, and is used medicinally as a general tonic and febrifuge; it is also used for curing diarrhoea, dysentery and fevers. Its decoction is used for gargles, vaginal infections and rheumatic inflammations. Wood is used for rafters, beams, posts, furniture, carving and turnery articles and the wood-pulp is used for the manufacture of wrapping paper.

Rohera – *see* Rugtrora.

Rohi (S) – *see* Rugtrora.

Rohini – *see* Kamela.

Rohisa (S) – *see* Gandhej ghas.

Rohituka (S) – *see* Harin-hara.

Ronj – *see* Safed kikar.

Rookmini – *see* Rangan.

Rousaghas; Bhutika (S) – *Cymbopogon schoenanthus* (L.) Spreng; Camel hay (E); Gramineae; many tillered fragrant grass. Plants are used as camel fodder. Leaves are the source of an essential oil which is used in perfumery. Leaf decoction is astringent and is used as a febrifuge.

Rowana – *Clausena pentaphylla* (Roxb.) DC.; Rutaceae; shrub. Plant is aromatic. Bark is used in poultices for wounds and sprains in veterinary medicine.

Rubber – *see* Rubberh-ka-paudha.

Rubberh-ka-paudha – *Hevea brasiliensis* (Willd. ex Adr. de Juss.) Muell.-Arg.; Para rubber tree (E); Euphorbiaceae; tall tree native to the Amazon valley of tropical America and successfully grown as a plantation crop in Assam, S. India and the Andaman islands. The plant is cultivated for its thick milky latex obtained by tapping the bark of the tree-trunks at certain intervals of time. The latex is used for the production of solid commercial rubber which is an indispensable item of modern life, and is used for the manufacture of innumerable products either directly or indirectly. Nearly 70 per cent of the rubber produced is consumed by the automobile industry for the production of tyres and tubes. The rest is utilised for the production of wire and cable insulation, foot-wear, hospital supplies, rubber sheets, foam rubber used for making mattresses, seats, cusions and pillows, rain-coats, water-proof cloth, frogmen's suits for divers, pressurised suits for special aircraft personnel, hoses, shock absorbers, hot-water bottles, gaskets, washers, belts, sports goods, rubber gloves, toys, erasers and a variety of other articles. Ebonite or vulcanite or hard rubber is used in various industries catering to electrical and radio engineering, as a protective lining in chemical plants and battery boxes and for the manufacture of many other products.

Rudraki – *see* Rudraksh.

Rudraksh, Rudraki; Rudraksha (S) – *Elaeocarpus sphaericus* (Gaertn.) K. Schum.; Utrasum bead-tree (E); Elaeocarpaceae; tree. Fruit is edible, and is used in epilepsy. Stones are hard and tubercled and are made into rosaries, bracelets and buttons. The plant is associated with Lord Shiva, one of the trinity Gods of the Hindus and the stone of the fruit called 'Rudraksh' is supposed to have originated from a tear in His eye and therefore, considered very sacred and worn as an amulet.

Rudraksha (S) – *see* Rudraksh.

Rudra pushpam (S) – *see* Gurhal.

Rudravanti – *Cressa cretica* L.; Convolvulaceae; undershrub. Plant is considered to be a stomachic, tonic and aphrodisiac.

Rugtoora – *Spathodea campanulata* Beauv.; African tulip tree (E); Fountain tree (E); Bignoniaceae; large tree. Cultivated as an ornamental avenue tree, or a live-shade tree in coffee plantations. Wood is used for general carpentry. Pulverized bark is used for skin ailments, and the bark decoction for gastro-intestinal and kidney trouble. Fruit pulp is used by tribals to poison birds and animals. Seeds are edible.

Rugtrora, Bohira, Rohera; Rohi (S) – *Tecomella undulata* (Sm.) Seem. (syn. *Bignonia undulata* Smith); Wave-leaved Bignonia (E); Rohida tree (E); Bignoniaceae; small tree with beautiful orange clusters of flowers. Often cultivated for hedges or as an ornamental tree. Wood is used for carving, and for making implements and furniture. Leaves are lopped for fodder.

Rui – *see* Kapas.

Rumi-mastaki – *Pistacia lentiscus* L.; Mastik tree (E); Pistaciaceae; evergreen small tree. Resinous exudation commercially traded as mastik is used in chewing gums, cordials and alcoholic beverages. Resin is chiefly used in transparent varnishes for coating paintings, retouching negatives and for lithographic processes. It is also considered as a stimulant, diuretic and carminative. Fruits and leaves are the source of an essential oil. Seeds yield an edible fatty oil. Leaves are also used as a source of tannin.

Rungru – *see* Haiza.

Rusmari – *Rosmarinus officinalis* L.; Rosemary (E); Labiatae; herb. Cultivated as an ornamental for its fragrant leaves and flowers. Leaves and flowering tops yield an essential oil called rosemary oil which is used in the preparation of scented soaps, hair oils, inhalants, and perfumes; it is also used for denaturing of alcohol. Leaf juice is antibacterial and leaf decoction abortifacient. Dried leaf fumes are inhaled for asthma. Leaves and flowering tops are used in remedies for treating paralysis and rheumatism. Plant infusion concentrate mixed with borax is used for curing premature baldness.

S

Saatar – *Zataria multiflora* Boiss.; Labiatae; small aromatic herb. All aerial parts are used in the drug marketed as 'saatar'. Plant is considered to be a tonic, stimulant, diuretic and stomachic, and is also used to treat premature labour pains. Aerial parts also yield an essential oil.

Sabbajaya, Keli; Devakili (S), Sarvajaya (S) – *Canna orientalis* Rosc.; Indian shot (E); Cannaceae; perennial herb. Cultivated as an ornamental for its beautiful flowers. Rhizomes are edible after cooking. Roots are the source of a fibre used for rough weaving and are also used in indigenous medicine as a diuretic and diaphoretic. Hard black seeds are used as beads for making necklaces.

Sabuni, Musna – *Saponaria vaccaria* L.; Caryophyllaceae; herb. Roots and leaves are rich in saponin, and are used for washing wool and silk. Roots are also used for making foam in beer. Mucilaginous sap is used medicinally for treating scabies and skin troubles. Herb is used as a tonic and febrifuge. Seed-saponin is haemolytic in activity.

Sada bahar, Sada sawagan – *Catharanthus roseus* Don; Madagascar periwinkle (E); Apocynaceae; small undershrub. Cultivated as an ornamental. Roots and basal part of stems contain about fifteen alkaloids of the drug rauvolfia group with hypotensive and sedative properties. Two other alkaloids are present *viz.*, vinblastine and vincristine which are being used in cancer therapy. Cultivation of the plant for medicinal extraction of drugs has been undertaken in Tamil Nadu and other states of India. Research is also being carried out in the regional Ayurvedic Research Centres on the side-effects of vincristine which is known to have anti-cancer properties.

Sadab – *Ruta graveolens* L.; Garden rue (E); Rutaceae; herb. Leaves are used as a condiment and the source of rue oil which is used mostly in veterinary medicine. Rue oil is anthelmintic, antispasmodic, rubefacient and antiepileptic. Herb extract is used for curing earache and toothache. Besides the essential oil, leaves also contain ample amounts of coumarins.

Sadah-dhatura, Kala dhatura; Dhustura (S) – *Datura metel* L.; Solanaceae; undershrub. Leaves and flowering tops act as an antispasmodic and narcotic, and are used in the treatment of asthma. Chief alkaloid present is scopolamine. Seeds contain a fixed oil.

Sadanatya – *see* Chaulai.

Sadaphal – *see* Chakotra.

Sada sawagan – *see* Sada bahar.

Sadodi – *see* Daudotpala.

Sadovani – *see* Jutuk.

Safeda – *see* Safed frast; *see also* Eucalyptus.

Safed-ak – *see* Akada.

Safed arand – *see* Bagbherenda.

Safed bach – *see* Bach.

Safed bombway, Safed terminalia – *Terminalia procera* Roxb.; White bombwe (E); Combretaceae; tree found in the Andaman islands. Wood is used for railway sleepers, construction work, bodies of lorries and their floor-boards, veneers, plywood and heavy packing boxes. Fruits are used for dyeing.

Safed champa – *Plumeria alba* L.; White frangipani (E); Apocynaceae; small tree. Cultivated as an ornamental for its beautiful glossy green foliage and white showy flowers arranged in clusters. Latex is used to treat ulcers.

Safed champak – *Michelia montana* Blume.; White champa (E); Magnoliaceae; tree chiefly grown in East India. Wood is used for construction work, furniture and bridges. Bark is bitter and is used as a febrifuge.

Safed chuglam – *Terminalia bialata* Steud.; White chuglam (E); Combretaceae; tree found in the Andaman islands. Silvery grey wood is used for decorative interior work, cabinet work, furniture and veneers.

Safed-damar, Barasal, Ral; Ajakarna (S) – *Vateria indica* L.; Indian copal tree (E), Piney varnish tree (E), White damar (E); Dipterocarpaceae; tree. Resin exuded from the tree known as dammar resin is soluble in turpentine and is used for making varnishes, and incense. It is considered to be an expectorant and used for combating chronic bronchitis, throat troubles, piles, diarrhoea and rheumatism in the indigenous systems of medicine. Seeds are also the source of a fat called piney tallow or dhupa fat, which is used for the manufacture of soaps and candles. Seed oil-cake is used as manure. Fruit shells yield tannin. The wood traded as malabar white pine is used for making packing cases and for the manufacture of plywood.

Safed frast, Jangli frast, Safeda – *Populus alba* L.; White poplar (E); Salicaceae; tree. Wood is used for cabinet work, packing boxes, turnery articles, match boxes and newsprint paper. Wood-wool is used for making cooling pads which are used in desert room-coolers. Bark is diuretic and antipyretic, and is used in remedies for fevers, neuralgia and rheumatism; its paste is also applied locally in skin ailments. Bark is rich in the glycosides salicin and populin.

Safed gulab; Bhringeshtha (S) – *Rosa alba* L.; White cottage rose (E), Common English dog rose (E); Rosaceae; undershrub. Cultivated as an ornamental. Flower petals yield an essential oil which is used for normalizing palpitation of the heart.

Safed kachnar; Sivamalli (S) – *Bauhinia acuminata* L.; Caesalpiniaceae; small tree. Cultivated as an ornamental and blooms profusely during summer. Flowers are edible and considered to be cooling. Decoction of the bark and leaves is administered in counteracting asthma, biliousness, stones in bladder and leprosy.

Safed kaddu, Kumra, Vilayati kaddu – *Cucurbita pepo* L.; Field pumpkin (E); Vegetable marrow (E); Cucurbitaceae; hairy, robust, annual herb. Cultivated for its raw fruits which are used as vegetable. Seeds are used as taeniacide.

Safed kadsumbal – *see* Bara sem.

Safed kikar, Arinj, Ronj; Arimeda (S) – *Acacia leucophloea* Willd.; Mimosaceae; tree characteristic of dry regions. Bark is the source of a fibre and tannin. It is used in the preparation of alcohol from palm juice and is also used in biliousness and bronchitis. Tree exudes a gum which is used as an emulsifier. Wood is used for agricultural implements and fire-wood. Leaves and pods are used as fodder.

Safed murgha, Sarwari; Vitunna (S) – *Celosia argentea* L.; Quail grass (E); Amaranthaceae; herb. Tender stems and leaves are used as vegetable. The decoction of seeds is used in treating sore mouth, diarrhoea and eye trouble.

Safed musli – *Asparagus adscendens* Roxb.; Liliaceae; small prickly shrub. Tubers are refrigerant, demulcent and tonic and are used as a remedy for general debility, diarrhoea and dysentery; they are also considered useful in impotency.

Safed rai, Ujli sarson; Swet sarisha (S) – *Brassica alba* (L.) Rabenh (syn. *Sinapis alba* L.); White mustard (E); Cruciferae; cultivated herb. Leaves and tender shoots are used as pot herb. Seeds are the source of a fatty edible oil called mustard oil. Seeds possess sinalbin a glycoside, which on hydrolysis with the enzyme myrosinase produces isothiocyanates imparting pungency to the mustard oil.

Safed sambhalu – *see* Pani-ka-sambhalu.

Safed senji – *Melilotus alba* Desr.; Hubam clover (E), White sweet clover (E); Papilionaceae; herb. Plant is used as fodder and silage, and is very rich in proteins. It is often cultivated and grows well even on poor soils. Seeds yield a semi drying fatty oil which is used in paints and varnishes.

Safed semul, Hattian; Sveta salmali (S) – *Ceiba pentandra* (L.) Gaertn.; Kapok (E), White silk cotton tree (E); Bombacaceae; tree. The plant is the source of kapok of commerce obtained from the silky floss on the inner wall of the mature capsule. The kapok fibre is very light, elastic, resilient, moisture proof and extremely buoyant and is in much demand for life belts, life jackets and other such devices. The fibre is also used in sound proofing, thermal insulation, upholstery, surgical bandages and for stuffing light pillows, cushions and mattresses. Seeds yield a fatty oil which is used in soap manufacture and on refining, used for edible purposes. Seed-cake is used as cattle-feed. Roots are considered to be diuretic and a gum obtained from the tree is used in treating bowel disorders.

Safed shahtoot – *see* Tut.

Safed siras – *Albizia procera* (Roxb.) Benth. (syn. *Mimosa procera* Roxb.); Mimosaceae; tree. Cultivated as an avenue tree. Wood is used for construction purposes, carriages, carts, tool handles, panelling and furniture. Wood pulp is used in the manufacture of printing paper and writing paper. Bark is considered to be poisonous and the tree serves as a host to lac insect.

Safed towdri – *Lepidium iberis* L. var. *alba*; Cruciferae; small herb. Plant yields a volatile oil which is rich in sulphur. Seeds are traded as 'towdri' and are used in treating bronchitis and dropsy.

Safedi-khus – *see* Ban piyazi.

Sag-angur – *see* Angurshefa.

Sagwan; Saka (S) – *Tectona grandis* L.f.; Verbenaceae; Teak (E); large tree. Wood is heavy termite-proof and very durable, and is used for construction work, panelling, bridges, ships, railway sleepers, furniture, cabinet work, musical instruments, carving and different grades of plywood and veneers. Wood waste is used for making chip-boards, particle boards, and fibre boards. Wood chips on distillation yield an oily material which is used to treat eczema. Kernels yield a fatty oil used in scabies and for promoting hair growth. Flowers and seeds are diuretic; flowers and bark are used in bronchitis. Leaves are rich in tannin and also yield a dye which is used for dyeing wool and silk.

Sahadevi – *see* Bhiunli.

Sahadevi (S) – *see* Daudotpala.

Sahadevi bari – *Sonchus arvensis* L.; Corn sow thistle (E); Compositae; erect herb. Roots are used in remedies for cough, bronchitis and asthma. Leaves are applied topically to inflamed parts. Seeds yield a fatty oil. Herb makes good fodder for cattle and horses.

Sain – *see* Asan.

Sainjna, Soanjna, Mungna; Shobhanjana (S) – *Moringa oleifera* Lamk.; Drumstick tree (E), Horse-radish tree (E); Moringaceae; moderate sized tree. Flowers and leaves are used as vegetable. Tender pods are added to curries and also pickled, and contain high concentrations of leucine. Flowers act as a tonic and diuretic, and seeds are antipyretic. Seeds yield the ben oil which is rubbed on painful joints in gout and rheumatism. The oil resembles olive oil and is also used as a lubricant in watches and other fine machinery. The oil-cake contains about 38 per cent protein and is suitable as cattle-feed. All parts are considered as circulatory stimulants. Roots are rubefacient and also used as a condiment. Wood is suitable for newsprint pulp and is also used for making shuttles used in textile mills.

Saj – *see* Asan.

Sajjibuti – *Salsola kali* L.; Glasswort (E), Prickly saltwort (E); Chenopodiaceae; spreading prickly herb, found in the hills. Plant is the source of 'sajji' used in the manufacture of glass, and is useful for reducing soil salinity. Herb is considered as an anthelmintic, diuretic and cathartic. Plant is also used as fodder.

Saka (S) – *see* Sagwan.

Sakalu, Sankalu – *Pachyrhizus erosus* (L.) Urb.; Yam bean (E); Papilionaceae; perennial herb. Cultivated for its young pods and tuberous roots which are used as vegetable. Tuberous roots can be eaten raw or cooked and made into chips. Mature root tubers are the source of good quality starch. Mature pods contain toxins and cause diarrhoea. Seeds are rich in rotenone and powdered seeds are used for insecticidal and piscicidal purposes. All parts of the plant are insecticidal in activity. Plant stems yield a fibre used for making fish-nets and seeds are used as a vermifuge and laxative.

Sakarkanda, Maravuli – *Manihot esculenta* Crantz. (syn. *M. utilissima* Pohl); Tapioca (E), Cassava (E), Manioc (E); Euphorbiaceae; small shrub. Cultivated for its root tubers which can be used after cooking or roasting. Starch extracted from the tubers is used as flour or converted into sago and samolina. Starch is widely used in laundry, cosmetics, adhesives, paper manufacture and as a sizing material in textiles. Starch is also used for puddings, confectionery, biscuits, preparation of an alcoholic beverage, and acetone.

Sakarkandi, Shakarkandi, Meetha alu – *Ipomoea batatas* (L.) Lamk.; Sweet potato (E); Convolvulaceae; spreading diffuse herb. Cultivated for its edible tuberous roots which are rich in sugars and starch. Tubers are consumed after baking, boiling, roasting or frying; they are also used in the manufacture of starch, glucose, syrups and industrial alcohol. The starch is used in the preparation of dextrins, adhesives, cosmetics, insulating fabrics, butanol, acetone, lactic acid, vinegar and as a sizing agent for paper and textiles. Spent pulp is used as a cattle feed. Leaves, stems, and tubers show bactericidal and fungicidal properties. Tender shoots and leaves are used as pot-herb.

Sakena – *see* Hakna.

Sakhu – *see* Sal.

Sakmunia – *Convolvulus scammonia* L.; Convolvulaceae; herb. Roots are the source of scammony resin which is used in the treatment of dropsy and anasarca. Resin is a hydragogue cathartic, in its activity.

Sal, Sakhu – *Shorea robusta* Gaertn. f.; Sal (E); Dipterocarpaceae; tree. Wood ranks next to teak in importance and is used chiefly for construction work, door and window frames, beams, rafters and railway sleepers. Bark is the source of tannin and the spent bark is used for boards, and as a filler in phenolic plastics. Tapping of the trunk yields an amber-coloured resin called 'ral', 'guggal', 'laldana', or saldammar, which is used in paints, varnishes, incense, and as one of the ingredients of 'samagri' burnt in various Hindu rituals and religious ceremonies to fumigate and purify the surroundings. The resin is also used for treating diarrhoea, dysentery, bleeding piles and in plasters and ointments for rheumatism and fractures, and medicinal oils for skin in the Ayurvedic system of medicine. The resin on distillation yields 'chua' oil used for flavouring tobacco and in perfumery. Saldammar resin is also used as a cementing medium for asbestos, plywood sheets and in wall and roof plasters. It is also employed for hardening softer waxes used in the preparation of typewriter ribbons, carbon-paper and shoe polishes. The tree serves as a host to the lac insect and the leaves are used to rear 'tassar' silkworm. Roasted seeds yield a fatty oil, called sal butter which is used as a cooking medium and as a substitute for cocoa butter in the manufacture of chocolates.

Salad-patti – *Lactuca sativa* L.; Lettuce (E); Compositae; herb. Cultivated for its large radical leaves eaten raw as salad or cooked as vegetable. Leaves are rich in minerals and vitamins and are the source of lactucarium which is used medicinally as a sedative in bronchitis and asthma.

Salai, Salai guggal; Sallaki (S) – *Boswellia serrata* Roxb.; Indian olibanum (E), Indian frankincense (E); Burseraceae; tree. Wood is used for packing cases, toys, carving, match sticks, newsprint, rayon-pulp, plywood and veneers. Tree exudes an oleo-gum-resin called 'salai guggal' or Indian frankincense chiefly used in the manufacture of incense. It yields three constituents *viz.*, a volatile oil similar to turpentine oil, a rosin used in high grade varnishes, lacquers and printing ink, and a gum used in calico printing and for sizing in textile industry. The gum is also a possible source of furfural and is used in the manufacture of plastics and nylon. It is considered to be an expectorant, diuretic and stomachic and is used in remedies for pulmonary infections, diarrhoea, dysentery and skin ailments.

Salai guggal – *see* Salai.

Salam – *see* Salibmisri.

Salap – *Orchis latifolia* L.; Orchis (E); Orchidaceae; perennial herb found at high altitudes. Dry scalded tubers yield the commercial salep which is highly mucilaginous and forms a jelly when soaked in water. Salep is used in diarrhoea, dysentery and fevers and is also considered as a tonic. Salep mucilage is also used as a sizing agent for silk fabrics. Tubers also contain a volatile oil and their infusion is administered to treat hoarseness of voice.

Salaree, Karas – *Apium graveolens* L. var. *dulce* (Mill.) DC; Garden celery (E); Umbelliferae; small aromatic herb. Cultivated for its long leaf-stalks which are used as salad and the ripe fruits used as a condiment. Seeds act as a stimulant, tonic, carminative and nerve soother. They yield a volatile oil called celery seed-oil which is used to flavour beverages, soups, food products and as a fixative in perfumes.

Salibmisri, Salam; Sudhamuli (S) – *Eulophia campestris* R. Br.; Orchidaceae; terrestrial herb, with irregular, oblong flattened rhizomes. Rhizomes are rich in mucilage and are highly esteemed as a tonic and aphrodisiac; they are used in medicines for stomatitis, cough, heart trouble, and piles. Tubers are usually traded in the form of dried rhizome powder and jelly.

Sallaki (S) – *see* Salai.

Salmali (S) – *see* Semul.

Salpan – *Maughania chappar* O. Kuntze.; Papilionaceae; undershrub. Roots are used to induce sleep and relieve pain, and are also used to treat hysteria and epilepsy.

Salparni – *see* Sarivan.

Salum – *Chrysopogon gryllus* (L.) Trin.; Gramineae; large profusely tillered perennial grass. Plants are used as fodder, and for thatching.

Salvia sefakuss, Seesti – *Salvia officinalis* L.; Sage (E) Labiatae; small shrub. Cultivated as an ornamental for its beautiful flowers. Leaves and flowering tops yield the sage oil which is used in the manufacture of perfumes, deodorants, and insecticides. Sage oil is also used in the treatment of thrush and gingivitis. Infusion of the leaves is used as a gargle in sore throat. Seeds are the source of a drying oil used in the manufacture of paints.

Salwan – *see* Sarivan.

Samak, Sanwak; Jalsamoka (S) – *Echinochloa crusgalli* (L.) Beauv.; Barnyard millet (E); Gramineae; annual grass. Cultivated for fodder and for its tiny white edible grains marketed as 'samak ke chaval' and consumed during special occasions.

Samandar-sokh, Ghabel, Samudrapalaka (S) – *Argyreia nervosa* (Burm. f.) Boj; Elephant creeper (E) Convolvulaceae; climbing shrub with whitish stem. Cultivated for its attractive flowers and foliage. Roots act as a diuretic and tonic, and are used in the treatment of nervous disorders and rheumatism. Leaf poultice is applied to eczema, itch and other skin ailments; leaves are also used as pot-herb. Seeds are spasmolytic and hypotensive and are also the source of a fatty oil. Herb is used in curing gonorrhoea and chronic ulcers.

Samarri – *see* Bodula.

Samber – *Desmodium tiliaefolium* G. Don. Papilionaceae; undershrub of sub-Himalayan region. Roots are carminative, diuretic and tonic and are used for counteracting biliousness. Leaves are lopped for fodder. Stem yields a rough fibre which is used for making ropes and baskets.

Sambhalu – *see* Nirgandi.

Sami – *see* Chaunkra.

Samp-ki-khumb – *Arisaema tortuosum* (Wall.) Schott; Cobra lily (E), Green dragons (E); Araceae; tall herb found in the hills with its spathe resembling the hood of a cobra. Root tubers are used to kill worms in cattle and are also used as an insecticide. Seeds are cooked and used as vegetable.

Samprani – *Kingiodendron pinnatum* (Roxb.) Harms. (syn. *Hardwickia pinnata* Roxb.); Caesalpiniaceae; evergreen tree. Wood is used for building purposes, planking, beams, rafters, furniture and billiard cues. Tapping of the tree trunk yields an oleoresin which on distillation gives a volatile oil which is used as a substitute for clove oil and the residual resin is used in varnishes.

Samudrapalaka (S) – *see* Samandar-sokh.

Samudraphala (S) – *see* Ijjul.

Samudulan, Punjki, Gobhi; Gojihva (S) – *Elephantopus scaber* L.; Compositae; herb. Root and leaf decoction is antipasmodic, and is used for checking stomach-ache, diarrhoea and dysentery. Roots are also used for relieving toothache and vomiting. Leaf paste is used externally for treating eczema and ulcers.

San – *Crotalaria mucronata* Desv.; Striped Crotalaria (E); Papilionaceae; herb. Cultivated as a green manure cover crop in rubber and coconut plantations. Stem is the source of a coarse fibre. Plant yields a black dye. Seeds are often substituted for coffee seeds.

Sana (S) – *see* Sannai-sunn.

Sandal – *see* Chandan.

Sandan, Panjan, Tinsa; Tinisha (S) – *Ougeinia oojeinensis* (Roxb.) Hochr.; Sandan (E); Papilionaceae; small tree. Wood is used for carts, axles, shafts, agricultural implements, oars, sugarcane crushers, construction work, rafters and heavy furniture. Wood is also used for making shuttles, spindles and bobbins. Bark is the source of tannin and is used as a febrifuge and to stupefy fish. Incised bark exudate is used in diarrhoea and dysentery.

Sandhor – *Bothriochloa intermedia* (R. Br.) A. Camus (syn. *Andropogon intermedius* R. Br.); Gramineae; tall grass. Young blades of grass are used as fodder. Mature blades yield good paper pulp.

Sandhur – *Bothriochloa pertusa* (Willd.) A. Camus (syn. *Andropogon pertusus* Willd.); Sour grass (E), Pitted blue grass (E); Gramineae; perennial grass. Plant is highly esteemed as fodder both in fresh and dry state.

Sandika (S) – *see* Khesari.

Sangkhi (S) – *see* Teanklo.

Sangkupi – *see* Lanjai.

Sanipat, Nepal nimb; Sannipat (S) – *Schweinfurthia sphaerocarpa* (Benth.) A. Br.; Scrophulariaceae; small herb found in the arid regions. Dry powdered leaves, stem, and broken pieces of fruit constitute the drug called 'sanipat' which is considered as a tonic and diuretic, and is used in Ayurvedic medicine for prolonged fevers involving intestinal infection. Leaves are also considered useful in combating diabetes.

Sanka – *see* Matamar.

Sankahuli, Sankapuspi – *Convolvulus pluricaulis* Choisy; Convolvulaceae; diffuse hairy twining herb. Rootstock is woody, perennial and is considered as a nerve tonic, stomachic, hypotensive and tranquilizer. Active principles present are convolvulin and sankhpuspine. Plant is used in many Ayurvedic preparations.

Sankalu – *see* Sakalu.

Sankapuspi – *see* Sankahuli.

Sankasura (S) – *see* Sankesar.

Sankesar; Sankasura (S) – *Delonix elata* (L.) Gamble; White gulmohar (E); Caesalpiniaceae; small tree. Cultivated as an ornamental for its beautiful foliage and yellow-white flowers. Wood is used for cabinet work and match boxes, and the leaves are used medicinally for flatulence and rheumatism.

Sankhaphuli; Sankhapushpi (S), Dandotpala (S) – *Canscora decussata* Schult.; Dankuni plant (E); Gentianaceae; herb. Leaves are used for cough and rheumatism. Fresh juice of aerial parts is used for controlling epilepsy, nervous debility and insanity. Plant is also considered to be anticancerous.

Sankhapushpi (S) – *see* Sankhaphuli.

Sankru, Gurlu; Jargadi (S) – *Coix lacryma-jobi* L.; Job's tears (E), Adlay (E); Gramineae; tall grass. Grain is enclosed in a tear-shaped hard shell, and is used for making rosaries, necklaces and bead-curtains. Grains are considered wholesome with high protein and fat content, and are used by the tribals as rice substitute, and to brew beer. Leaves and culms are used for fodder.

Sannai-sunn; Sana (S) – *Crotalaria juncea* L.; Sunnhemp (E); Papilionaceae; tall shrub. Cultivated for a coarse, strong fibre called sunnhemp obtained from its stems. Fibre is considered to be good for the manufacture of cigarette-paper as it is high in cellulose and low in ash content. Fibre is also used for making ropes, twines, fishing nets, coarse bags, matting and canvas. All aerial parts are used for green manuring. Seed is also rich in gum content.

Sannipat (S) – *see* Sanipat.

Sansaru, Siaru – *Debregeasia longifolia* (Burm. f.) Wedd.; Wild rhea (E); Urticaceae; large shrub or small tree. Fruits are edible. Wood is used for making charcoal. Stem fibre is used for making ropes and twines. Another species *D. hypoleuca* Wedd. is also known by the same Hindi name.

Sant; Punarnava (S) – *Boerhaavia diffusa* L.; Hogweed (E), Horse-purslane (E); Nyctaginaceae; spreading prostrate herb. Whole plant yields the Ayurvedic drug called 'punarnava', with its chief active principle being punarnavine. Herb acts as an astringent, carminative, stimulant, intoxicant (it exerts nicotine-like action), and nervine tonic. Roots are diuretic, expectorant and laxative and are used in combating asthma, dropsy and urinary disorders. Green kernels are very rich in tannin and the nuts are used as a masticatory.

Santara, Narangi – *Citrus reticulata* Blanco; Mandarin (E), Loose-skinned orange (E), Tangerine (E); Rutaceae; small tree. Cultivated for its delicious fruit rich in vitamins, specially vitamin C; peeled fruit is eaten fresh or preserved as marmalade and juice. Citrus pulp is also used for the preparation of molasses which can be fermented to prepare alcohol. Residual pulp after extraction of orange juice and exhausted peels make excellent cattle feed. Peels yield an essential oil called citrus oil or mandarin oil, used in toiletries, pharmaceutical preparations and confectionery. Peels are also used in cakes, puddings and marmalades, and the exhausted peels are used as boiler fuel. Peels are also a rich source of pectins, carotenes and vitamin A. Fresh peel pulp is used for softening the skin and as a germicide. Dry peel, crushed and mixed with tea soothes sore throat. Oil extracted from the peel is a natural pesticide and is not harmful to humans. It can be used for pest control in house-hold fumigating, food handling and disinfecting livestock of external parasites. Seeds yield a fatty oil. Petit-grain oil is extracted from the leaves and twigs.

Santhi – *see* Lal sabuni.

Sanwa, Sawa; Shyamaka (S) – *Echinochloa frumentacea* (Roxb.) Link.; Japanese barnyard millet (E); Gramineae; annual grass. Cultivated for the leaves and culms which serve as forage and for its grains which are used for food and for making a very potent beer. Grains are rich in fibre content and are considered good for getting rid of constipation and biliousness.

Sanwak – *see* Samak.

Sanwani, Bari sanwani – *Lagerstroemia thorelii* Gagnep.; Queen's flower (E); Lythraceae; small tree. Cultivated as an ornamental for its beautiful foliage and white, pink or mauve flowers; it is also grown as a hedge plant.

Saona – *see* Arlu.

Sapota – *see* Chiku.

Saptala – *see* Muta-bela.

Saptaparni (S) -- *see* Chatian.

Sara, Sarkanda – *Erianthus arundinaceus* (Retz.) Jesw. ex Heyne (syn. *Saccharum arundinaceus* Retz.); Gramineae; tall perennial grass. Cultivated for its sturdy stems which are used for making screens, stools, baskets and walls of thatched houses. Leaf-sheaths are the source of a fibre used for making ropes and twines and are also suitable for paper pulp and production of furfural. Leaf buds are eaten raw as salad.

Sarahati – *Ophiorrhiza mungos* L.; Mongoose plant (E); Rubiaceae; herb or undershrub, found in Khasi hills. Roots are tonic, and are used as an antidote against bites of venomous snakes; they are also considered useful in cancer treatment. Leaves are used as dressing on ulcers by tribals. Root, leaf and bark decoction acts as a stomachic.

Sarai, Amladandi – *Polygonum polystachyum* Wall. ex Meissn.; Polygonaceae; herb. Stalks are soft and fleshy, and are used either raw or peeled and cooked. Young leaves are used as pot-herb. Plant is also used as fodder.

Sarala (S) – *see* Chir.

Sarangum – *see* Matazor.

Saras – *see* Saru.

Sariva – *see* Anantamul.

Sarivan, Salparni, Salwan; Shalaparni (S) – *Desmodium gageticum* (L.) DC.; Tick trefoil (E); Papilionaceae; perennial herb. Roots are febrifuge, diuretic and expectorant, and are used as one of the ingredients of 'Dasamula', an Ayurvedic medicine. Roots and seeds are also used for catarrh.

Sarkanda – *see* Munj; *see also* Sara.

Sarkhara – *see* Ulla.

Sarnali – *see* Kalmisag.

Sarpagandha, Asrel, Chandrabhaga, Chhota-chand; Sarpagandha (S) – *Rauvolfia serpentina* (L.) Benth ex Kurz.; Serpentine root (E); Apocynaceae; undershrub. Dried roots constitute the drug commercially known as 'sarpagandha' or rauvolfia and have been used in India for centuries for curing hypertension, nervous disorders and epilepsy. The drug is now used in modern allopathic medicine in the preparation of hypertensives and sedatives. Several alkaloids have been isolated of which the principal one is reserpine. Rauvolfia preparations are widely used to treat various disorders of central nervous system including insanity, insomnia and schizophrenia. Root extract along with other plant mixtures is used for treating colic and fever. Root extract is also considered to be helpful in child-birth, by stimulating uterine contractions.

Sarpagandha (S) – *see* Sarpagandha.

Sarphonka, Bal-nil, Dhamasia; Sharapunkha – *Tephrosia purpurea* (L.) Pers.; Purple Tephrosia (E); Papilionaceae; herb. Often cultivated as a green manure and cover crop. Leaves contain rutin and also a dye. Pulverized roots and dry powdered leaves are smoked for providing relief in asthma and cough. Root decoction is used in combating diarrhoea, urinary disorders, dyspepsia, asthma and rheumatism. Roots and seeds are piscicidal and insecticidal in activity. Seeds yield a fatty oil which is used to treat eczema, itch, scabies, and other skin ailments. Extract of the herb is reported to be useful in liver cirrhosis.

Sarsan-banda, Bhatua ghas, Tokra – *Orobanche aegyptiaca* Pers.; Orobanchaceae; total root parasite. Small colourless plant considered as a cure for boils in the throat of cattle.

Sarsapa (S) – *see* Sarson.

Sarson, Peeli sarson; Sarsapa (S) – *Brassica napus* L. var. *glauca* (Roxb.) Schulz. (syn. *B. campestris* var. *sarson* Prain); Yellow sarson (E), Indian colza (E); Cruciferae; herb. Cultivated as an oil-seed crop. Oil is commonly used for edible purposes; it is also used for body massage and when mixed with camphor is applied to rheumatic joints. Oil-cake is used as cattle feed. Tender shoots and leaves are used as pot-herb. Seeds are used as a condiment to flavour many dishes. Mustard oil is rich in monounsaturated fatty acids, protein and calcium, but the content of polyunsaturated fatty acids is low as compared to many other popular edible oils. The oil, however, is rich in α-linolenic and linoleic fatty acids and the content of omega-3 fatty acids varies from 9-15 per cent, which is much higher than most other edible oils, the n-6 : n-3 ratio being within 4:5. According to recent researches this desirable quality coupled with its very low content of saturated fatty acid makes this oil more effective in reducing the risk of coronary heart diseases as compared to other edible oils. Seeds are rich in the glycoside sinigrin which on hydrolysis with the enzyme myrosinase yields an essential oil that imparts the typical pungency and aroma to mustard oil.

Saru, Saras; Surahva (S) – *Cupressus sempervirens* L.; Italian cypress (E), Mediterranean cypress (E); Cupressaceae; tall evergreen tree. Cultivated as an ornamental in parks. Leaves are the source of an essential oil known as oil of cypress which is used in perfumery and for scenting soaps.

Sarvajaya (S) – *see* Sabbajaya.

Sarvad, Bedina – *Mussaenda glabrata* (Hook. f.) Hutch.; Paperchase tree (E); Rubiaceae; small tree. Cultivated as an ornamental.

Sarwari – *see* Safed murgha.

Satamuli, Satawar – *Asparagus racemosus* Willd. var. *javanicus* Baker.; Wild Asparagus (E); Liliaceae; spiny scandent shrub. Cultivated as a climbing shrub. Underground small white tuberous root-stocks are considered to be anti-dysenteric, anti-spasmodic, carminative, demulcent, astringent, diuretic, tonic and nervine tonic, and are used in combating diarrhoea, dysentery, urinary and pulmonary complaints and rheumatism; they are also used widely in medicated oils for nervousness and rheumatism.

Satapushpi (S) – *see* Sowa.

Satari – *see* Pismarum.

Satavari – *Eulophia pratensis* Lindl. Orchidaceae; terrestrial herb with fleshy tubers. Tubers are anthelmintic; they are also used to cure scrofulous glandular swellings in the neck.

Satawar – *see* Ṡatamuli.

Sathra – *Origanum vulgare* L.; Potmarjorum (E), Wild marjorum (E); Labiatae; perennial aromatic herb found in the hills. Leaves and young flowering tops contain a volatile oil used for flavouring. The oil called origanum oil is considered as a diuretic, carminative and stomachic; it is also used externally for getting relief from toothache, earache, rheumatism, bronchitis and whooping cough. Oil is further used to scent soaps and cosmetics.

Sati – *see* Kachura.

Satila (S) – *see* Matar.

Satpura, Setburosa, Mahadev-ka-phul – *Daphne papyracea* Wall. ex Steud.; Nepal paper plant (E); Thymelaeaceae; evergreen shrub found in the temperate Himalayas. Stem bark yields a fibre used for making ropes and a special paper called Nepal paper. Flower is considered sacred and is used in religious ceremonies.

Satwin – *see* Chatian.

Saunf, Sonp; Madhurica (S) – *Foeniculum vulgare* Mill.; Fennel (E); Umbelliferae; aromatic annual herb. Cultivated for its fruits used as a spice and condiment for flavouring various sweet and savoury dishes, confectionery and pickles. Fruits are carminative, diuretic, expectorant, digestive, stimulant and tonic, and are used in remedies for renal, gastric and chest disorders. Fruit extract forms an important component of griping mixtures. Fruits contain an essential oil which is medicinally carminative and also used to flavour liqueurs, confectionery, candy and many a cuisine. The residue left after distillation of the volatile oil from the fruits, is used as a cattle feed. Leaves are used to cure gastric disorders, rheumatism and cramps. Roots are considered to be purgative.

Saurif – *see* Badian.

Sawa – *see* Sanwa.

Sawala – *see* Jallil.

Sawank – *see* Jangli sawuk.

Saya – *see* Chirval.

Seb, Sev, Seba (S) – *Malus pumila* Mill.; Apple (E); Rosaceae; small tree. Cultivated in the hills for its edible fruits used either fresh as dessert or preserved into jam, jelly, marmalade, juice, syrup and cider. Fruit is rich in vitamins, minerals specially iron, and organic acids which are present in high concentrations just below the skin. Wood is used for small wooden articles and turnery. Root bark is considered to be anthelmintic, and cooling.

Seba (S) – *see* Seb.

Sedwa, Pavna – *Sehima nervosum* (Rottl.) Stapf. (syn. *Andropogon nervosum* Rottl.); Gramineae; perennial grass. Aerial parts are used for thatching and for fodder which is prepared in the form of both hay and silage.

Seesti – *see* Salvia sefakuss.

Seet muli – *see* Halyun.

Sehund, Thohar; Snuhi (S), Vajra (S) – *Euphorbia neriifolia* Auct. Pl. non L.; Thorny milk hedge (E); Euphorbiaceae; succulent shrub with sharp stipular thorns. Cultivated either for making a boundary fence or as an ornamental on rockeries. Milky juice is laxative, stomachic, febrifuge, expectorant, digestive and rubefacient, and is used for treating colic, dyspepsia, flatulence, intermittent fever, insect bites, cutaneous ailments, dropsy, asthma and rheumatism.

Seja – *see* Dhaura.

Sem – *Dolichos lablab* L. var. *typicus* Prain. [syn. *Lablab purpureus* (L.) Sweet.]; Lablab bean (E), Hyacinth bean (E); Papilionaceae; perennial twining herb. Cultivated for its tender pods and seeds which are used as vegetable. Fried seeds are considered a delicacy. Seeds are considered to be antispasmodic, stomachic, aphrodisiac and febrifuge. Plants are also cultivated for fodder, green manuring, and to check soil erosion.

Semla – *see* Kandla.

Semul, Semur; Salmali (S) – *Bombax ceiba* L. [syn. *Salmalia malabarica* (DC.) Schott & Endl.]; Red silk-cotton tree (E); Bombacaceae; large tree. Cultivated as an ornamental for its beautiful, showy red flowers. Wood is light, and is used for making canoes, toys, handles, pencils, frames, plywood, match-sticks, and match-boxes. Silky fibres called floss, obtained from the inner wall of the fruit are used for stuffing cushions, pillows, life belts, quilts and upholstery. Fibres are also used for sound proofing and insulation purposes. Flower buds and fleshy calyces are used as vegetable. Tree is the source of mocharus gum which is used as an adhesive. Seeds yield an edible fatty oil which is also used for the manufacture of soaps. Oil cake is used as fodder.

Semur – *see* Semul.

Sena – *see* Hindi-sana.

Senai – *see* Hindi-sana.

Senji, Banmethi – *Melilotus indica* (L.) All.; Sweet clover (E); Papilionaceae; herb. Often cultivated for green manuring and for improving saline soils. The plant is used for fodder as an admixture with other stock-feed. Seeds are used for curing infantile diarrhoea and bowel disorders.

Sentha – *see* Munj.

Sephalika (S) – *see* Harsinghar.

Seri; Pithari (S) – *Glossocardia bosvallia* DC.; Compositae; herb, with fennel-like odour. The plant is used as an emmenagogue.

Setburosa – *see* Satpura.

Sev – *see* Seb.

Sevanti (S) – *see* Guldaudi.

Sewan – *Lasiurus hirsutus* (Forsk.) Boiss. (syn. *Elionurus hirsutus* Munro ex Benth.); Gramineae; perennial grass found in desert areas. Plants are used as fodder both fresh and stacked; they are also used for thatching.

Sewati (S) – *see* Kuji.

Shaftal – *Trifolium resupinatum* L.; Persian clover (E); Papilionaceae; pasture herb. Cultivated for fodder, and provides a feed rich in protein, calcium and phosphorus combined with easy digestibility. Plants are better suited as hay. Another species *T. repens* L., or White clover is also known by the same Hindi name.

Shaftalu – *see* Aru.

Shahterah – *see* Pitpapara.

Shahtoot, Krishna toot – *Morus nigra* L.; Black mulberry (E); Moraceae; tree. Cultivated for its sweet and delicious fruits consumed either fresh or preserved into jam and cordials. Fruit is laxative in action and bark is purgative and vermifuge. The infusion of leaves is useful as a hypotensive.

Shah-zirah – *see* Kala-zira.

Shakakul – *Asparagus gonocladus* Baker; Liliaceae; undershrub. Roots are boiled in oil and their paste is used for skin ailments.

Shakarkandi – *see* Sakarkandi.

Shakarpitan – *see* Thor.

Shakhotaka (S) – *see* Daheya.

Shakri-phalsa – *see* Phalsa.

Shalapara, Guliajaib – *Hibiscus mutabilis* L.; Cotton rose (E); Changeable Hibiscus (E); Confederate rose (E); Malvaceae; tomentose shrub. Cultivated for hedges and as an ornamental. Bark is the source of a coarse but strong fibre used for making ropes. Leaves are used for getting rid of cough and leaf juice is used on scalds and burns. Flower infusion is used in pulmonary complaints.

Shalaparni (S) – *see* Sarivan.

Shaljum – *Brassica rapa* L.; Turnip (E); Cruciferae; annual herb. Cultivated for its tuberous roots which are used as vegetable or made into soup and pickle. Aerial greens are rich in calcium and vitamin C and are used as fodder. Leaves are stomachic in action. Turnips are also used in the treatment of tumours and carcinoma. Seeds yield a fatty oil, which is mixed with camphor and then applied to rheumatic joints and muscular pains. Oil is also used for the manufacture of soaps and as a lubricant.

Shambhaluka bui – *Piper wallichii* Hand-Mazz.; Piperaceae; stout climber. Fruit is bitter acrid and refrigerant and is used as a diuretic.

Shami (S) – *see* Chaunkra.

Shanarghandika (S) – *see* Ghunghunian.

Shanasokha (S) – *see* Chirpoti.

Shankhahuli – *see* Gaozaban.

Sharapunkha (S) – *see* Sarphonka.

Sharifa; Sitaphal (S) – *Annona squamosa* L.; Custard apple (E); Sweet-sop (E); Sweet apple (E); Annonaceae; small tree. Cultivated for its fruits, used as dessert. Ripe fruits with sweet, creamy white flesh are used fresh or made into liquor. Powdered seeds and leaves are insecticidal. Seeds are the source of a fatty oil and the green leaves yield an essential oil. Roots are considered to be purgative.

Shatapatri (S) – *see* Fasli gulab.

Shavaka (S) – *see* Jhau.

Shavan, Kutki – *Panicum sumatrense* Roth. ex Roem. & Schult.; Little millet (E); Gramineae; annual grass. Cultivated for its grains cooked like rice or made into flour and used for puddings. Leaves are used as fodder and are rich in carotene.

Shea, Sheva – *Lonicera glauca* Hook. f. & Thoms.; Caprifoliaceae; scandent shrub, found in the hills. Flowers and leaves are used in venereal diseases. Seeds are used for treating colic in horses in veterinary medicine.

Sheetal chini – *see* Kabab chini.

Shetapushapa (S) – *see* Badian.

Sheva – *see* Shea.

Shevra – *Alysicarpus glumaceus* (Vahl.) DC.; Papilionaceae, herb. Plant is used as a stock-feed.

Shiah-kanta – *Mimosa himalayana* Gamble.; Mimosaceae; straggling shrub. Cultivated for making hedges.

Shia-jira, Vilayati zirah; Sushavi (S) – *Carum carvi* L.; Caraway (E); Umbelliferae; herb. Cultivated for its dry mature fruits which are used as a spice and condiment, and also to flavour cheese and liqueurs. Fruits are carminative and stomachic and are used in flatulent colic. Fruits yield an essential oil called oleum carvi, which is used to flavour medicines, soaps, and mouth washes and also used in perfumery. Caraway water is used for gripe mixtures and as a remedy for flatulent colic in infants.

Shialkanta – *see* Bharband.

Shikakai, Kochi – *Acacia rugata* (Lamk.) Ham. (syn. *A. concina* DC.); Soap pod (E); Mimosaceae; scandent shrub. Extract of the mature and dried fruits soaked in water overnight is used as a herbal hair-shampoo and for washing delicate silks and woollens. Tender leaves are acidic and used in chutneys. Roasted seeds are edible. Bark is the source of a tan used for fishing lines. Decoction of the pods is used to relieve biliousness, and is also used as a purgative. Plant serves as a host to lac insect.

Shikha-mula (S) – *see* Gajar.

Shikhi (S) – *see* Chaupatia.

Shilapushpa (S) – *see* Pathar phori.

Shilaras, Silaras; Silhaka (S) – *Liquidambar orientalis* Mill.; Oriental sweet gum (E); Altingiaceae; tree. Plant yields styrax, a fragrant gum-resin which is used as an ingredient of pharmaceuticals, fumigating powders and perfumes; it is also used for adding flavour to tobacco and toiletries.

Shingrota – *see* Ambarvel.

Shinshapa (S) – *see* Shisham.

Shirkhist – *Fraxinus ornus* L.; Oleaceae; small deciduous tree. Stem tapping yields an exudate which is used as a mild laxative for children.

Shisham; Aguru (S), Shinshapa (S) – *Dalbergia sissoo* Roxb.; Sissoo (E); Papilionaceae; large tree. Cultivated along the roadsides and in the parks for providing shade. Timber is highly esteemed for cabinet work, furniture, boats, railway sleepers, carving, calico printing-blocks, keys of musical instruments like 'sitar', picture, door and window frames, and tool handles. Wood also yields good quality charcoal, and the wood pulp is suitable for good quality paper.

Shishapa (S) – *see* Kala-shisham.

Shiulik – *Elaeagnus angustifolia* L.; Oleaster (E); Elaeagnaceae; small tree found in the hills. Wood is used for fencing. Fruits are edible. Dried fruits are used for brewing liquor. Seed is the source of an oil used in bronchial ailments. Flower infusion is used as a febrifuge.

Shivala (S) – *see* Sivara.

Shobhanjana (S) – *see* Sainjna.

Shoti, Chiluchi – *Iris nepalensis* D. Don; Iridaceae; perennial herb. Roots act as an aperient and diuretic, and are used in counteracting bilious obstruction.

Shumeo – *see* Tagger.

Shurval – *see* Kumeria.

Shveta-dhataki (S) – *see* Kokaraye.

Shveta-punarnava (S) – *see* Lal-sabuni.

Shvetpushpi (S) – *see* Lal-indrayan.

Shwasvalk – *Machilus macrantha* Nees.; Machilus (E); Lauraceae; large tree found in the hills of S. India. Wood is used for construction work, rafters, canoes, boats, packing cases, plywood and matches industry. Roots are the source of a volatile oil. Bark is used for combating asthma, consumption and rheumatism, and the leaves for treating ulcers.

Shyamaka (S) – *see* Sanwa.

Shyama kranta – *see* Vishnu-kranti.

Shyonaka (S) – *see* Arlu.

Siali – *see* Bankumra.

Siamlata – *see* Kali dudhi.

Siaru – *see* Sansaru.

Sicka – *see* Chetihola.

Sidhoul – *see* Chandramula.

Sidi – *see* Dhaura.

Silapoma – *Engelhardtia spicata* Bl.; Juglandaceae; tree. Wood is used for building purposes, carving, planking and tea-chests. Bark is the source of a resin which is used as a fumigant and tannin used for tanning and to stupefy fish.

Silaras – *Altingia excelsa* Noron.; Altingiaceae; tall tree found in East India. Stem yields an aromatic resin traded as 'rasamala' which is considered to be stomachic, carminative, antipyretic and expectorant, and is used for cough, pulmonary disorders and kidney-trouble; it is also used for treating scabies, leucoderma and lumbago. The resin is also substituted for styrax and used in perfumery. *See also* 'Shilaras'.

Silhaka (S) – *see* Shilaras.

Sinatha – *see* Aliar.

Sindur – *see* Kamela.

Sinduria, Latkan – *Bixa orellana* L.; Annatto (E), Urucu (E); Bixaceae; small tree. Seeds are the source of a vegetable dye called annatto which is found as a thick pigment cover around each seed. The chief constituent of annatto is bixin, which is used for colouring ice creams, chocolates, dairy and bakery products, foods, and edible oils. The dye is also used in the manufacture of nail polish, shoe polish, wood polish, flooring wax, and hair oils.

Singhara; Jalaphala (S), Sringataka (S) – *Trapa natans* L. var. *bispinosa* (Roxb.) Makino.; Caltrops (E), Water chestnut (E); Trapaceae; aquatic herb. Cultivated for its edible tender fruit-kernels, used fresh or boiled or roasted. Dry kernels on grinding yield flour which is used for preparing pancakes and snacks.

Singri, Mungra – *Raphanus caudatus* L.; Rat-tail radish (E); Cruciferae; tall herb. Tender long and slender fruits are used as vegetable and are also pickled.

Siora – *see* Daheya.

Siran – *see* Kanujera.

Siras, Siris, Sirisha (S) – *Albizia lebbeck* (L.) Benth.; Kokko (E), East Indian walnut (E); Mimosaceae; large tree. Cultivated on the roadsides for providing shade, and also for erecting shelter-belts and wind-breaks. Wood yields excellent timber which is used for furniture, panelling, railway carriages, bridges and agricultural implements. Wood pulp is suitable for good quality paper. The tree yields a gum which is used as gum-arabic and the bark yields tannin.

Siratro – *Phaseolus atropurpureus* Moc & Sesse. emend Hassler.; Papilionaceae; herb introduced successfully in arid regions of Rajasthan, India. Plants are drought-resistant, rich in protein and can withstand frequent grazing.

Siris – *see* Siras.

Sirisha (S) – *see* Siras.

Sirpon – *Calophyllum elatum* Bedd.; Sirpoon tree (E), Poonspar tree (E); Guttiferae; tall tree found in South India. Wood is the source of a timber traded as poonspar which is used for rafters, masts, cheap furniture, planking and general construction work. Seeds are the source of a fatty oil used as an illuminant.

Siru – *see* Dabh.

Sitaphal – *see* Kaddu; *see also* Mitha kaddu.

Sitaphal (S) – *see* Sharifa.

Sitruti – *see* Kapur kachri.

Sivamalli (S) – *see* Safed-kachnar.

Sivanimba (S) – *see* Ratakohomba.

Sivara; Shivala (S) – *Ceratophyllum demersum* L.; Ceratophyllaceae; slender, submerged aquatic herb. Plants are considered to be refrigerant and useful in biliousness. Plant hair possess microphyllin.

Sneta khadira – *see* Kumta.

Snuhi (S) – *see* Sehund.

Soanjna – *see* Sainjna.

Sodh – *see* Bholia.

Sola – *Aeschynomene aspera* L.; Sola pith plant (E); Papilionaceae; perennial undershrub found along margins of lakes and ponds. Soft and light pith of the plant has insulating properties and is employed for making solar hats, toys, models, artistic decorative wall hangings and ear ornaments worn by tribals. Pith is also used for making life-belts and swimming jackets and as a substitute for bottle cork sheets. Leaves are edible.

Soltraj; Baghanulla – *Cyanotis axillaris* Roem. & Schult. f.; Commelinaceae; herb. Plant is used in the treatment of tympanitis and dropsy.

Soma (S) – *see* Somlata.

Somaraji – *see* Gandhali.

Somlata; Som (S)–*Sarcostemma acidum* (Roxb.) Voigt.; Asclepiadaceae; much branched leafless shrub, found in arid regions. Decoction of the dried stems is used for inducing vomiting. Plant is also used to eliminate termites from the fields.

Somraj – *see* Kalijiri.

Somraji (S) – *see* Kalijiri.

Sonchala – *see* Khubasi.

Son champa – *see* Khair champa.

Son khair, Kaiger – *Acacia ferruginea* DC.; Mimosaceae; tree. Wood is used for making fence posts, beams, and agricultural implements. Tender branches are used as fodder. Tree is the source of a gum.

Sonp – *see* Saunf.

Son-patti – *see* Arlu.

Sosun, Irsia – *Iris ensata* Thunb.; Iridaceae; herb found in the hills. Roots are considered to be useful in the treatment of dropsy and liver disorders. Plant yields a fibre. Leaves are woven into mats and baskets.

Sowa, Soya, Satapushpi (S) – *Anethum sowa* Kurz; Indian dill (E); Umbelliferae; aromatic herb. Cultivated for its aromatic leaves and fruits. Leaves are used for flavouring. Dry fruits are stomachic and carminative and yield an essential oil called dill-seed oil which is used in pharmaceuticals and perfumery and for flavouring food. Fresh aerial parts on distillation yield another essential oil called dill-herb oil. Dill water is used to cure gastric flatulence in infants.

Soya – *see* Sowa.

Soya bean – *see* Bhat.

Srigalakoli (S) – *see* Makoh.

Srihastini (S) – *see* Hati-sura.

Sringataka (S) – *see* Singhara.

Sriphala (S) – *see* Bael.

Sritalam (S) – *see* Bajarbattu.

Sthalapushpa (S) – *see* Genda.

Sthal-padma – *Hydrangea paniculata* Sieb. var. *grandiflora* Sieb.; Hydrangeaceae; perennial undershrub. Cultivated in the hills as an ornamental for its beautiful blossoms. Flowers are rich in rutin and are used to treat capillary fragility, particularly in hypertension.

Subabul; Vilayati baral – *Leucaena leucocephala* (Lamk.) de Wit.; Horse tamarind (E), White popinac (E); Mimosaceae; tree. Often cultivated as a cover crop to provide shade in coffee, rubber, and tea plantations. Tender pods and seeds are edible. Leaves and pods are lopped for fodder.

Subhar (S) – *see* Machola.

Sudhamuli (S) – *see* Salibmisri.

Sudhavriksha (S) – *see* Baikal.

Sugandha-bala; Hribera (S) – *Pavonia odorata* Willd.; Malvaceae.; aromatic undershrub. Cultivated in the gardens for its fragrant flowers. Roots with musky odour yield an essential oil which is used in perfumery. They are stomachic, antipyretic and refrigerant and are used in intestinal haemorrhage and dysentery. Plant is used for the treatment of rheumatism, and also yields a short-length, soft, fine fibre similar to mesta fibre.

Sugandhakantak (S) – *see* Babchi.

Sugandha-mantri – *Homalomena aromatica* (Roxb.) Schott. (syn. *Calla aromatica* Roxb.); Araceae; aromatic perennial herb found in East India. Rhizomes yield an essential oil which is used in the preparation of otto of henna. Powdered dry rhizomes are used to flavour tobacco and snuffs. Plant is used to cure skin ailments.

Sugandha-rohisha – *see* Agin ghas.

Sugandha-vacha (S) – *see* Chandramula.

Sugandhi-mula (S) – *see* Khas-khas.

Sugandh kokila; Kakoli (S) – *Luvunga scandens* (Roxb.) Buch. Ham. ex Wight; Rutaceae; thorny woody climber found in East India.

The dried fruits are the source of an essential oil which is used in perfumery and medicinal oils. Fruits and roots are also used as a remedy for scorpion stings. Seeds yield a fatty oil.

Sukasa (S) – *see* Khira.

Sukhdarshan; Vishamandala (S) – *Crinum defixum* Ker-Gawl.; Amaryllidaceae; large evergreen bulbous herb. Cultivated as an ornamental. Bulbs are used for the treatment of carbuncles, burns and whitlow.

Sukshamaphala (S) – *see* Jharberi.

Sukulbet – *see* Baishi.

Sultan champa, Surpan – *Calophyllum inophyllum* L.; Indian laurel (E); Guttiferae; evergreen tree found in coastal regions. Cultivated as an ornamental and avenue tree. Wood is used for making beams, posts, keels of ships, boats, furniture, packing-boxes, plywood and veneers. Bark yields tannin. Pounded bark juice is used as a purgative and its decoction is used topically on ulcers. Seeds yield a fatty oil called poonseed or laurel-nut oil which is used for making soaps and varnishes. Oil is also applied locally to treat painful rheumatic joints and skin infections.

Sundri – *Heritiera fomes* Buch.-Ham.; Sundri (E); Sterculiaceae; evergreen tree found in the Sundarbans. Wood is extremely hard and heavy, and is used for construction work, boats, oars, masts, carriages, carts, agricultural implements and railway keys. Bark and the leaves yield tannin. Gum exuded from the bark is used as an adhesive. The Sundarbans are named after the 'Sundri' trees.

Supari; Poogiphalam (S), Puga (S) – *Areca catechu* L.; Betel-nut (E); Areca nut (E); Palmae; erect palm, with slender stem. Cultivated for its fruit, with the edible part formed by endosperm. Kernels from ripe fruits are separated from the husk, sliced and then chewed with 'pan' or betel leaf as a masticatory. The nut is considered sacred by the Hindus and included as an offering in many rituals and religious ceremonies. Juice of tender nuts is laxative and the fresh fruits are intoxicating. Ripe nuts contain the alkaloid Arecoline, which is used as a taenicide and vermifuge for expelling tapeworm in veterinary medicine and also as an ophthalmic. Ripe, sliced kernels are boiled and made into a tannin-rich cutch, a by-product of the areca-nut industry which is employed in the manufacture of a surface coating resin. Husks are used for making activated charcoal, hard board and brown wrapping paper.

Supota – *see* Khorial.

Sura – *see* Kumeria.

Surabhininiba (S) – *see* Mitha neem.

Surahva – *see* Saru.

Surajmukhi; Surya-mukhi (S), Adityavalli (S) – *Helianthus annuus* L.; Sunflower (E); Compositae; herb. Cultivated as an ornamental, for fodder and as an oil-seed crop. Seeds yield a fatty oil with high content of polyunsaturated fatty acids and is used as a cooking medium, illuminant, lubricant, salad oil, and in the manufacture of margarine, soaps, paints and varnishes. Oil-cake is rich in high-grade proteins and is used as stock-feed. Aerial parts are also used as fodder both fresh and ensilaged. Seeds act as an expectorant and diuretic, are considered to be nutritious and are eaten raw, roasted and salted.

Surake – *see* Chakwat.

Suran – *see* Zamin-kand.

Surasa – *see* Chhota kulpha.

Sureta – *Polycarpon prostratum* (Forsk.) Aschers. & Schweinf.; Caryophyllaceae; perennial herb. Roasted leaf infusion is administered for curing cough following fevers and measles.

Surguja – *see* Kala til.

Suria – *see* Jambu.

Surinjan – *see* Hirantutiya.

Surmainil; Kalaklitaka (S) – *Indigofera articulata* Gouan.; Arabian indigo (E), Egyptian indigo (E); Papilionaceae; shrub. Cultivated as a fodder plant. Seeds are considered to be anthelmintic, and the roots and leaves are used as tonic.

Surna (S) – *see* Diva.

Surpan – *see* Sultan champa.

Surra – *see* Pashan bhedak.

Surwala – *see* Lampa.

Surya-mukhi (S) – *see* Surajmukhi.

Sushavi (S) – *see* Shiajira.

Susnialu – *Dioscorea esculenta* (Lour.) Burkil; Karen potato (E); Lesser yam (E); Dioscoreaceae; prickly woody climber. Tubers are starchy and edible. They possess weak concentrations of diosgenin and can be exploited for precursors of steroids. Grated tubers are used as an analgesic on painful inflamed swellings.

Sutei-gul – *see* Babuna.

Sutejasi (S) – *see* Badrang.

Suthara – *see* Kheu.

Sutri, Ghurush – *Vigna umbellata* (Thunb.) Ohwi & Ohashi (syn. *Dolichos umbellatus* Thunb.); Rice bean (E); Papilionaceae; perennial herb. Often cultivated for its tender edible pods and seeds which are consumed after cooking. Tender shoots and leaves are rich in proteins, minerals and vitamin C, and are used as a stock-feed.

Suvaha (S) – *see* Goali lata.

Suvarnaka (S) – *see* Amaltas.

Suvasa tulsi (S) – *see* Tulsi.

Svarnajuthica (S) – *see* Peeli chameli.

Sveta salmali (S) – *see* Safed semal.

Svethuli – *Zeuxine strateumatica* Schlechter (syn. *Z. sulcata* Lindl.); Orchidaceae; small perennial, terrestrial, rhizomatous herb. Creeping, fleshy rhizomes are used as salep.

Svet jaba – *Hibiscus syriacus* L.; Shrubby Althea (E), Rose of sharon (E); Malvaceae; shrub. Cultivated as an ornamental for its beautiful flowers. Flower decoction is diuretic and is applied topically to itch and skin diseases. Seeds are used for getting rid of colds and headache. Roots and stem bark are used in diarrhoea and dysentery.

Swarn-gandhmadini – *Matricaria aurea* Boiss. (syn. *Cotula aurea* L.); Compositae; herb. Flowers act as a diaphoretic and tonic and are used to treat colic and hysteria.

Swet sarisha (S) – *see* Safed rai.

Syala – *see* Jallil.

Syali (S) – *see* Chaval.

T

Tadrelu – *Barleria cristata* L.; Acanthaceae; undershrub. Cultivated as an ornamental for its beautiful flowers and foliage.

Tagar – *see* Chandni, *see also* Mushkwalee.

Tagara (S) – *see* Chandni

Tagarmul–*see* Ghainchu.

Tagger, Shumeo – *Valeriana hardwickii* Wall.; Valerianaceae; herb found in the hills. Rhizomes and roots are traded as 'mushkbala', and 'mushkwalee' respectively, and are considered to be a good substitute for the drug valerian; they are also used as incense and for scenting hair and hair oils.

Takapana – *see* Jalkhumbi.

Takmak – *see* Meki.

Takoli – *see* Bithua.

Takopat – *Livistona jenkinsiana* Griff.; Palmae; tall palm found in East India. Cultivated as an ornamental also. Leaves are very durable and tough, and are used for thatching and for making hats.

Takri, Takria – *Brachiaria paspaloides* (Presl.) C.E. Hub.; Crab grass (E); Gramineae; perennial grass. Cultivated as a turf grass. Plants are used as fodder either fresh or as hay. *see also* Takria.

Takria, Takri – *Digitaria adscendens* (H.B. & K.) Henr.; Gramineae; perennial grass. It is considered to be good for fodder. *See also* Takri.

Tal (S) – *see* Tar.

Tali (S)–*see* Bajarbattu.

Taliaparnam (S) – *see* Chandan.

Talier – *see* Tara.

Talimakhana; Kokilaksha (S) – *Hygrophila auriculata* (Schum.) Heine [syn. *Asteracantha longifolia* (L.) Nees.]. Acanthaceae; tall hispid herb found near water. Seeds, leaves and roots act as a diuretic, and are used in combating urinary disorders, rheumatism, jaundice and dropsy. Seeds are a rich source of a semi-drying fatty oil.

Talisha (S) – *see* Paniamla.

Talispatri – *Abies spectabilis* (D.Don.) G. Don.; East Himalayan silver fir (E); Pinaceae; tall evergreen tree. Leaves are considered to be tonic, expectorant, diuretic and carminative in small doses, and are used in treating asthma, cough, bronchitis, dyspepsia and epilepsy. Tree yields a resin and the cones are the source of a violet dye. *See also* Paniamla and Thuno which are also known by the same Hindi name.

Tamaku – *see* Tambaku.

Tamal; Tamala (S) – *Garcinia morella* Desr.; Indian gamboge tree (E); Guttiferae; large tree. Stem on scrapping yields a yellow gum resin commercially termed gamboge, which is used in water colours, spirit varnishes for metals, and in dyeing of silks; it is also used in indigenous system of medicine for treating constipation, dropsy and rapid lowering of blood pressure in cerebral congestion. Seeds are the source of a fat which is used in candles, confectionery and as a cooking medium. Fruit rind is used for tanning.

Tamala (S) – *see* Tamal.

Tamalaka (S) – *see* Tejpat.

Tamalapatra (S) – *see* Dalchini.

Tamatar, Vilayati baigan – *Lycopersicon lycopersicum* (L.) Karst. (syn. *Lycopersicum esculentum* Mill.); Tomato (E); Solanaceae; annual herb. Cultivated for its fleshy, nutritious and delicious fruits which are used either raw as salad or cooked to make vegetable, curries, soups, ketchup, sauce and juice. Fruits are rich in minerals, vitamins, and carotenoids specially the pigment lycopene (lycopersicin) which is reported to help lower the risk of colon and prostate cancers. Seeds are the source of a semi-drying oil which is used in the manufacture of soaps and paints, and on refining used as a salad oil. Oil-cake is used as fodder and fertilizer.

Tambaku, Tamaku – *Nicotiana tabacum* L.; Tobacco (E); Solanaceae; herb. Cultivated for its leaves which are used in the manufacture of cured and processed tobacco of various types, *viz*., cigarette, cigar, cheroot, hookah, snuff and chewing tobacco. The leaves contain several alkaloids of which nicotine is important and habit-forming; it is also used medicinally as a sedative, in gastro-intestinal disorders and locally applied on skin diseases. Extract of tobacco dust and inferior grade leaves which are rich in nicotine sulphate are used as an insecticide for the elimination of ticks and lice in animals and also in agriculture. Leaves are also used to prepare tobacco-absolute which is used for improving aroma of lower grade tobacco. Seeds are the source of a semi-drying oil used for the manufacture of soaps and paints. The oil-cake is free from nicotine and is used as fodder. *See also* Vilayati tambaku.

Tambula (S) – *see* Pan.

Tambuli – *see* Pan.

Tamthar – *Grewia villosa* Willd.; Tiliaceae; shrub. Fruits are edible and the seeds yield a fatty oil. Stem is used for making bows and walking-sticks. Bark is the source of a fibre which is used for cordage. Roots are considered to be useful in controlling diarrhoea.

Tandlen, Chiriya-ka-dana – *Sporobolus diander* (Retz.) Beauv.; Gramineae; perennial grass. Plants are used as fodder for cattle and horses, and also considered to be good as a sand binder. Culms are used for making brooms.

Tandula (S) – *see* Chaval.

Tanduliya (S) – *see* Kataili chaulai. *see also* Jangli chaulai.

Tankari – *see* Rasbhari.

Tantee – *see* Karer.

Tapasya-priya (S) – *see* Chironji.

Tapinijha (S) – *see* Dampel.

Tar; Tal (S) – *Borassus flabellifer* L.; Palmyra palm (E); Palmae; tall palm found in coastal regions of India. Fruit pulp and seeds are edible. Tapping of the inflorescence yields a sap which is used for the production of palm-sugar or jaggery. Sap of the peduncles yields toddy, which is used fresh or fermented as arrack and also used for the production of palm-sugar. Leaves are used for thatching, basketry, and for making bags, mats, fans and hats. Leaf stalks are the source of a fibre used for making brushes and for the manufacture of paper. Tree yields a black gum and the trunk is used for posts, pillars and rafters.

Tara, Talier – *Corypha taliera* Roxb.; Palmae; stout palm found along Tamil Nadu coast of peninsular India. Leaves are used for making mats and baskets and are also used for thatching.

Tarai – *Melocanna baccifera* (Roxb.) Kurz; Tarai bamboo (E); Gramineae; stout perennial grass found in East Indian hills. Leaves are used for making baskets and mats. Plants are used for the manufacture of paper.

Tarali – *see* Kundri.

Taramira; Daradharsh (S), Bhutaghna (S) – *Eruca vesicaria* (L.) Cav. ssp. *sativa* (Mill.) Thell; Taramira (E), Roquette (E); Cruciferae; herb. Cultivated as an oil seed crop in North India. Seeds yield a pungent fatty oil, used as an illuminant and for making pickles. Oil-cake and young plants are used as stock-feed. Seeds are acrid, and seed-paste is anti-bacterial. Tender shoots and leaves are used as vegetable. Leaves are considered as stomachic, diuretic and stimulant.

Tarbooz – *Citrullus lanatus* (Thunb.) Mansf. (syn. *Citrullus vulgaris* Schrad.); Watermelon (E); Cucurbitaceae; annual trailing herb. Cultivated for its big, juicy, nutritious and refreshing fruit which is used fresh. Fruit juice is diuretic and cooling. Seeds are edible and yield a fatty oil which can be used for cooking and illumination. Seeds are also considered to be a tonic, stimulant and diuretic.

Tarcharbi – *see* Pippalyang.

Tarla – *Heteropanax fragrans* (D. Don.) Seem; Araliaceae; small tree found in the sub-Himalayan tract. Leaves are used for rearing 'eri' silkworms. Wood is used for making walking-sticks and handles.

Tarwar – *Cassia auriculata* L.; Tanners Cassia (E), Avaram (E); Caesalpiniaceae; shrub. Bark forms the main source of an indigenous tannin which is used in the South Indian tanneries and is also an astringent. Roots are used for treating skin ailments. Fruits and leaves are anthelmintic, and seeds are used in eye trouble.

Tatara – *see* Haiza.

Tatri – *Rhus chinensis* Mill.; Anacardiaceae; tree found in the hills. Leaf galls provide high grade concentrated tannin and gallic acid. Galls are used medicinally for curing diarrhoea, dysentery, colic and in ointments for the treatment of wounds and inflammations. Fruits are edible, and are used as a rennet substitute for curdling of milk to make cheese; they also serve as the source of a vegetable wax which is used in the manufacture of candles.

Tavakshira (S) – *see* Tikora.

Teanklo; Sangkhi (S) – *Catharanthus pusillus* (Murr.) G. Don.; Apocynaceae; wild herb with white flowers. Dried plant decoction made in oil is used for massage in lumbago.

Tejpat; Tejpatra (S), Tamalaka (S) – *Cinnamomum tamala* (Buch.-Ham.) Nees & Eberm; Indian Cassia-lignea (E): Lauraceae; small tree found in the hills. Leaves are used as a spice and condiment. Bark and leaves are aromatic, and serve as the source of an essential oil which is used for flavouring.

Tejpatra (S) – *see* Tejpat.

Tejphal – *see* Timur; *see also* Tumru.

Telingachina – *see* Pharash.

Temru – *see* Kendu.

Tendu, Timburni; Dirghapatraka (S) - *Diospyros melanoxylon* Roxb.; Coromandal ebony persimmon (E); Ebenaceae; large tree. Leaves are highly valued as wrappers for 'beedis' a cheap substitute of cigarette which are very popular amongst the rural masses in India. Dark coloured black heart-wood is the source of timber called Coromandal ebony which is used for carving, turnery, tool handles, toys and miscellaneous other purposes. Ripe fruits are edible. Raw fruits and bark is used for tanning. Decoction of the bark is used for treating diarrhoea and indigestion. Dried flower decoction is used in urinary and skin disorders.

Tepari – *Abutilon persicum* (Burm. f.) Merr.; Malvaceae; undershrub. Stem is the source of a coarse fibre used for cordage.

Tesu – *see* Dhak.

Thakal – *see* Jangli khajur.

Thanella – *see* Ghurgia.

Tharbal – *see* Bamora.

Thelu, Bettar – *Juniperus recurva* Buch.-Ham.; Weeping blue juniper (E); Cupressaceae; evergreen small tree. Wood and leaves are used as incense. Wood is also suitable for making pencils. Fruiting bodies are the source of an essential oil which is used for flavouring.

Thohar – *see* Sehund.

Thoonia loth, Bhoree loth – *Combretum pilosum* Roxb.; Combretaceae; large climber found in East India. Leaves act as an anthelmintic and are used specifically for getting rid of roundworm infection.

Thor, Shakarpitan – *Euphorbia royleana* Boiss.; Euphorbiaceae; succulent shrub. Often planted on the boundary for fencing. Latex is anthelmintic and purgative.

Thuno, Birmi, Talispatri; Manduparni (S) – *Taxus baccata* L. ssp. *wallichiana* (Zucck.) Pilger; Common yew (E); Taxaceae; tree found in the hills. Wood is used for furniture, panelling, cabinet work, fancy articles, carving, pencils and veneers. Leaves act as an expectorant, antispasmodic, sedative and antiseptic and are used in small doses for the treatment of asthma, bronchitis, hiccups, diarrhoea, dyspepsia, headache, hysteria, epilepsy and nervousness. In larger doses the drug works as a heart poison. The leaves also have cancer fighting property and are used in the manufacture of taxol and baccatine. They are marketed by the trade name of 'talispatra'; the active principles present are taxine, taxinine and traces of ephedrine.

Tikhar – *Breynia rhamnoides* Muell-Arg.; Euphorbiaceae; shrub. Leaves are used as vegetable. Dry leaf-fumes are inhaled for tonsilitis. Fresh leaf-poultice is applied to abscesses to hasten suppuration. Leaf juice is used to prevent haemorrhage after child-birth.

Tikhor – *see* Ararut.

Tikhur – *Hitchenia caulina* (Grah.) Baker (syn. *Curcuma caulina* Grah.); Indian arrowroot (E); Zingiberaceae; large perennial herb. Tuberous starchy root stocks are edible. Starch is also used as a sizing material and in the manufacture of glues. Leaves are used in the manufacture of paper. *See also* Tikora.

Tikora, Tikhur; Tavakshira (S) – *Curcuma angustifolia* Roxb.; East Indian arrowroot (E); Zingiberaceae; perennial herb with tuberous rootstock. Plant is often cultivated. Tubers are starchy, edible and easily digestible. Starch is used like arrowroot.

Til; Tila (S) – *Sesamum indicum* L.; Sesame (E), Gingelly (E); Pedaliaceae; herb. Cultivated as an oil-seed crop. Oil is edible and has high content of both mono- and polyunsaturated fatty acids. Seeds are edible and nutritious, and are used in confectionery as topping or they are roasted and made into candy. Seeds considered to be auspicious are included in many Hindu religious ceremonies. Oil from the seeds called gingelly or sesame-oil is used for preserving mango and other pickles, and as an important ingredient of many snacks and sweetmeats.

Oil is also used for cooking purposes, and in the manufacture of hair oils, pharmaceuticals, cosmetics, insecticides and soaps. Oil-cake is rich in proteins and is used as a stock-feed. Oil-cake after processing yields a protein-rich flour which is suitable for human consumption. Fresh leaves are used in renal and bladder disorders and fresh leaf juice is applied to skin infections. Mucilaginous juice of the plant is used for getting rid of hair lice.

Tila (S) – *see* Til.

Tilaunja – *Populus ciliata* Wall.; Salicaceae; tree found in the hills. Wood is used for packing-cases, turnery articles, cricket bats, veneers and match industry. Wood pulp is used for the manufacture of printing and writing paper. Bark is considered to be a stimulant and tonic. Leaves are lopped for fodder.

Tilki – *see* Birsa.

Tilluk – *see* Khilut.

Timar, Mazenga – *Fagara oxyphylla* (Edgew.) Engl. (syn. *Zanthoxylum oxyphyllum* Edgew.); Rutaceae; shrub. Tender shoots and leaves are used as vegetable.

Timburni – see Tendu.

Timla, Tirmal – *Ficus auriculata* Lour.; Eve's apron (E); Moraceae; tree found in East India. Fruits are edible and are used in the preparation of jams and curries.

Timur, Darmar, Nepali dhaniya, Tejphal – *Zanthoxylum acanthopodium* DC.; Rutaceae; aromatic shrub found in the hills. All parts are aromatic with coriander-like flavour and are used as a spice and condiment. Seeds are rich in an essential oil and yield the 'attar of henna' or otto of 'henna'. Seeds are also used widely to flavour tobacco, pharmaceuticals and tooth powders. Dried flowers yield another essential oil known commercially as wartara oil, rich in a compound called linalool which is in great demand in perfumery. Wartara oil is antiseptic, and is used in the manufacture of toothpastes, mouth-washes, deodorants and soaps. Plant exhibits insecticidal properties, and the seed decoction is used as a fever reducing agent.

Tinda – *Citrullus lanatus* (Thunb.) Mansf. var. *fistulosus* (Stocks) Mansf. [syn. *C. vulgaris* Schrad. var. *fistulosus* (Stocks) Duth. & Full.]; Round gourd (E); Cucurbitaceae; trailing herb with fistulous petioles and stems. Cultivated for its tender small green fruits which are used as a vegetable.

Tenduka (S) – *see* Gab.

Tinisha (S) – *see* Sandan.

Tinsa – *see* Sandan.

Tipari – *see* Rasbhari.

Tirmal – *see* Timla.

Tisi – *see* Alsi.

Titapat – *see* Pat.

Titbaigan, Ranbaigan, Bhurat – *Solanum torvum* Swartz; Solanaceae; undershrub or herb with spines. Fruits are used as vegetable, and considered to be specially useful in spleen and liver enlargement. Plant acts as a tonic, expectorant, digestive, diuretic and sedative. Fruit decoction is used for relieving cough and burning seed-fumes are inhaled for curing toothache. Leaves are considered as haemostatic.

Titlia – *Launaea aspleniifolia* Hook. f.; Compositae; perennial wild herb. Root is used as a constituent of galactagogue drugs.

Titlokia – *Veronica anagallis-aquatica* L.; Scrophulariaceae; annual herb. Tender shoots and leaves are used as salad and pot-herb. Herb is diuretic, appetizer and antiscorbutic and is used for bladder and skin disorders. Roots are used for the preparation of gargles.

Titmuliya – *Viburnum coriaceum* Blume; Caprifoliaceae; shrub found in the hills. Seeds are the source of a fatty edible oil which is also used as an illuminant. Ethanolic extract of the aerial parts is reported to exhibit activity against *Entamoeba hystolytica*.

Titri – *Rhus punjabensis* J.L. Stew ex Brand; Anacardiaceae; small tree. Fresh ripe fruits are edible, and are also used for the preparation of a refreshing drink. Wood is used for cabinet work, tobacco pipes and ornamental inlay-work. Leaves are used as a tan. Plant juice is irritating to the skin and is blister-forming.

Tivar – *see* Bina.

Tivra – *Mentha aquatica* L.; Marsh mint (E), Water mint (E); Labiatae; herb. Often cultivated for its aromatic leaves in Indian gardens. Leaves are rich in an essential oil which is used for the treatment of headaches and vomiting. Plant infusion is carminative, stimulant, digestive and cooling and is used in treating dyspepsia and rheumatism.

Todri-safed – *Matthiola incana* R. Br.; Stock (E), Gilli flower (E); Cruciferae; annual herb. Cultivated as an ornamental for its beautiful white, pink and purple flowers. Seeds are expectorant, tonic, stomachic and diuretic; they also serve as the source of a volatile oil and a fatty oil.

Todri-surkh – *Cheiranthus cheiri* L.; Wall flower (E); Cruciferae; annual herb. Cultivated as an ornamental for forming low border with very striking, showy, yellow and deep maroon coloured flowers. Seeds act as a tonic, diuretic and stomachic and contain cheirotoxin, a cardiac glycoside. Flowers are aromatic, source of an essential oil, and considered as an emmenogogue and stimulant.

Tohar sem – *see* Kumach.

Tokra – *see* Sarsan-banda.

Tongus – *see* Jiti.

Toom – *see* Ghogar.

Toon, Mahanim; Nandavriksha (S) – *Toona ciliata* M.J. Roem. (syn. *Cedrella toona* Roxb. ex Rottl. & Willd.); Cedrela tree (E), Red cedar tree (E); Meliaceae; tree. Often cultivated as an avenue tree. Flowers are the source of an orange-red dye called 'gunari' which is used for dyeing cottons. Wood is used for flooring, doors and windows, furniture, packing cases, cigar-boxes and manufacture of plywood. Bark is rich in tannin and is used for curing dysentery in infants and as a topical application on ulcers. Wood also yields an essential oil.

Tope gola – *Couroupita guianensis* Aubl.; Cannon ball tree (E); Lecythidaceae; tree. Cultivated in Indian gardens as an introduced ornamental plant, and bears white, yellow or rose-purple flowers and very striking fruits with woody shells resembling a canon-ball. Fruit-pulp is edible.

Tori, Ghiya tori; Rajakoshataki (S) – *Luffa cylindrica* (L.) M.J. Roem; Sponge gourd (E), Vegetable sponge (E); Cucurbitaceae; climbing annual herb. Cultivated for its tender fruits which are used as vegetable; they are also considered digestive and diuretic. Pulverized mature fruits are anthelmintic, purgative and carminative. Seeds act as an emetic and cathartic. Dry spongy fibrous vascular network of fruit is widely used as a scrubber and its fibre is used as a stuffing material for mattresses. The fibre also makes good sound-proofing, heat-proofing, shock absorbency and packing material. Seeds yield a fatty oil which is used as olive oil substitute.

Toria – *Brassica campestris* L. var. *toria* Duth & Full.; Indian rape; Cruciferae; herb. Cultivated as an oil-seed crop. Seeds are the source of an edible fatty oil. Oil-cake makes good fodder and fertilizer. Leaves are used as pot-herb. Roots act as a diuretic and root paste is used to soften the skin. Seeds are also used as bird-feed.

Torki – *Indigofera linifolia* Retz. Papilionaceae; annual herb. Plant infusion is used to treat febrile eruptions. Plant decoction is also used for expelling intestinal worms.

Toriva – *see* Kali sarson.

Trayamaana (S) – *see* Asbarg.

Tredhara sehund, Vajrakantaka (S), Vajri (S) – *Euphorbia antiquorum* L.; Euphorbiaceae; shrub with succulent spiny stems. Often cultivated for protective fencing as a hedge. Latex is used as a fish poison and also used topically on wounds. Stem juice is applied to warts and cutaneous infections and is also used internally for dropsy and nervine disorders. Decoction of stem is purgative and digestive, and is used as a remedy for gout.

Trepakashee (S) – *see* Tripungki.

Trepatra – *Trifolium pratense* L.; Red clover (E); Papilionaceae; small herb good for pastures. Cultivated for protein-rich fodder which is either used fresh or made into hay and silage. Flower-infusion is used as a sedative and flower-extract is used on ulcers and corns.

Trikantaka (S) – *see* Konpal sehund.

Trinpoli; Palanggini (S) – *Rytilix granularis* (L.) Skeels [syn. *Hackelochloa granularis* (L.) O. Kuntze., and *Manisuris granularis* L.f.]; Gramineae; annual grass. Plant is used for fodder and is also used medicinally in liver and spleen disorders.

Tripungki; Trepakashee (S) – *Coldenia procumbens* L.; Ehretiaceae; prostrate wild herb. Fresh leaf paste is used for treating painful rheumatic inflammation.

Trivrit (S) – *see* Nisoth.

Tukh-malanga, Gharei kashmalu – *Lallemantia royleana* (Wall. ex Benth.) Benth.; Labiatae; perennial herb found in the hills. Soaked seed-coats become mucilaginous and are then used for flatulence and constipation. Seeds possess cooling, diuretic and sedative properties. Seed poultice is applied to boils and inflammations, and seeds are also the source of a semi-drying fatty oil.

Tula (S) – *see* Tut.

Tulati patti, Papotan – *Physalis minima* L.; Sunberry (E); Solanaceae; annual wild herb. Fruits are edible. Fruits and leaves act as a diuretic, laxative and tonic. Fruits of *P. minima* L. var. *indica* C.B. Clarke., form one of the components of a medicinal oil used for spleen disorders.

Tulsi, Brinda; Ajaka (S), Manjari (S), Suvasa tulsi (S) – *Ocimum sanctum* L.; Holy basil (E), Sacred basil (E); Labiatae; strongly scented undershrub. Cultivated as a sacred plant in all Hindu homes and temples. Leaf infusion in the form of medicated tea is considered to be anti-catarrhal, expectorant, digestive, diuretic and febrifuge, and is used for treating colds, cough, bronchitis, and liver, gastric and bladder complaints. Leaf juice and leaf paste is used for topical application on ringworm and other skin diseases. Root decoction is administered for fevers including malaria. Seeds act as a demulcent, and are used in urinary complaints. Leaves are the source of an essential oil, rich in eugenol, methyl eugenol and cavacrol, exhibiting insecticidal and bactericidal properties. The plant has many legends associated with it and is revered as 'Mother Tulsi' and as 'Haripriya' or Goddess Lakshmi. According to the 'Tulsi mantra' the plant has been worshipped by the great saints since eternity, as the 'Vedas' reside in the upper part, the 'Devtas' in the central and the pilgrimages in the bottom part of its leaves. It is quite obvious that the plant's medicinal and other uses were known to our sages since very ancient times.

Tumala (S) – *see* Bistendu.

Tumra – *see* Tung.

Tumri – *Pittosporum floribundum* Wight & Arn.; Pittosporaceae; tree. Bark is considered to be a febrifuge and expectorant and is used for chronic bronchitis, and leprosy; it is also considered as an antidote to snake-poison. Root paste is used on rheumatic and dropsical inflammation. Wood is used for making toys, and is also the source of an essential oil which is used internally for combating rheumatism, leprosy and skin disorders, and externally for topical application on cuts, bruises, sprains, inflammatory rheumatic joints, chest infections and ophthalmia. Flowers also yield an essential oil which is used in perfumery.

Tumru, Darmar, Nepali dhaniya, Tejphal – *Zanthoxylum armatum* DC., Wingleaf prickly ash (E); Rutaceae; small prickly tree. Aromatic bark, fruits and seeds are medicinal. They are considered as an anthelmintic, stomachic, carminative, stimulant, astringent, digestive, diuretic and expectorant, and are used in the treatment of colds, cough, asthma, dyspepsia, piles, nervous debility and for expelling worms. Root-bark is used as an aromatic masticatory with betel leaf. Fruit tubercles contain an oleo-resin, and are aromatic and pungent in taste. Fruits are used for toothache and for tenderizing meat and fish. Dry fruits also yield an essential oil used in tooth-powders. Aromatic seeds are stimulating and tonic. Wood is used for making walking-sticks.

Tumul – *see* Dampel.

Tung, Tumra, Raitung – *Rhus parviflora* Roxb.; Anacardiaceae; shrub or small tree. Ripe fruits are consumed both fresh and dried. Fruit juice is a vermifuge. Plant is considered to be very useful for afforestation. Wood is used for tool handles and turnery articles. Dried leaves are used either as a substitute for tobacco or are mixed with tobacco.

Tunga, Tungla – *Cotinus coggygria* Scop. (syn. *Rhus cotinus* L.); Indian sumach (E), Smoke tree (E), Wig tree (E); Anacardiaceae; small tree found in N.W. Himalayas as an undergrowth with pines. Stem and large branches constitute a yellow wood commercially known as Young-fustic. Wood is the source of a yellow dye which is used in leather and textile industry. Wood is also used for picture frames, inlay-work and carving. Bark and powdered leaves are used for tanning of soft leather. Twigs are used for basketry and tender twigs yield an aromatic essential oil.

Tungla – *see* Tunga.

Tur – *see* Arhar.

Turanj – *see* Bijaura.

Turmas – *Lupinus albus* L.; White lupine (E); Papilionaceae; herb. Cultivated for fodder and green manuring. Seeds are soaked in water to remove the toxic alkaloids before being used as food and cattle-feed. Seeds act as a carminative, deobstruent and anthelmintic and yield a fatty oil which can be used for cooking only after refining. Stems and seedlings are a rich source of asparagine.

Tut, Tutri, Safed shahtoot; Tula (S) – *Morus alba* L.; White mulberry (E); Moraceae; fast growing tree. Cultivated for its fruit, shade, and the leaves which are rich in calcium and vitamin C and are used mainly for feeding silkworms. Wood is used chiefly for making hockey sticks, cricket bats, stumps, rackets along with their presses and other sports goods; it is also used for turnery articles, shafts, spokes, agricultural implements and the manufacture of printing and writing paper. Fruits are edible, and also made into syrups which are considered useful for curing sore throat and indigestion. Roots are anthelmintic. Bark is purgative and the bark fibre is used for the manufacture of paper-pulp. Leaves are lopped for fodder.

Tutri – *see* Tut.

Tuvari (S) – *see* Arhar.

Tuvrak (S) – *see* Chaulmoogra.

U

Ubdie-narikaylum (S) – *see* Darya-ka-naryal.

Udajati – *Ecbolium linneanum* Kurz var. *dentata* (Klein) Clarke; Acanthaceae; shrub. Cultivated in the gardens as an ornamental for its beautiful flowers. Leaf decoction is used for stricture, an abnormal constriction of ducts in the body (e.g. esophagus). Roots are used for treating rheumatism, jaundice and menorrhagia.

Udal, Udar – *Sterculia villosa* Roxb.; Sterculiaceae; large spreading tree. Wood is used chiefly for packing-cases, match industry and plywood. Bark yields a rough fibre which is used for cordage and the gum exudate from the bark is used in veterinary medicine and also as an adhesive. Seeds are edible after they are cooked or roasted.

Uddalaka (S) – *see* Lasora.

Udis – *see* Utis.

Udi–sambhalu – *see* Neeli nargandi.

Ud-salap – *Paeonia emodi* Wall. ex Royle; Himalayan Peony (E); Paeoniaceae; herb found in W. Himalayas. Tuberous fleshy roots act a blood purifier and are used for treating hysteria, convulsions, epilepsy, dropsy, uterine ailments, biliousness and colic; excessive usage and high doses are harmful and can cause vomiting, headache and other side-effects. Roots are rich in an essential oil. Flower infusion is used for checking diarrhoea. Seeds are emetic and laxative.

Udumbara (S) – *see* Gular.

Ugragandha (S) – *see* Bhaulan.

Ujli sarson – *see* Safed rai.

Ukh, Ganna – *Saccharum sinense* Roxb. (syn. *S. barberi* Jesw.); North Indian cane (E); Gramineae; tall perennial grass with juicy and jointed stems. Cultivated in India from very ancient times, as a source of sugar, jaggery, and 'khansari'. Important by-products include molasses and bagasse or fibre left after extraction of the juice. Molascuit, a mixture of bagasse and molasses is used as fodder. Bagasse is also used for fodder, fuel and the manufacture of paper. Molasses are used for the preparation of industrial alcohol, rum and synthetic rubber.

Ulatkambal, Kumal, Olak; Bharadvaji (S) – *Abroma augusta* (L.) L.f. (syn. *Theobroma augusta* L.); Devil's cotton (E), Perennial Indian hemp (E); Sterculiaceae; small tree often cultivated in gardens. Stem bark serves as the source of a coarse, but soft and lustrous fibre suitable for mixing with jute, and also used as a cordage fibre. Dried root bark is used medicinally as a uterine tonic and fresh juice of root bark is administered in neuralgic and congestive dysmenorrhoea. Leaf infusion is used in combating diabetes, sinusitis, rheumatism and uterine disorders. Seeds yield a fatty oil reported to lower down the cholesterol level in blood.

Ulla, Sarkhara – *Themeda arundinacea* (Roxb.) Ridley [syn. *Anthistiria gigantea* Hack. ssp. *arundinacea* (Roxb.) Hack.]; Ulla grass (E); Gramineae; perennial grass. Plant is the source of paper-pulp used for the manufacture of printing, writing and wrapping paper. Culms are also used for making the walls of mud-huts and as a source of fibre used for cordage. Plant is also used as hay for cattle.

Ulu – *see* Dabh.

Umar – *see* Gular.

Umtao – *Antidesma ghesaembilla* Gaertn.; Black currant (E); Stilaginaceae; small tree. Fruits are edible and are used for seasoning non-vegetarian dishes. Stem bark is used for making ropes.

Undarbibi, Jangli-erandi; Nikumba (S) – *Jatropha glandulifera* Roxb.; Euphorbiaceae; shrub. Fresh root paste mixed with water is administered to children with liver enlargement and also used to reduce glandular swellings. Seed oil is used topically on rheumatic and paralytic parts, and internally as a purgative.

Unga – *see* Bachita.

Unmatta (S) – *see* Dhatura.

Unnab, Ban baer, Pitni baer – *Ziziphus sativa* Gaertn. (syn. *Z. vulgaris* Lamk.); Rhamnaceae, thorny tree. Fruit is considered to be an anodyne, tonic and cooling and is used to check vomiting and nausea. Fruit constitutes one of the ingredients of an Ayurvedic preparation called 'Joshanda' which is used to cure colds. Bark is the source of tannin.

Urad, Urd, Mah; Masha (S) – *Vigna mungo* (L.) Hepper (syn. *Phaseolus mungo* L., non Roxb. & Auct.); Black gram (E); Papilionaceae; herb. Cultivated as an important pulse crop. Seeds which are rich in proteins and phosphorus are consumed as 'dal' or pulse and very widely used in the Indian cuisine for miscellaneous food preparations. The pulse acts as a diuretic and its intake is advised in dropsy, and in hepatic and nervous ailments. Roots are narcotic and are prescribed for aching bones. Aerial parts after harvesting the pods are used as fodder and green manure.

Urd – *see* Urad.

Urni – *see* Bhutia-badam.

Uruvaka (S) – *see* Errandi.

Usar-ki-ghas – *Sporobolus maderaspatanus* Bor.; Gramineae; common perennial herb. The plant is used for reclamation of 'usar' or waste lands where the salts have seeped up to the soil surface. Plants serve as good fodder for cattle and horses, both in fresh state and as hay.

Ustabunda – *see* Agetha.

Ustarkhar – *see* Damahan.

Utakanta; Kantalu (S), Utati (S) – *Echinops echinatus* Roxb.; Compositae; herb. Plant acts as a nerve tonic, stimulant and diuretic and is used in indigestion, cough and ophthalmia. Powdered roots possess larvicidal and insecticidal properties and are used to kill lice, and maggots in cattle wounds.

Utati (S) – *see* Utakanta.

Utigun – *Laportea crenulata* (Roxb.) Gaud.; Devil nettle (E), Fever nettle (E); Urticaceae; stout shrub found in the hills. Flowers are used in curries. Seeds are used as condiment and as a carminative. Root juice is used as a febrifuge in chronic fevers. Bark provides a strong coarse fibre which is used by the tribals for cordage and coarse cloth.

Utis, Udis – *Alnus nepalensis* D. Don.; Indian alder (E); Betulaceae; tree. Wood is used for general carpentry, house-construction, tea chests, pencils and for the manufacture of writing and printing paper. Bark is rich in tannin, and is used for deepening the colour of the dye 'manjit' or Indian madder.

Utran – *see* Jutuk.

Uttanjan – *see* Chaupatia.

Uttaravaruni (S) – *see* Jutuk.

V

Vacha (S) – *see* Bach.

Vahisi (S) – *see* Jangli karela.

Vajra (S) – *see* Sehund.

Vajradruma (S) – *see* Konpal sehund.

Vajrakantaka (S) – *see* Tredhara sehund.

Vajri (S) – *see* Tredhara sehund.

Vakavryksha (S) – *see* Dhawa.

Vakeri-mul – *Caesalpinia digyna* Rottler; Teri pods (E); Caesalpiniaceae; large prickly shrub. Fruit-wall or shell of pods marketed by the trade name teri, are high in tannin content and are used for tanning. Seeds are used as cattle feed and the roots are used in treating diabetes and phthisis.

Valuka (S) – *see* Balu-ka-sag.

Vana-bhenda (S) – *see* Bachita.

Vana-haridra – *see* Jangli haldi.

Vanajai – *see* Lanjai.

Vanamalli (S) – *see* Nwari.

Vanamallika (S) – *Jasminum rottlerianum* Wall.; Oleaceae. Climbing or erect shrub, found in the W. peninsular part of India. Leaves are used to treat eczema.

Vananimbuka (S) – *see* Ban nimbu.

Vanapandan (S) – *see* Ban piyazi.

Vanardraka (S) – *see* Jangli adrak.

Vanatiktika (S) – *see* Nimuka.

Vanayamini (S) – *see* Banajowan.

Vanda – *see* Rasna.

Vanda (S) – *see* Banda.

Van natya; Alpa marisha (S) – *Amaranthus blitum* L. Amaranthaceae; wild herb. Tender shoots and leaves are used as pot-herb.

Vansh (S) – *see* Bans.

Vansha (S) – *see* Bans-kaban.

Vapusha (S) – *see* Abhal.

Varaguna (S) – *see* Jangli madan-mast-ka-phul.

Varaka (S) – *see* Cheen.

Vartaka (S) – *see* Baigan.

Varuna (S) – *see* Bilasi; *see also* Baishi.

Varvara (S) – *see* Marua.

Vasaka (S) – *see* Arusha.

Vasanta (S) – *see* Kundphul.

Vasuka (S) – *see* Latahai.

Vaṭa (S) – *see* Barh.

Vatadalla (S) – *Ziziphus glabrata* Heyne.; Rhamnaceae; tree. Leaves are used in the indigenous system of medicine to treat venereal diseases.

Vetasa – *see* Bet.

Vetra (S) – *see* Bet.

Vibhitaka (S) – *see* Bahera.

Vidari (S) – *see* Bilaikand; *see also* Chichora.

Vidhara – *Rourea minor* (Gaertn.) Alston; Connaraceae; large woody climber. Fresh arils of the fruits are edible. Roots and twigs are used for combating diabetes, pulmonary disorders, rheumatism and scurvy; they are also applied as a topical preparation for skin ailments and ulcers. The decoction of wood is given after childbirth and also used as a febrifuge.

Vijaya (S) – *see* Bhang.

Vikangata (S) – *see* Baikal.

Vikarini (S) – *see* Badhara.

Vilayati afsanthin; Damar (S), Indhana (S) – *Artemisia absinthium* L.; Absinthe (E), Wormwood (E); Compositae; herb found in the hills. Inflorescence (capitula) and leaves, are the source of the drug afsanteen considered to be a stimulant and tonic, and used in chronic fevers and inflammation of liver. Herb yields an essential oil called wormwood oil which is used as a digestive stimulant and tonic, and is also applied to painful rheumatic joints. Seeds are the source of a fatty oil.

Vilayati anchhu – *Rubus fruticosus* L.; European black berry (E); Rosaceae; shrub. Cultivated in some parts of the hills. Fruits are edible, and are used for making wine and for colouring other liqueurs.

Vilayati baral – *see* Subabul.

Vilayati baigan – *see* Tamatar.

Vilayati bel – *see* Bilayati bel.

Vilayati bhendi – *see* Ranbhendi.

Vilayati gab – *see* Bilayati gab.

Vilayati gawuth, Hol – *Medicago sativa* L.; Alfalfa (E), Lucerne (E); Papilionaceae; perennial herb. Cultivated in the temperate regions for pastures, and is mostly used as green fodder for horses; it also forms nutritious silage and hay. Plant is used as a commercial source of chlorophyll, and vitamins A, C and E. Seeds yield a drying oil which is used for the manufacture of paints and varnishes, and are also the source of a yellow dye.

Vilayati imli – *see* Jangal Jalebi.

Vilayati kaddu – *see* Safed kaddu.

Vilayati kangai – *see* Gulkhair.

Vilayati kikar – *Prosopis juliflora* (Sw.) DC.; Mesquite (E), Algaroba (E); Mimosaceae; medium-sized tree. Plant very hardy, and has been successfully introduced into India and now forms the characteristic landscape of scrub vegetation. It is considered to be very useful as a wind-break plant and in afforesting dry and degraded lands and shifting sand-dunes. Wood is used for making fence-posts, hardboard and furniture. Leaves and pods are used as a stock-feed. All parts are rich in tannin and the gum from the tree is used in confectionery and as an emulsifier. Another species *Parkinsonia aculeata* L. is also known by the same Hindi name.

Vilayati kikar – *Parkinsonia aculeata* L.; Jerusalem thorn (E), Ratama (E); Caesalpiniaceae; small tree. Cultivated for making hedges, and as a shelter-belt and wind-break plant. Bark yields a fibre which is suitable for paper-pulp. Seeds are edible and are rich in the proteins albumin and glutelin. Leaves and twigs are lopped for fodder.

Vilayati lassan, Kirath – *Allium ampeloprasum* L. var. *porrum* (L.) Gay.; Leek (E); Alliaceae; stout herb, with weak bulbs. Cultivated for stems and leaves which are used blanched and in soups.

Vilayati mehndi – *see* Murad.

Vilayati nil – *Indigofera suffruticosa* Mill.; Anil indigo (E), West Indian Indigo (E); Papilionaceae; introduced into India from tropical America. Root decoction is reported to be useful in treating ulcers and urinary tract diseases. Herb is considered to be a stomachic, diuretic and febrifuge, and is used in remedies for treating syphilis and epilepsy.

Vilayati Panas – *Artocarpus altilis* (Park.) Fosb.; Bread fruit (E); Moraceae; small tree. Cultivated for its fruits which are starchy and are used as vegetable. Bark yields a fibre used for cordage and a thick white gum which is used for caulking boats and canoes. Wood is used for posts, beams and rafters and leaves are lopped for fodder.

Vilayati pudina – *Mentha piperita* L.; Peppermint (E); Labiatae; perennial herb. Cultivated for its aromatic leaves which are used as a condiment and as the source of an essential oil used medicinally to check vomiting and nausea, and in the manufacture of ointments and drops for headaches and rheumatism; they are also used in the manufacture of cough lozenges, inhalers, breath freshners and mouth-washes. The oil is also used in perfumery and soap industry.

Vilayati sem – *see* Frash bean.

Vilayati siras – *Samanea saman* Merr.; Monkey-pod tree (E), Rain-tree (E); Mimosaceae; large handsome tree. Cultivated as an avenue or shade tree. Leaves and green tender pods are used as cattle feed. Tree is the source of a gum which when in contact with water swells up into a tough cartilage-like mass.

Vilayati shisham – *see* Pippalyang.

Vilayati tambaku – *Nicotiana rustica* L.; East Indian or Turkish tobacco (E); Solanaceae; herb. Cultivated for its leaves which have high nicotine content. They are used in the manufacture of insecticides and for 'hookah', chewing and snuff tobacco and also as a filler for 'beedis'.

Vilayati tulsi – *see* Bilayati tulsi.

Vilayati zirah – *see* Shia-jira.

Vingar – *see* Baikal.

Virtuli, Kunlai – *Dichrostachys cinerea* (L.) Wight & Arn. (syn. *Mimosa cinerea* L.); Mimosaceae; thorny small tree. Wood is used for making tent-pegs and walking-sticks. Bark is used for tanning.

Roots are used in remedies for kidney disorders and rheumatism. Leaves are lopped for fodder.

Visha – *see* Bish.

Vishagna (S) – *see* Jangli chaulai.

Vishala (S) – *see* Bhakura.

Vishamandala (S) – *see* Sukhdarshan.

Vishambil – *see* Kokam.

Vishamushti (S) – *see* Kuchla.

Vishnugandhi (S) – *see* Vishnu-kranti.

Vishnu-kranti, Shyamakranta; Vishnugandhi (S) – *Evolvulus alsinoides* L.; Convolvulaceae; prostrate herb. Plant is considered to be a tonic, febrifuge, anthelmintic, stomachic and nerve tonic and is useful in treating skin diseases.

Vitunna (S) – *see* Safed murgha.

Vrahikanda – *Tacca integrifolia* Ker-Gawl; Taccaceae; herb. Cultivated for its tubers formed by underground rhizomes which are sweet, easily digestible and nutritive; they are also used in the treatment of leprosy and hemorrhagic diathesis.

Vrana patta; Rakta-skandana (S) – *Anaphalis neelgerriana* DC.; Compositae; perennial herb or undershrub, found on the Nilgiri mountain slopes. Fresh bruised leaves are applied topically to treat wounds and cuts.

Vriddu-tulsi (S) – *see* Ram tulsi.

Vrihati (S) – *see* Birhatta.

Vriksharuha (S) – *see* Banda.

Vrishanasana (S) – *see* Baberang.

Vrishchikali (S) – *see* Barhanta.

W

Warras – *see* Pullung.

Watpan – *Tussilago farfara* L.; Colt's foot (E), Coughwort (E); Compositae, perennial herb found in the hills. Leaves and tender shoots are used as vegetable. Leaves act as a diuretic, expectorant and sudorific, and are used in cough, colds and asthma. They are also used in combating diarrhoea, indigestion, rheumatism and nerve disorders. Leaves yield an essential oil and tannin. Rhizomes also contain an essential oil. The decoction of flower is used for gargles.

Wawrung – *see* Baberang.

Wumb – *see* Anshphal.

Yasti-madhu (S) – *see* Mulhatti.

Yava (S) – *see* Jau.

Yeshul – *Rubus rosaefolius* Sm.; Mauritius raspberry (E); Rosaceae; shrub. Cultivated in the hilly regions for its edible fruits which are either eaten fresh or made into jam.

Yuthuka-parni (S) – *see* Palak juhi.

Z

Zafran – *see* Kesar.

Zaitoon, Jaitoon – *Olea europaea* L.; Olive (E); Oleaceae; small tree. Cultivated as an introduced plant in N. India for its fruits. Mature fruits are the source of olive oil which is employed chiefly as a salad oil and as an emollient for softening the skin; it is also used for the manufacture of soaps, textile lubricants and sulphonated oils. Fruits though bitter when fresh can be used stuffed and pickled. Leaves and fruits are reported to possess principles for lowering high levels of cholestrol and blood-pressure.

Zaitun – *Gyrocarpus jacquini* Gaertn; Gyrocarpaceae; tree found in West Bengal, Orissa and the peninsular regions of India and Andaman Islands. Wood is soft and light and is in great demand for making catamarans; it is also used for making toys, light furniture, frames, fancy articles and for carving.

Zakhm-haiyat, Pathur-chatta – *Bryophyllum pinnatum* (Lam.) Kurz.; Crassulaceae; perennial herb. Cultivated as an ornamental in pots for its beautiful, succulent and evergreen foliage. Toasted leaves are applied locally to treat bruises, boils, wounds and insect bites; they are also used in poultice form on sloughing ulcers.

Zamin-kand, Balukand, Suran; Arsaghna (S) – *Amorphophallus campanulatus* (Roxb.) Blume ex Dcne.; Elephant-foot yam (E); Telugu potato (E); Araceae; perennial herb with large underground stems called corms. Cultivated for its corms which are used as vegetable after proper boiling or pressure cooking. Corms are also used in the treatment of piles, dysentery and acute rheumatism.

Zardalu – *see* Khubani.

Zarga, Apang – *Dichanthium annulatum* (Forssk.) Stapf.; Marvel grass (E); Gramineae; perennial grass. Plants are relished by cattle and thus highly valued as a wild fodder grass both when young and in mature flowering stage.

Zeera – *see* Jira.

Zergul – *Calendula officinalis* L.; Potmarigold (E); Compositae; herb. Cultivated as an ornamental in flower beds and pots for its beautiful bright turmeric yellow flower-heads. Capitula act as a stimulant, diuretic and diaphoretic, and are used for the treatment of internal and external ulcers. The active principle present is calendulin. Petals are often used as an adulterant of 'kesar' or saffron.

Zufah – *Hyssopus officinalis* L.; Hyssop (E); Labiatae; aromatic undershrub found in W. Himalayas. Leaves are considered to be a stimulant, stomachic and carminative. Leaf infusion in the form of tea is used medicinally for curing cough, colds, asthma and also uterine, urinary, digestive and nervous disorders. Leaves are the source of an essential oil called hyssop oil which is used for adding flavour to liqueurs. Leaf juice is used for expelling roundworms.

Glossary of Some Medical Terms

Abortifacient–an agent that induces abortion.

Abscess–localized collection of pus anywhere in the body walled off by damaged and inflamed tissues.

Addiction–inability to resist habitual indulgence especially strong dependence on a drug, or alcohol.

Allergy–an exaggerated reaction or sensitivity of the body cells to specific substances such as antigens and allergens.

Alopecia–falling of hair.

Amenorrhoea–stopping of menstrual periods during pregnancy and lactation and after menopause.

Analgesic–anodyne or a pain reliever.

Anasarca – massive swelling of legs, trunk and genetalia due to retention of fluid in congestive heart failure and some forms of renal failure.

Anemia (or anaemia)–a condition in which the equilibrium between blood production and blood loss is disturbed, causing reduction either in the number of erythrocytes, the quantity of haemoglobin or the volume of packed red blood cells.

Anesthesia – induction of the loss of feeling or sensation, especially of pain in a part or whole of the body.

Anodyne – analgesic.

Anthelmintic – a drug which is used for combating intestinal parasitic worms.

Anticoagulant – an agent which prevents blood from clotting.

Anticonvulsant – agent that prevents or stops convulsion (muscle relaxant).

Antipyretic – a drug that relieves or reduces fever.

Antiscorbutic – agent that relieves scurvy.

Antispasmodic – a drug which relieves muscular spasm and has a sedative effect on the nerves.

Antitussive – agent that prevents or relieves cough.

Apperient – substance employed to evacuate the bowels; includes laxative (mild purgative like mineral oil) and cathartics (powerful purgative such as castor oil).

Aphrodisiac – a drug which arouses sexual desire.

Arteriosclerosis (= atherosclerosis) – a condition characterised by thickening and hardening of the walls of the arteries as a result of accumulation of lipoid substances and progressive diminution in the size of the lumen.

Arthritis – inflammation of joints.

Ascitis – accumulation of fluid in the peritoneal cavity causing abdominal swelling.

Atonic – state in which muscles lack in their normal elasticity.

Asthma – inflammation of the bronchial tubes.

Attenuant – agent bringing about attenuation i.e. reduce the virulence of a bacterium or virus, by chemical treatment, heating or other means.

Astringent – an agent which shrinks and hardens tissues, thereby lessening secretion.

Bilious – affected by disorder of bile.

Blennorrhagia – copious discharge of mucus, particularly from the urethra.

Bronchitis – an inflammation of the air passages.

Cachexia – abnormally low weight, weakness and general body decline associated with chronic disease.

Calculus – hard pebble like mass formed within body anywhere in urinary tract or gall bladder.

Cancer – any malignant growth.

Carcinogen – any physical or chemical agent that tends to produce a cancer.

Caries – bacterial infection of the enamel and dentin of the tooth leading to the formation of cavities.

Cephalagia – pain in head.

Carminative – any substance that promotes expulsion of gas or reduces formation of gas in the stomach.

Catarrh – the discharge from inflammed mucous membranes, such as those lining the nasal cavity.

Cathartic – a fairly powerful purgative or agent used to evacuate the bowels.

Cerebral haemorrhage – a stroke resulting from the bleeding of a vessel in the brain.

Cerebral thrombosis – stroke resulting from a blood clot blocking a cerebral vessel.

Cholagogue – drug that stimulates the flow of bile from gall bladder and bile ducts into the duodenum.

Colic – pain due to spasmodic contraction of the abdomen.

Croup – laryngitis in children with harsh cough and difficulty in breathing.

Deliruim – an extreme mental disturbance marked by excitement, restlessness and rapid succession of confused and unconnected ideas.

Demulcent – a drug having a soothing action on the skin and mucous membranes.

Deobstruent – agent that opens up the natural passages or pores of the body to aid excretion or secretion process.

Depressant – an agent that reduces the functional activity; a sedative.

Dermatitis – inflammation of the skin.

Diaphoretic – a drug which tends to induce copious perspiration.

Diarrhoea – abnormal frequency and fluidity of faecal discharges.

Diathesis – higher than average tendency to acquire certain diseases such as allergies, rheumatism and gout.

Diuretic – a drug that increases the secretion and discharge of urine.

Dropsy – a disease marked by an excessive collection of a watery fluid in body tissues or cavities.

Dysentry – an infectious disease, causing acute diarrhoea and discharge of mucus and blood.

Dysmenorrhoea – painful menstruation.

Dyspepsia – the impaired digestion of food.

Dysuria – difficult or painful urination.

Emetic – an agent that induces vomiting.

Emmenogogue – agent that promotes menstruation.

Emollient – an agent that allays irritation of the skin and softens it.

Expectorant – a drug that helps the removal of phlegm from the bronchial tubes.

Febrifuge (= antipyretic) – an agent which reduces fever.

Febrile – affected with fever.

Flatulence –excessive accumulation of gas in the alimentary canal.

Galactogogue – agent that stimulates secretion of milk.

Gangrene – tissue death resulting from inadequate blood supply, direct injury or infection.

Goitre – a chronic enlargement of the thyroid gland.

Gout – painful disease affecting the joints, resulting in accumulation of excess of uric acid from faulty purine metabolism.

Haemolysis – the breakdown of red blood cells.

Haemoptysis – severe cough associated with spitting of blood from lungs.

Haemorrhage – Flow of blood from a ruptured blood vessel externally or internally.

Haemostatic (styptic) – agent that prevents or stops haemorrhage.

Hemicrania – headache affecting only one side of the head usually migraine.

Hemiplegia – paralysis of one side of the body.

Hydrogogue – an agent that acts as a laxative producing watery stools.

Hydrothorax – fluid in the pleural cavity.

Hypertension – abnormally high tension in blood vessels; usually recorded as high blood pressure.

Hypnotic – sleep inducing drug, same as soporific.

Hypoglycemia – deficiency of glucose in the blood stream causing muscular weakness, sweating and mental confusion.

Hypotension – a state of abnormally low blood pressure.

Infusion – an extract obtained by steeping the drug in water.

Lactogogue – agent stimulating secretion of milk, same as galactogogue.

Laxative – a mild purgative.

Liniment – a liquid pharmaceutical preparation for external use, usually oily and applied by rubbing.

Menorrhagia – abnormally heavy bleeding during menstruation.

Micturition – urination.

Migraine – periodic severe attacks of headache, commonly affecting only one side of the head.

Narcotic – an agent capable of causing a depression in the central nervous system.

Nausea – feeling that vomiting is about to begin.

Necrosis – death of tissues, usually in localised areas.

Neuralgia – nerve pain.

Neuritis – nerve inflammation.

Ophthalmia – inflammation of the eye, particularly the conjunctiva.

Orchitis – inflammation of testicles.

Oxytocic – hastening childbirth.

Panacea – universal remedy or cure all.

Paralysis – loss of power of voluntary movement in any part of the body.

Parturition – childbirth.

Pectoral – a drug to cure chest infection.

Phthiriasis – infestation of pubic- and armpit hair in humans by crab or pubic louse causing intense itching.

Phthisis – another name for pulmonary tuberculosis or any disease resulting in wasting of tissues.

Piles – an inflammed condition of the veins in the region of rectum.

Prolapse – descending of an organ from normal position.

Psychotomimetic – an agent which produces conditions that mimic mental disorders.

Purgative – an agent that stimulates peristaltic action and bowel evacuation.

Pyorrhoea – a disease marked by purulent discharge from the gums.

Rheumatism – a term used for pain in the muscles, joints and certain tissues.

Rubefacient – agent that causes warming of the skin and often used for relief of muscular pain.

Scabies – an itching skin disease caused by a mite.

Scrobutic – affected with scurvy.

Scurvy – a deficiency disease caused by lack of vitamin C in the diet, and is characterised by multiple haemorrhage, especially of the gums, gastro-intestinal disturbances and loss of teeth.

Sedative – a drug that has a soothing and sleep-producing action.

Soporific – a drug that induces sleep.

Spasm – an intense, uncontrolled muscular contraction.

Spermatorrhoea – the involuntary discharge of semen.

Stomatitis – inflammation of the mouth.

Stomachic – a drug that stimulates the appetite, thereby promoting the functional activity of the stomach.

Stricture – narrowing of any tubular structure in the body such as esophagus, bowel, ureter or urethra.

Stypic – an agent which checks bleeding.

Sudorific – drug that causes an increase in sweating; same as diaphoretic.

Suppuration – formation of pus.

Topical – external local application of the drug directly on the part being treated.

Tranquiliser – a drug used to calm down a person without inducing sleep.

Ulcer – an open sore.

Vermifuge – a drug that expels intestinal worms.

Vertigo – dizziness.

Vesicant – an irritating substance producing blisters on the skin.

Bibliography

Aiyadurai, S.G. 1966. A Review of Research on Spices and Cashewnut in India. Regional Office (Spices and Cashewnut), ICAR, Ernakulum, India.

Anonymous. 1970. Pulse Crops of India. Indian Coun. agric. Res., New Delhi, India.

Anonymous. 1970, 1972. Indian Forest Utilization. Vol. I 1970; II 1972. Manager of Publications, Govt. of India, New Delhi, India.

Anonymous. 1976. Medicinal Plants of India. Vol. I. Indian Coun. med. Res., New Delhi, India.

Anonymous. 1989, 1999, 2001. The Ayurvedic Pharmacopoeia of India. Part I, Vol. I 1989; II 1999; III 2001. Ministry of Health and Family Welfare, Govt. of India, New Delhi, India.

Anonymous. 1996. Pharmacopoeia of India, (The Indian Pharmacopoeia) Vols. I & II, 4th edn., Manager of Publications, Govt. of India, New Delhi, India.

Anonymous. 1998, 1999. Indian Herbal Pharmacopoeia. Vol. I 1998; II 1999. RRL, Jammu and IDMA, Bombay, India.

Anonymous. 2000. CITES-Listed Medicinal Plants of India – An Identification Manual. TRAFFIC. India/WWF- India, New Delhi, India.

Atchison, J.E. 1974. Present status and future potential for utilization of non-wood plant fibres : A world-wide review. Indian Pulp Pap. **28**(8): 10-17.

Babu, C.R. 1977. Herbaceous Flora of Dehra Dun. Coun. sci. Ind. Res., New Delhi, India.

Bailey, L.H. 1950. The Standard Cyclopaedia of Horticulture. Vols I, II and III. The Macmillan Co., New York, USA.

Bailey, L.H. 1971. Manual of Cultivated Plants. The Macmillan Co., New York, USA.

Baker, H.G. 1978. Plants and Civilization. 3rd edn. Macmillan: London, London, England.

Balfour, E. 1862. The Timber Trees, Timber and Fancy Woods, as also the Forests of India and of Eastern and Southern Asia. 2nd edn. Madras, India.

Banerji, S.C. 1980. Flora and Fauna in Sanskrit Literature. Naya Prokash, Calcutta, India.

Bender, A.E. 1965. Dictionary of Nutrition and Food Technology. 2nd edn. Butterworths, London, England.

Benthall, A.P. 1946. The Trees of Calcutta and Its Neighbourhood. Thacker, Spink & Co., Ltd., Calcutta, India.

Berger, J. 1969. The World's Major Fibre Crops: Their Cultivation and Manuring. Centre d'Etude de L'Azote, Zurich, Switzerland.

Beri, R.M. 1977. Wood as raw material for chemical industries. Indian Pulp Pap. **31**(5): 3-8.

Bhandari, M.M. 1974. Famine foods in the Rajasthan desert. Econ. Bot. **28**(1): 73-81.

Bhandari, M.M. 1978. Flora of the Indian Desert. Scientific Publishers, Jodhpur, India.

Bhatia, S.L. 1977. A History of Medicine with Special Reference to the Orient. Medical Coun. India, New Delhi, India.

Biswas, K. 1956. Common Medicinal Plants of Darjeeling and the Sikkim Himalayas. Govt. Press, Calcutta, W. Bengal, India.

Biswas, K. 1966. Plants of Darjeeling and the Sikkim Himalayas. Vol. I. Govt. Press, Calcutta, W. Bengal, India.

Blatter, E. 1926. Palms of British India and Ceylon. Oxford University Press, London, England.

Bodding, P.O. 1925-1940 (Reprinted 1986). Studies in Santal Medicine and Connected Folklore. Asiatic Soc. Bengal, Calcutta, India.

Bor, N.L. 1953. Manual of Indian Forest Botany. Oxford University Press, London, England.

Bor, N.L. 1960. The Grasses of Burma, Ceylon, India and Pakistan (excluding Bambuseae). Pergamon Press, Oxford, England.

Bor, N.L. and Raizada, M.B. 1954. Some Beautiful Indian Climbers and Shrubs. The Bombay Natural History Society, Bombay, India.

Bose, D.M., Sen, S.N. and Subbarayappa, B.V. 1971. A Concise History of Science in India. Indian National Science Academy, New Delhi, India.

Braudel, F. 1985. The Structures of Everyday Life – The Limits of the Possible. (Translation from French, revised edn.). Fontana Paperbacks, London, England.

Brickell, C. *et al.* (eds.) 1994. New Encyclopedia of Plants and Flowers. The Royal Hort. Society. Dorling Kindersley Ltd., London, England.

Chadha, Y.R. 1971. Indian rubber industry. Res. & Ind. **16**(1): 1-14.

Chandel, K.P.S. and Singh, B.M. 1984. Some of our under-utilized plants. Indian Fmg. **34**(2): 23-29.

Chandel, K.P.S. *et al.* 1996. Medicinal Plants of India. NBPGR. Indian Coun. agric. Res., New Delhi, India.

Chatterjee, D. and Randhawa, G.S. 1952a. Standardized names of cultivated plants in India. I. Fruits. Indian J. Hort. **9**: 24-36.

Chatterjee, D. and Randhawa, G.S. 1952b. Standardized names of cultivated plants in India. II. Cereals, Pulses, Vegetables and Spices. Indian J. Hort. **9**: 64-85.

Chaturvedi, O.H. *et al.* 1999. Siris: A multipurpose fodder tree. Yojana **43**: 36-38.

Chopra, R.N., Badhwar, R.L. and Ghosh, S. 1965. Poisonous Plants of India. Vols I & II. 2nd revised and enlarged edn. Indian Coun. agric. Res., New Delhi, India.

Chopra, R.N., Chopra, I.C., Handa, K.L. and Kapur, L.D. 1958. Indigenous Drugs of India. 2nd edn. U.N. Dhur & Sons Private Ltd., Calcutta, India.

Chopra, R.N., Chopra, I.C. and Varma, B.S. 1969. Supplement to Glossary of Indian Medicinal Plants. Coun. sci. ind. Res., New Delhi, India.

Chopra, R.N., Nayar, S.L. and Chopra, I.C. 1956. Glossary of Indian Medicinal Plants. Coun. sci. ind. Res., New Delhi, India.

Choudhury, B. 1967. Vegetables. National Book Trust of India, New Delhi, India.

Conway, D. 1973. The Magic of Herbs. Jonathan Cape, London, England.

CSIR. 1948-1976. The Wealth of India – Raw Materials. A Dictionary of Indian Raw Materials and Industrial Products. Vol. I-XI. Shastri, B.N. *et al.* (eds.). Coun. sci. ind. Res., New Delhi, India.

CSIR. 1986. The Useful Plants of India. Ambasta, S.P. *et al.* (eds.). Coun. sci. ind. Res. New Delhi, India.

CSIR. 1991. The Treatise on Indian Medicinal Plants. Vol. I. Chatterjee, Asima *et al.* (eds.). Coun. sci. ind. Res., New Delhi, India.

Dahanukar, S. and Hazara, A. 1995. Heal with Herbs. Coun. sci. ind. Res., New Delhi, India.

Das, D.N. 1972. Avenues and avenue planting. Indian Hort. **17** (2): 21-22.

Dastur, J.F. 1964. Useful Plants of India and Pakistan. 2nd edn., D.B. Taraporewala Sons & Co. Pvt. Ltd. Bombay, India.

Dastur, J.F. 1970. Medicinal Plants of India and Pakistan. 3rd edn., D.B. Taraporewala Sons & Co. Pvt. Ltd. Bombay, India.

Desai, B.L. 1970. Seasonal Flowers. Revised edn. Indian Coun. agric. Res., New Delhi, India.

De, Amit Krishna 1992. A chilli a day. Science Reporter, **29** (5): 15-18.

Dey, A.C. 1980. Indian Medicinal Plants used in Ayurvedic Preparations. Bishen Singh Mohinderpal Singh, Dehradun, India.

Dhamaney, C.P., Joshi, H.C. and Nautiyal, S.N. 1973. Studies on hardboard preparation : Part II – Nagaland forest waste for hardboards. Indian Pulp Pap. **28** (6): 17-19.

Downer, A.W.E. 1973. The application of flavours in the soft drinks industry. Flavour Ind. **4** (11): 488-490.

Duke, J.A. 1973. Utilization of *Papaver*. Econ. Bot **27** (4): 390-400.

Dutta, S. 1966. Horticulture in the eastern region of India. Farm Information Unit, Directorate of Extension, Ministry of Food and Agriculture, New Delhi, India.

Enas, A.E. 1996. Cooking oil, cholestrol and CAD: Facts and myths. IHJ – July-Aug.: 423-427.

Farooqui, M.I.H. and Kapoor, L.D. 1968. Some Indian plant gums – Their botany, chemistry and utilization. Indian For. **94** (9): 662-666.

Farooqi, M.I.H. and Sharma, V.N. 1972. *Sesbania aculeata* Pers. Seeds – A new source for gum. Res. & Ind. **17** (3): 94-95.

Fernandez, R.R. 1964. Gums and Resins. Indian For. Leafl. No. 174, FRI, Dehra Dun, India.

Firminger, W.K. 1957. Manual of Gardening for India. 8th edn. Thacker, Spink & Co., Calcutta, India.

Gamble, J.S. 1922. A Manual of Indian Timbers. 2nd edn. Sampson Low, Marston & Col. Ltd, London, England.

Ghosh, P.C. 1973. Some interesting trees in Delhi gardens. Indian Hort. **18** (2): 19-23.

Ghosh, T. 1977. Some useful plants. Indian Fmg **26** (11): 93-94.

Guha, S.R.D. 1977. Raw materials for paper. Indian Pulp Pap. **31** (6): 7-15.

Gupta, R. 1972a. Grow Palmarosa oil-grass for rose-like perfume. Indian Fmg **22** (1): 17-20.

Gupta, R. 1972b. Vital drugs and essential oil-bearing plants as future cash crops in India. Indian Fmg **22** (6): 67-75.

Gupta, R. 1973. 'Kuth' has many uses. Indian Fmg **23** (6): 11-13.

Gupta, R. 1977a. Medicinal plants components of Indian forests. Indian Fmg **26** (11): 96-98.

Gupta, R. 1977b. Periwinkle produces anti-cancer drug. Indian Fmg **27** (4): 11-13.

Gupta, R. 1993. Emerging medicinal plants in world pharmaceutical industry. Indian Hort. **38** (1): 43-46.

Gupta, R., Sethi, M.L. and Atal, C.K. 1961. *Jurinea macrocephala* Benth., the commercial source of 'dhoop'. Indian For. **87**: 104-115.

Gurr, M. 1992. Dietary lipid and coronary heart disease. Prop. In Lipid Research **31**: 195-243.

Harlan, J.R. 1975. Crops and Man. Crops Science Soc. America, Wisconsin, USA.

Hawkes, A.D. 1965. Encyclopaedia of Cultivated Orchids. Faber and Faber Ltd., London, England.

Hayes, W.B. 1957. Fruit Growing in India. 3rd edn. Kitabistan, Allahabad, India.

Hill, A.F. 1952. Economic Botany: A Textbook of Useful Plants and Plant Products. 2nd edn. McGraw-Hill Book Co., Inc., New York, USA.

Hooker, J.D. 1875-1897. Flora of British India Vol. 1-7. Reeve and Co., London, England.

Howes, F.N. 1974. A Dictionary of Useful and Everyday Plants and their Common Names. Univ. Press, Cambridge, England.

Hussain, Akhtar *et al*. 1992. Dictionary of Indian Medicinal Plants. CIMAP., Lucknow, India.

Hutchinson, J. 1959. Families of Flowering Plants. 2 Vols. Clarendon Press, Oxford, England.

Jain, S.K. 1963. Studies in Indian Ethnobotany: Less known uses of 50 common plants from tribal areas of Madhya Pradesh. Bull. Bot. Survey India. **5**: 223-226.

Jain, S.K. 1967. Vanaspati Kosh – A Hindi-Latin Dictionary of Economic Plants of India. Rajkamal Prakashan, Delhi, India.

Jain, S.K. 1975. Medicinal Plants. 2nd edn. National Book Trust of India, New Delhi, India.

Jain, S.K. (ed.) 1981. Glimpses of Indian Ethnobotany. Oxford and IBH, New Delhi, India.

Jain, S.K. 1989. A Manual of Ethnobotany. Scientific Publishers, Jodhpur, India.

Jain, S.K. and Tarafder, C.R. 1970. Medicinal plant-lore of the Santals. Econ. Bot. **24** (3): 241-278.

Jain, S.K. *et al* 1984. Bibliography of Ethnobotany. Botanical Survey of India, Calcutta, India.

Jindal, S.L. 1968. Ornamental Bulbous Plants. Indian Coun. agric. Res., New Delhi, India.

Johri, B.M. and Srivastava, Sheela 1978. Famous Plants. Indian national Science Academy, New Delhi, India.

Joshi, S.G. 2000. Medicinal Plants. Oxford and IBH, New Delhi, India.

Katyal, S.L. 1972. Twenty-five years of research on fruit crops. Indian Fmg **22** (6): 14-16.

Kempanna, C. 1974. Prospects for medicinal plants in Indian agriculture. World Crops **26** (4): 166-168.

Kirby, R.H. 1963. Vegetable Fibres: Botany, Cultivation and Utilization. Leonard Hill (Books) Ltd., London, England.

Kirtikar, K.R. and Basu, B.D. 1933. Indian Medicinal Plants. 2nd edn. Lalit Mohan Basu, Allahabad, India.

Kochhar, S.L. 1998. Economic Botany in the Tropics. 2nd edn. Macmillan India Ltd., New Delhi, India.

Krishnamurthi, S. (ed.) 1953. Horticultural and Economic Plants of the Nilgiris. Govt. Botanic Gardens, Ootacamund, India.

Lamba, S.S. 1970. Indian piscicidal plants. Econ. Bot. **24** (2): 134-136.

Lubomir, O and Volak, J. 2000. Healing Plants (English edn.). Silverdale Books, Leicester, England.

Mahendru, S. 1975. Cashewnut shell liquid – A historical survey of its development. Indian Cashew J. **9** (4): 7-9.

Maheshwari, J.K. 1963. The Flora of Delhi. Coun. sci. ind. Res., New Delhi, India.

Maheshwari, P. and Singh, H. 1960. Economic importance of conifers. J. Univ. Gauhati **11**: 1-28.

Maheshwari, P. and Umrao Singh, 1965. Dictionary of Economic Plants in India. Indian Coun. agric. Res., New Delhi, India.

Mani, V. 1975. Puranic Encyclopedia. Motilal Banarsidas, Varanasi, India.

McCann, C. 1959. 100 Beautiful Trees of India. A Descriptive and Pictorial Handbook. D.B. Taraporevala Sons & Co. Pvt. Ltd., Bombay, India.

McClure, F.A. 1966. The Bamboos, A Fresh Perspective. Cambridge, England.

Mehra, K.L., Kanodia, K.C. and Srivastava, R.N. 1975. Folk uses of plants for adornment in India. Econ. Bot. **29** (1): 39-46.

Menon, K.P.G. 1975. Indian turmeric wins world market. Indian Spices **12** (2): 6-13.

Menon, A.K. 1960. Indian Essential Oils: A Review. Coun. sci. ind. Res., New Delhi, India.

Mortensen, E. and Bullard, E.T. 1964. Handbook of Tropical and Sub-tropical Horticulture. Washington, D.C., USA.

Mukerji, B. 1953. Indian Pharmaceutical Codex. Vol. I. Coun. sci. ind. Res., New Delhi, India.

Mukherjee, S.K. 1969. Survey of plant resources of India and its use. Bull. Bot. Surv. India **11** (3, 4): 217-223.

Nadkarni, K.M. 1954. Indian Materia Medica. Vols I & II, 3rd edn., revised and enlarged by A.K. Nadkarni. Popular Book Depot, Bombay, India.

Naik, K.C. 1958. Horticulture in South India. Ministry of Food and Agriculture, New Delhi, India.

Nambisan, Bala, Sundaresan, S. and Padmaja, G. 1984. Tuber crops in human nutrition. Indian Fmg. **33** (12): 67-71.

Narayanan, T.R. and Dabadghao, P.M. 1972. Forage Crops of India. Indian Coun. agric. Res., New Delhi, India.

Nayar, M.P., Ramamurthy, K. and Agarwala, V.S. 1989. Economic Plants of India. Vol. 1. Botanical Survey of India, Calcutta, India.

Negi, S.S. 1977. Fodder trees in Himachal Pradesh. Indian For. **103** (9): 616-622.

Pal, B.P. 1960. Beautiful Climbers of India. Indian Coun. agric. Res., New Delhi, India.

Pal, B.P. and Krishnamurthi, S. 1967. Flowering Shrubs. Indian Coun. agric. Res., New Delhi, India.

Pandey, R.M. 1993. More hybrids of mango. Indian Hort., **38** (2): 4-5.

Parry, J.W. 1969. Spices. 2 vols. Chemical Publishing Co., Inc., New York, USA.

Pathak, P.S., Deb Roy, R. and Patil, B.D. 1977. Koo babool has varied uses. Indian Fmg **27** (5): 16-17.

Paulose, T.T. 1970. Development of ginger in India. Indian Spices **7** (2): 2-4.

Pearson, R.S. and Brown, H.P. 1932. Commercial Timbers of India. Vols I & II. Govt. Press, Calcutta, India.

Prabhakar, V.S., Sarin, Y.K. and Atal, C.K. 1971. Utilization of wild Daturas of N.-W. India for commercial production of hyoscine. Indian J. Pharm. **33** (2): 35-36.

Prakash, Ved 1998. Indian medicinal plants – current status. Ethnobotany, **10**: 112-121.

Purseglove, J.W. 1968. Tropical Crops: Dicotyledons. Vols I & II. Longmans, London, England.

Purseglove, J.W. 1972. Tropical Crops: Monocotyledons. Vols I & II. Longmans, London, England.

Pushkarnath 1969. Potato in India : Varieties. Indian Coun. agric. Res., New Delhi, India.

Radwanski, S. 1977. Neem tree: Part I. Commercial potential, characteristics and distribution. World Crops **29** (2): 62-66.

Raizada, M.B. 1968. Some name changes in the flora of India. Indian For. **94** (6): 432-462.

Rajan, B.K.C. 1977. The sandal tree. Indian Fmg **26** (11): 94-95.

Ramakrishnan, P.S. *et al.* (eds.) 1998. Conserving the Sacred for Biodiversity Management. UNESCO and Oxford and IBH., New Delhi, India.

Randhawa, M.S. 1957. Flowering Trees in India. Indian Coun. agric. Res., New Delhi, India.

Randhawa, M.S. 1971. Beautiful Gardens. Indian Coun. agric. Res., New Delhi, India.

Randhawa, M.S. 1983. Flowering Trees. 7th edn. National Book Trust of India, New Delhi, India.

Rathore, J.S. 1972. *Diospyros melanoxylon*, a bread-winner tree of India. Econ. Bot. **26** (4): 333-339.

Ray, P. and Gupta, H.N. 1980. 'Caraka Samhita' – A Scientific Synopsis. Indian National Science Academy, New Delhi, India.

Roy, R.D. and Arora, G.D. 1971. Vilayati babool – Ideal for afforestation of arid, semi-arid areas. Indian Fmg **20** (10): 26.

Sagreiya, K.P. 1994. Forests and Forestry. 5th edn. National Book Trust of India, New Delhi, India.

Samarawira, I. 1972. Cardamom. World Crops **24** (2): 76-78.

Santapau, H. 1966. Common Trees. National Book Trust of India, New Delhi, India.

Santapau, H. and Henry, A.N. 1973. A Dictionary of the Flowering Plants in India. Coun. sci. ind. Res., New Delhi, India.

Sarin, Y.K. 1996. Illustrated Manual of Herbal Drugs. Coun. Sci. ind. Res. and Indian Coun. med. Res., New Delhi, India.

Schery, R.W. 1972. Plants for Man. 2nd edn. Prentice-Hall, Inc., Englewood Cliffs N.J., USA.

Sensarma, P. 1988. Plants in the Indian Puranas: An Ethnobotanical Investigation. Naya Prokash, Calcutta, India.

Shah, N.C. and Joshi, M.C. 1970. Folk-lore and aromatic plants of Kumaon Hills. Flavour Ind. **1** (12): 851-855.

Sharma, O.P. 1977. Fodder trees of Himachal Pradesh. Indian Fmg **26** (11): 88-89.

Sholto Douglas, J. 1971. Growing medicinal plants for essential oils and flavours. Flavour Ind. **2** (12): 697-698.

Sholto Douglas, J. 1972. Tree crops for food, forage and cash. Part I. World Crops **24** (1): 15-19.

Singh, A. and Mehra, K.L. 1971. New varieties of legume fodders. Indian Fmg **21** (8): 43-44.

Singh, K.M. *et al*. 1994. Cultivation of gorgon fruit is remunerative. Indian Hort. **39** (1): 35-36.

Singh, R. 1969. Fruits. National Book Trust of India, New Delhi, India.

Singh, R.V. 1969. Coniferous raw material potential of Himachal forests for pulp and paper industry. Indian Pulp Pap. **23** (7): 417-420.

Singh, S., Krishnamurthi, S. and Katyal, S.L. 1967. Fruit Culture in India. Revised edn. Indian Coun. agric. Res., New Delhi, India.

Singh, U., Wadhwani, A.M. and Johri, B.M. 1983. Dictionary of Economic Plants of India. 2nd edn. Indian Coun. agric. Res., New Delhi, India.

Singh, V. and Singh, C. 1972. Sunflower cultivation. Indian Fmg **22** (4): 34-35.

Sood, V.K. 1974. Indian essential oils: Review of work at Forest Research Institute. Indian For. **100** (4): 259-264.

Subramanyam, K. 1962. Aquatic Angiosperms. Botanical Monograph No. 3, Coun. sci. ind. Res., New Delhi, India.

Sundararaj, D.D. and Balasubramanyam, Girija 1959. Guide to the Economic Plants of South India. Amudha Nilayam Private Ltd., Madras, India.

Swaminathan, M.S. and Kochhar, S.L. (eds.) 1989. Plants and Society. Macmillan: London, London, England.

Swaminathan, M.S. and Kochhar, S.L. 2003. Groves of Beauty and Plenty: An Atlas of Major Flowering Trees in India. Macmillan India Ltd., New Delhi, India.

Swarup, V. 1967. Garden Flowers. National Book Trust of India, New Delhi, India.

Tiwari, K.M. 1968. The resin industry in India and some suggestions for its improvement. Indian For. **94** (5): 363-372.

Trotter, H. 1940. Manual of Indian Forest Utilization. Oxford University Press, London, England.

Trotter, H. 1960. The Common Commercial Timbers of India and Their Uses. Manager of Publications, Government of India, Delhi.

Uphof, J.C.Th. 1959. Dictionary of Economic Plants. Hafner Publishing Co., New York, USA.

Uphof, J.C.Th. 1968. Dictionary of Economic Plants. 2nd edn. Verlag von J. Cramer, Lehre, Germany.

Usher, G. 1974. A Dictionary of Plants Used by Man. Constable, London, England.

Vaughan, J.G. 1970. The Structure and Utilization of Oilseeds. Chapman and Hall Ltd., London, England.

Venkateswarlu, J. and Chaganti, R.S.K. 1973. Job's-Tears (*Coix lacryma-jobi* L.). Indian Coun. agric. Res. Bull. No. 44.

Verma, N. 1970. Opportunities for the large-scale cultivation of aromatic and medicinal plants in the province of Uttar Pradesh (India). Flavour India. **1** (5): 332-334.

Vimal, O.P. 1975. Utilization of agro-industrial byproducts: Part I – Paddy husk. Res. & Ind. **20** (3): 113-120.

Vimal, O.P. and Adsule, P.G. 1976. Utilization of fruit and vegetable waste. Res. & Ind. **21** (1): 1-7.

Watt, G. 1889-1893. A Dictionary of the Economic Products of India. Vols I-VI. Govt. Press, Calcutta, India.

Watt, G. 1908. The Commercial Products of India. John Murray, London, England.

Weiss, E.A. 1971. Castor, Sesame and Safflower. Leonard Hill, London, England.

Whyte, R.O. 1957. The Grassland and Fodder Resources of India. Indian Coun. agric. Res., New Delhi, India.

Wilkes, H.G. 1968. Interesting beverages of the eastern Himalayas. Econ. Bot. **22** (4): 347-353.

Willis, J.C. 1973. A Dictionary of the Flowering Plants and Ferns. 8th edn, revised by H.K. Airy Shaw. University Press, Cambridge, England.

Warrier, P.K. *et al* (eds.) 1996. Indian Medicinal Plants. Orient Longman, Hyderabad, India.

Yawalkar, K.S. 1969. Vegetable Crops of India. Agri-Horticultural Publishing House, Nagpur, India.

Index of Latin Botanical Names (Including Synonyms)

C

I

M

N

Q

R

T

U

Index of Common English Names

C

G

J

Q

R

V

W